DATE DUE

CLINICAL APPLICATIONS
OF DOPPLER ULTRASOUND

Clinical Applications
of Doppler Ultrasound

Editors

Kenneth J. W. Taylor, M.D., Ph.D., F.A.C.P.
Professor of Diagnostic Radiology
Chief, Ultrasound Section
Yale University School of Medicine
New Haven, Connecticut

Peter N. Burns, Ph.D., M.Inst.P.
Assistant Professor of Radiology
Department of Diagnostic Radiology
Yale University School of Medicine
New Haven, Connecticut

Peter N. T. Wells, Ph.D., D.Sc., F.Eng.
Chief Physicist
Department of Medical Physics
Bristol and Weston Health Authority
Honorary Professor in Radiodiagnosis
University of Bristol
Bristol, England

Raven Press ✒ New York

Raven Press, 1185 Avenue of the Americas, New York, New York 10036

Made in the United States of America

The material contained in this volume was submitted as previously unpublished material, except in the instances in which credit has been given to the source from which some of the illustrative material was derived.

Great care has been taken to maintain the accuracy of the information contained in the volume. However, neither Raven Press nor the editors can be held responsible for errors or for any consequences arising from the use of the information contained herein.

Materials appearing in this book prepared by individuals as part of their official duties as U.S. Government employees are not covered by the above-mentioned copyright.

9 8 7 6 5 4 3 2

Library of Congress Cataloging-in-Publication Data

Clinical applications of Doppler ultrasound.

Includes bibliographies and index.
1. Diagnosis, Ultrasonic. I. Taylor, Kenneth
J. W., 1939–   . II. Burns, Peter N.
III. Wells, P. N. T. (Peter Neil Temple)
[DNLM: 1. Ultrasonic Diagnosis—methods. WB 289 C6405]
RC78.7.U4C57 1988   616.07'543   85-43361
ISBN 0-88167-355-2

Preface

Doppler ultrasound has been in use, mainly by vascular surgeons, for peripheral and cerebrovascular diagnosis for the past 30 years. Recently, however, the addition of an image in duplex scanning has aroused the interest of diagnostic imagers. With duplex instruments now available in many imaging departments, the duplex Doppler technique has been applied to more and more diagnostic problems.

In this book, the principles upon which Doppler diagnoses are based are explained. The current role of Doppler in carotid disease is reviewed and some new applications in limbs, the abdomen, pelvis, and obstetrics and gynecology are described.

This book is intended for radiologists, surgeons, obstetricians, gastroenterologists and sonographers who are interested in applying the Doppler technique to the clinical problems in their subspecialties. In a relatively small volume, we have attempted to introduce the neophyte to Doppler techniques, to explain how to perform them and to indicate the clinical results that may be expected.

It is easy for those whose background is in the interpretation of images to overlook the physiological significance of Doppler information. Here, perhaps more than in the other areas, an appreciation of the physical principles upon which Doppler technique is based is indispensible. We believe that the time spent on the chapters describing these principles, the instrumentation and introducing the somewhat intimidating subject of hemodynamics will be rewarded by a better understanding of results of clinical studies. We hope that the inclusion of a glossary of some of the burgeoning number of technical terms associated with Doppler will be helpful.

The amount of clinical material in this book was determined by our personal view of each area of application. We have minimized material which has little or no current clinical application and concentrated on areas of clinical utility and those we believe to be fertile for new application. This is, however, a rapidly changing field and we recognize that this balance will inevitably change as experimental techniques mature and new applications emerge.

> *Kenneth J. W. Taylor*
> *Peter N. Burns*
> Yale University School of Medicine
>
> *P. N. T. Wells*
> University of Bristol, U.K.

v

Acknowledgments

We are grateful to Raven Press, and in particular Mary Rogers, who facilitated the rapid production of this book on a time schedule envied by most journals. We thank Tom McCarthy for the quality of the illustrations and Quantum for provision of excellent color figures. We are most grateful to our co-authors from other institutions who provided their material in succinct style and timely manner. We also thank Beatrice Cavaliere and Jill Scognamillo for typing the manuscripts, and Cheryl Wilcox for editing them.

Contents

Contributors

Peter N. Burns, Ph.D. *Department of Diagnostic Radiology, Yale University School of Medicine, New Haven, Connecticut 06510*

M. R. Drayton, M.B. *Department of Neonatal Medicine, Bristol Maternity Hospital, Bristol BS1 6SY England*

Robert A. Kane, M.D. *Department of Radiology, New England Deaconess Hospital, Boston, Massachusetts 02215*

Marsha M. Neumyer, B.S., R.V.T. *Vascular Studies Section, Department of Surgery, The Milton S. Hershey Medical Center, The Pennsylvania State University, Hershey, Pennsylvania 17033*

Daniel H. O'Leary, M.D. *Department of Radiology, New England Deaconess Hospital, Boston, Massachusetts 02215*

Christopher M. Rigsby, M.D. *Department of Diagnostic Radiology, Yale University School of Medicine, New Haven, Connecticut 06510; Presently, Department of Radiology, Fairfax Hospital, Falls Church, Virginia*

Kenneth J. W. Taylor, M.D., Ph.D. *Department of Diagnostic Radiology, Yale University School of Medicine, New Haven, Connecticut 06510*

Brian L. Thiele, M.D. *Vascular Studies Section, Department of Surgery, The Milton S. Hershey Medical Center, The Pennsylvania State University, Hershey, Pennsylvania 17033*

P. N. T. Wells, Ph.D., D.Sc. *Department of Medical Physics, Bristol and Weston Health Authority, Bristol BS1 6SY, England*

1 / *Basic Principles and Doppler Physics*

P. N. T. Wells

Department of Medical Physics, Bristol General Hospital, Bristol BS1 6SY, England

> *Shall I refuse my dinner because I do not fully understand the process of digestion?*
> —OLIVER HEAVISIDE

THE DOPPLER EFFECT

A Qualitative Explanation

The Doppler effect is the phenomenon by which the frequency of a wave received after reflection by a moving target is shifted from that of the source. In fact, the Doppler effect can be observed in a great variety of situations. For example, a stationary listener perceives a different sound frequency depending on whether a source of fixed-frequency sound is approaching or receding. Radio waves reflected from a moving aircraft are shifted in frequency by the Doppler effect. Thus, the Doppler effect occurs whenever the effective distance between the observer and the source is changing with time, and the phenomenon can be explained by considering the compression of transmitted waves into a contracting space and vice versa.

In order to understand the Doppler effect in relation to medical ultrasound, consider first the situations illustrated in Fig. 1. In Fig. 1A, the source and the receiver are stationary; waves travel from the source to the receiver at the speed of ultrasound through the medium and, in any fixed period of time (say 1 sec), the number of cycles of the wave detected by the receiver is obviously the same as the number of cycles transmitted by the source (equal to the frequency of the wave if the period of measurement is 1 sec). In Fig. 1B, the receiver is moving toward the stationary source; it is obvious that the receiver encounters more cycles of the wave in any fixed period of time than it would have done if it had been stationary, and so the received frequency is shifted upward from that of the source. The opposite situation is illustrated in Fig. 1C; here the receiver is moving away from the source, and it is again obvious that fewer cycles of the wave are detected in any fixed period than

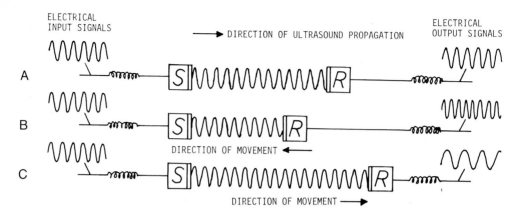

FIG. 1. Doppler effect caused by a moving receiver. **A:** The source (S) and the receiver (R) are stationary, and the frequencies of the input and output signals are equal. **B:** The receiver is moving toward the source, causing an upward shift in the received frequency. **C:** The receiver is moving away from the source, causing a downward shift in the received frequency.

would have been the case with a stationary receiver, so the received frequency is shifted downward.

The situation with a stationary receiver and a moving source is conceptually a little more difficult. Consider Fig. 2; Fig. 2A represents the situation in which both the source and the receiver are stationary, and, as in Fig. 1A, the frequency of the received wave is equal to that of the source. In Fig. 2B, however, the source is moving toward the receiver; the number of wave cycles emitted per second by the source is equal to the frequency of the source, but the waves are compressed in space (that is, their wavelengths are shortened) because, once the waves have left the source, they can only travel at the speed of ultrasound through the medium. (Obviously, the waves cannot travel faster than the speed of ultrasound despite the fact that they have been transmitted from a source moving in the same direction as the ultrasound is being propagated.) As far as the receiver is concerned, the received frequency is shifted upward from that of the source. The opposite situation is illustrated in Fig. 2C; the receiver is moving away from the source, fewer wave cycles are detected per second, and the received frequency is shifted downward.

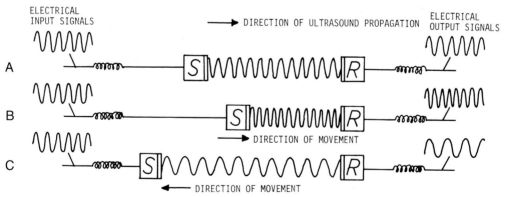

FIG. 2. Doppler effect caused by a moving source. **A:** The source (S) and receiver (R) are stationary, and the frequencies of the input and output signals are equal. **B:** The source is moving towards the receiver, causing an upward shift in the received frequency. **C:** The source is moving away from the receiver, causing a downward shift in the received frequency.

Most medical applications of the ultrasonic Doppler effect involve stationary and more-or-less coincident transducers for transmitting and receiving the ultrasonic waves. The waves travel from the source to the receiver by reflection; if there is movement of the reflector toward the transducers, the received frequency is shifted upward by the Doppler effect and vice versa. One way of explaining the process is to consider that a movement of the reflector toward the transducers is equivalent to having a stationary source and a receiver moving towards the source at twice the velocity of the reflector (because the reflected beam is folded back on its original path and so the ultrasonic go-and-return path length is reduced by a distance equal to twice the distance moved by the reflector). More usefully, however, the reflector can be considered to take a more active role: the concept is that the reflector receives the waves from the source and then reradiates the waves back to the receiver, the reflector itself acting as a secondary source of waves. Thus, as far as the transmitting transducer is concerned, the reflector can be considered to be a moving receiver behaving as illustrated in Fig. 1; the reflector simultaneously acts as a moving source, as illustrated in Fig. 2, by reradiating Doppler-frequency-shifted waves to the receiving transducer.

A Mathematical Approach

Consider Fig. 3, which represents coincident transmitting and receiving transducers and a moving reflector returning the transmitted wave from the source to the receiver. The speed of ultrasound in the medium is c, and the velocity of the reflector toward the transducers is v_r. If f is the transmitted frequency, the wavelength λ_s of the waves traveling from the source to the reflector is given by

$$\lambda_s = c/f \qquad [1]$$

Next, consider the changes that take place in a period of time t. During this time, the reflector moves a distance $v_r t$ toward the source, and so it encounters $v_r t/\lambda_s$ more cycles than it would have done if it had been stationary; if it had been stationary, ct/λ cycles would have reached the reflector. Thus, the total number of cycles en-

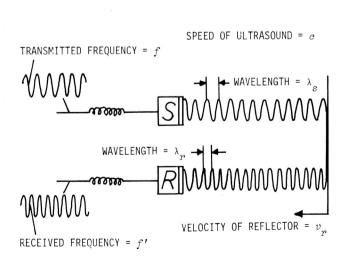

SPEED OF ULTRASOUND = c

TRANSMITTED FREQUENCY = f

WAVELENGTH = λ_s

WAVELENGTH = λ_r

VELOCITY OF REFLECTOR = v_r

RECEIVED FREQUENCY = f'

FIG. 3. Doppler effect caused by a moving reflector. The source (S) and the receiver (R) are coincident (they are shown displaced in the diagram for clarity) and stationary. Movement of the reflector towards the transducers causes an upward shift in the frequency of the received signal by a two-stage process in which the reflector behaves simultaneously as a receiver moving toward the source transducer and as a source moving toward the receiving transducer while reradiating Doppler frequency-shifted signals received from the source transducer. Conversely, movement of the reflector away from the transducers causes a downward shift in the received frequency.

countered by the reflector if $t = 1$ sec (that is, the frequency f_r of ultrasound at the reflector) is given by

$$f_r = c/\lambda_s + v_r/\lambda_s \qquad [2]$$

and, by substituting $f = c/\lambda_s$ (from Eq. 1),

$$f_r = f + v_r/\lambda_s \qquad [3]$$

The next step is to consider what happens when the reflector, moving toward the receiver at velocity v_r, reradiates ultrasound at the frequency f_r. In time t, the reflector moves toward the receiver by a distance $v_r t$, and, consequently, the receiver detects $v_r t/\lambda_r$ more cycles than it would have done had the reflector been stationary, where

$$\lambda_r = c/f_r \qquad [4]$$

Thus, the total number of cycles detected by the receiver if $t = 1$ sec (that is, the frequency f' of ultrasound at the receiver) is given by

$$f' = f_r + v_r/\lambda_r \qquad [5]$$

Notice the similarity of Eqs. 3 and 5, in agreement with the idea that the Doppler frequency shift results from a two-stage process in which the reflector acts both as a moving receiver and as a reradiating moving source.

It is the difference between the received and transmitted frequencies at the transducers that is the important quantity in the context of medical ultrasonic Doppler techniques. The next step in the derivation of this difference frequency, f_D (which is equal to $f' - f$), is to calculate f' by substitution in Eq. 5. If you have followed the math so far, do not give up now; considered step by step, the rest is easy:

$$f' = f_r + v_r/\lambda_r \quad (\text{Eq. 5})$$

$$\begin{aligned}
&\quad\;(\text{Eq. 3}) \\[2pt]
&= f + v_r/\lambda_s + v_r/\lambda_r \\[2pt]
&\qquad\;(\text{Eq. 1}) \quad (\text{Eq. 4}) \\[2pt]
&= f + v_r f/c + v_r f_r/c \\[2pt]
&= f + (v_r/c)(f + f_r) \\[2pt]
&\qquad\qquad\qquad (\text{Eq. 3}) \\[2pt]
&= f + (v_r/c)(f + f + v_r/\lambda_s) \\[2pt]
&\qquad\qquad\qquad\quad (\text{Eq. 1}) \\[2pt]
&= f + (v_r/c)(2f + v_r f/c) \\[2pt]
&= f + 2f v_r/c + f(v_r/c)^2 \qquad [6]
\end{aligned}$$

There are now only two more steps to follow. First, the Doppler shift frequency f_D = $f' - f$, so from Eq. 6,

$$\text{(Eq. 6)}$$

$$f_D = f' - f = \overbrace{f + 2fv_r/c + f(v_r/c)^2 - f}$$

$$= \overline{2fv_r/c + f(v_r/c)^2} \qquad [7]$$

and the final step depends on substituting some typical values in Eq. 7 to demonstrate that the term $f(v_r/c)^2$ can be neglected. For medical Doppler ultrasound, typical values might be as follows: ultrasonic frequency f = 3 MHz, reflector velocity v_r = 1 m/sec, and speed of sound c = 1,500 m/sec. Substituting these values in Eq. 7 reveals that, in this specific example,

$$f_D = \frac{2 \times 3{,}000{,}000 \times 1}{1{,}500} + 3{,}000{,}000 \left(\frac{1}{1{,}500}\right)^2$$

$$= (4{,}000 + 1.333) \text{ Hz}$$

Thus, $f(v_r/c)^2$ is tiny in comparison with $2fv_r/c$ and therefore may be neglected without introducing any significant error. (Mathematics say that the term may be neglected provided that $v_r \ll c$, as is always the case in medical Doppler ultrasound.) Therefore, we arrive at the result

$$f_D = 2fv_r/c \qquad [8]$$

This result applies to the situation illustrated in Fig. 3; the Doppler difference frequency (or "Doppler shift frequency") is positive because the reflector is moving toward the transducers. If the reflector is moving away from the transducers, the received frequency f' is lower than the transmitted frequency f and, mathematically, the Doppler shift frequency f_D has a negative value. For any given geometry and reflector velocity, the magnitude of the Doppler shift frequency is the same; the direction of movement of the reflector determines whether the frequency shift is positive (for movement toward the transducers) or negative (for movement away from the transducers).

The Velocity Vector Problem

In practice, it is seldom the case that the reflector moves exactly along the effective direction of the ultrasonic beam. It is only when this is the case that Eq. 8 is valid. Figure 4A illustrates the more general situation, where the directions of movement of the reflector and of the ultrasonic beam are at some angle θ, the "angle of attack." The Doppler frequency shift then arises because the reflector has an effective component of velocity—the vector velocity v_{eff}—along the direction of the ultrasonic beam. The magnitude of this velocity vector can be calculated by resolving the velocity v_r as shown in Fig. 4B. According to the well-known trigonometric relationship,

$$v_{eff} = v_r \cos \theta \qquad [9]$$

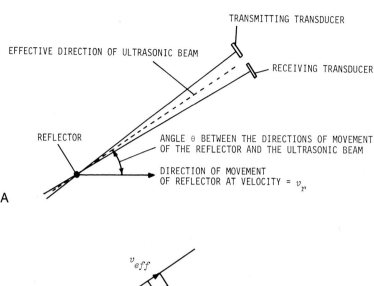

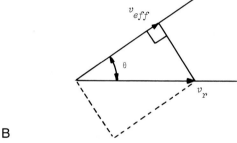

FIG. 4. The effect of the angle between the effective direction of the ultrasonic beam and the direction of movement of the reflector. **A:** Diagram showing the relative positions of the transducers and the moving reflector. **B:** Vector diagram showing how the effective velocity v_{eff} of the reflector is related to the velocity of the reflector v_r by the angle of attack θ.

Thus, for the special case in which the directions of movement and of the beam are coincident, $\theta = 0°$ and so $\cos \theta = 1$, so that $v_r = v_{\text{eff}}$. In general, however, it is the effective value of reflector velocity that needs to be substituted from Eq. 9 into Eq. 8, so that the Doppler shift frequency is given by

$$f_{\text{D}} = (2fv_r \cos \theta)/c \qquad\qquad [10]$$

Figure 5 is a nomogram, based on Eq. 10, from which the Doppler shift frequency, reflector velocity, angle of attack, or ultrasonic frequency can be derived, provided that the values of the other three parameters are known, for the ranges of values commonly involved in medical applications.

A Fortunate Coincidence

Although not a prerequisite for success, it is indeed a happy accident that the Doppler shift frequencies in most medical applications happen to lie in the audible range. For example, with an ultrasonic frequency of 5 MHz and an angle of attack of 60°, blood flowing at 10 cm/sec gives rise to a Doppler shift frequency of about 300 Hz. It should be realized that this satisfactory result—satisfactory because the signals can be heard and interpreted by ear—is not the result of any deliberate choice

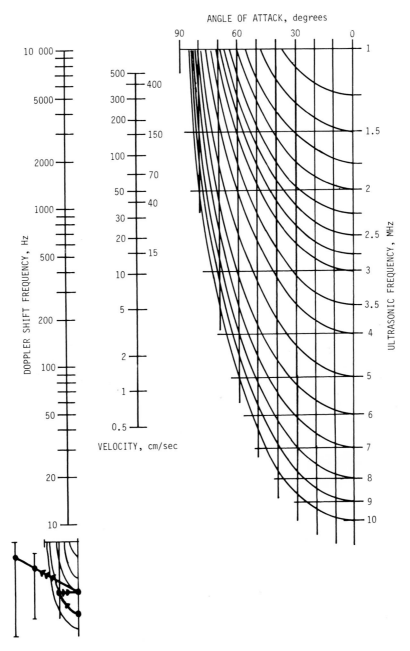

FIG. 5. Nomogram showing the relationships among reflector velocity, Doppler shift frequency, and ultrasonic frequency for various angles of attack. The diagram in the lower left-hand corner indicates the sequence for reading the nomogram. Values calculated for blood, velocity = 1,570 m/sec.

of operating conditions but results from the physics of the Doppler effect and the constraints on the choice of ultrasonic frequency as discussed in the next section.

THE CHOICE OF THE ULTRASONIC FREQUENCY

Scattering Targets

So far, we have considered the situation in which the ultrasound is reflected from the transmitting transducer to the receiving transducer by a reflector of the specular type: this is a reflector that is flat and large in relation to the ultrasonic wavelength. This quite closely approximates the situation with the moving fetal heart, the pulsating walls of a large blood vessel, or the motion of a cardiac valve leaflet, but it is not a good model of the situation with flowing blood.

Although blood is a complex fluid, ultrasonically it behaves like a suspension of small particles (mainly the red cells), each one of which scatters incident ultrasonic waves more-or-less independently. It is the energy scattered back towards the receiving transducer—the backscattered energy when the transmitting and receiving transducers are effectively coincident—that is important from the point of view of medical ultrasonic Doppler techniques. For a given size of scatterer, the backscattered energy is proportional to the fourth power of the frequency provided that the scatterer is small in relation to the wavelength (a condition that is easily satisfied, the wavelength being in the range 1,500 to 150 μm—corresponding to frequencies of 1 to 10 MHz—whereas the maximum diameter of a red cell is about 12 μm). Thus, other things being equal, increasing the ultrasonic frequency from 3 to 6 MHz would result in an increase by a factor of 16 (equivalent to $+12$ dB) in the backscattered energy from blood.

Figure 6A illustrates the situation with a single small scatterer (such as a red cell) irradiated by a plane ultrasonic wave (which is a reasonable approximation to the waves in the beam produced by a medical ultrasonic transducer). Although the situation is straightforward, only a minute fraction of the incident wave is backscattered to the receiving transducer, partly because the effective cross-sectional area of the scatterer is only a tiny fraction of the total beam cross section and partly because the scattered energy is radiated approximately uniformly in all directions (that is, as spherical wavelets). In reality, of course, blood can be considered to be an ensemble of scatterers as illustrated in Fig. 6B. In order to understand the way in which the backscattered components of the wavelets combine, it is necessary to introduce the concept of interference. First, consider the wavelets scattered by only two obstacles. If at some point in space—and, in particular, at the surface of the receiving transducer—the maxima of the two wavelets arrive simultaneously, followed simultaneously by the zeroes and the minima, the wavelets are said to be in phase, and the resultant combination wave has an amplitude corresponding to the sum of the separate amplitudes of the two waves. (The actual relationship is that the square of the amplitude of the combination wave is equal to the sum of the squares of the amplitudes of the two waves.) This process is called "constructive interference." On the other hand, if the maximum of one wavelet coincides with minimum of the other, the wavelets are said to be in antiphase, and the combination wave has an

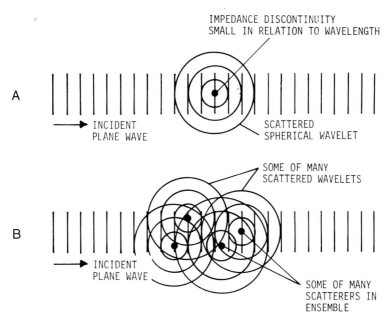

FIG. 6. Diagrams illustrating the scattering of ultrasound. **A:** A single small scatterer irradiated by a plane ultrasonic wave reradiates the incident wave energy as a spherical wavelet. **B:** An ensemble of small scatterers (e.g., blood) produces a backscattered wave amplitude that depends on the interference among all the individual scattered spherical wavelets.

amplitude depending on the difference between the individual amplitudes of the two wavelets (zero if the two wavelets are of equal amplitude). This is called "destructive interference." The relationship between the two wavelets can be expressed in terms of a phase angle. There are 360° in a complete wave cycle; wavelets are in phase if their relative phase angle is 0°, 360°, and so on, and in antiphase if it is 180°, 540°, etc.

Situations in which the wavelets are neither exactly in phase nor exactly in antiphase can be resolved by taking all the individual phase angles and amplitudes into account. Now consider again the ensemble of scatterers illustrated in Fig. 6B. The receiving transducer detects the wavelets backscattered by all the individual scatterers lying in the ultrasonic beam. Because the transducer is sensitive to phase as well as amplitude (as opposed to being a power detector), the output from the transducer depends on the spatial relationships of the scatterers as well as on the number of scatterers in the ultrasonic beam. Averaged over a suitably long period of time, the amplitude does depend on the density of scatterers (the actual relationship is that the power is proportional to the total number of scatterers in the interrogated volume and thus to the density of scatterers, so the amplitude is proportional to the square root of the total number of scatterers).

Because the entire interference pattern moves with the flowing blood, the instantaneous value of the amplitude fluctuates with time, and this should be remembered when the analysis of Doppler signals is being considered. Apart from this complication (which, in any case, fortunately can usually be neglected), flowing blood can be considered to behave in the same way as a simple moving reflector in giving rise to the Doppler effect, and, in particular, Eq. 10 can be applied without modification.

Up to now, we have been assuming that the Doppler effect occurs because the ultrasonic beam is reflected (or backscattered) by a moving reflector (or ensemble of scattering targets). Fortunately, this assumption leads to useful results in medical Doppler applications. It is worth noting, however, that it is only seldom that either reflectors or scatterers move independently of their surrounding media. Certainly in the case of blood, for example, the blood cells are carried along by the motion of the liquid in which they are suspended. Strictly speaking, the ''Doppler effect'' that is observed is the result of the ultrasonic waves being accelerated or decelerated in the moving medium relative to the fixed transducers and the speed the ultrasound would have if the medium were stationary; the reflector (or ensemble of scatterers) has the purely passive role of reradiating the wave without actually introducing any Dopler frequency shift. The analysis of this situation is really quite difficult, and so it is indeed fortunate that this effect can, at least for practical purposes, be neglected and Eq. 10 can be applied without introducing significant error.

Attenuation in Intervening Media

Medical applications of ultrasound based on reflection techniques depend on the echo amplitude from the structure of interest being large enough to be detected. In pulse-echo imaging of soft tissues, a reasonably good working rule is to expect that satisfactory echoes can be obtained with a penetration of up to about 200 wavelengths. This limitation arises because of the attenuation of ultrasound in tissues, which increases with the ultrasonic frequency. The wavelength is about 1.5 mm at a frequency of 1 MHz, corresponding to a maximum penetration of about 300 mm; at 3 MHz the maximum penetration is reduced to about 100 mm, at 5 MHz to about 60 mm, and so on. The echo amplitude from blood (caused mainly by backscattering of the red cells) is much lower than that from most soft tissue boundaries, but it has already been explained that the backscattered power is proportional to the fourth power of the frequency (so the amplitude is proportional to the square of the frequency). Since the attenuation in the intervening media (the attenuation in the media between the transducers and the blood that it is desired to study) also increases with frequency, the choice of the optimum frequency (i.e., the frequency that gives the maximum echo amplitude) has to be based on the optimum compromise. A working rule is that

$$f_{opt} \simeq 90/d \qquad [11]$$

where f_{opt} is the optimum ultrasonic frequency (in megahertz), and d is the soft-tissue distance (in millimeters) between the transducers and the blood. Most blood flow studies are made at distances between 5 and 100 mm, and substitution in Eq. 11 indicates that the corresponding optimum frequencies would be in the range between 20 and 1 MHz. In practice, frequencies of between 10 and 2 MHz are generally used, mainly because there are a number of other constraints (such as the need for transducers to be used for imaging and for Doppler, the desirable Doppler frequency shift range, and the problem of aliasing, which are discussed later).

ULTRASONIC BEAMS FOR DOPPLER APPLICATIONS

Dynamic Range

In almost all of the familiar pulse-echo ultrasonic imaging techniques, the same transducer is employed both to transmit the ultrasound and to receive the ultrasonic echoes. It is possible for the same transducer to be used for both purposes because the two functions are separated in time: the transducer is not required to receive low-level ultrasonic echoes at the same time as it is being excited to transmit by a high-level electrical pulse. Similarly with pulsed Doppler techniques, the same transducer can be used both as transmitter and receiver, at least to the extent that the problem of the masking of weak echo signals by the transmitting pulse does not arise.

The situation is different with continuous-wave (CW) Doppler techniques. In a CW Doppler system, the transmitter operates continuously, and if the same transducer were to be used both as transmitter and receiver, it would be inevitable that the high-level electrical output exciting the transmitting transducer to emit ultrasound would also be applied continuously to the receiver circuit. The receiver circuit would be required to detect the tiny echo signals superimposed on the transmitting signal, although they would typically be 70 to 90 dB below the amplitude of the transmitting signal. Electronic engineers would say that the receiving circuit would need to be able to handle a dynamic range of more than 90 dB; such performance is at the limit of technical possibility. An analogy may help in understanding the problem: it is like trying to see the inside of a room by looking through a window reflecting the full glare of the sun into the eye of the observer. In this analogy, one solution is to illuminate the inside of the room by allowing the sun to shine through one window and to view the contents of the room through another window shielded from the sun. Likewise with CW Doppler techniques, one solution to the dynamic range problem is to use one transducer as the transmitter and another transducer, as close as possible to the transmitting transducer but ultrasonically isolated from direct coupling with it, as the receiver.

A Qualitative Approach to the Ultrasonic Field

In pulse-echo imaging, usually one of the objectives is to have the best possible spatial resolution. As far as resolution normal to the ultrasonic beam axis is concerned, this means that the width of the beam (which controls the lateral resolution within the scan plane) and the thickness of the beam (which controls the thickness of the scan plane) are both made as small as possible. This involves optimizing the choices of ultrasonic frequency, transducer dimensions, and focusing arrangements. For example, Fig. 7 shows the main components of a single-element disk transducer probe with a concave plastic lens designed to focus the ultrasonic beam to give the best possible resolution over a fixed and limited depth of focus. When such a transducer is used for imaging, reflecting and backscattering targets lying within the ultrasonic beam may be detected; satisfactory performance depends on targets outside the beam not being detected. For pulsed Doppler operation, the same considerations

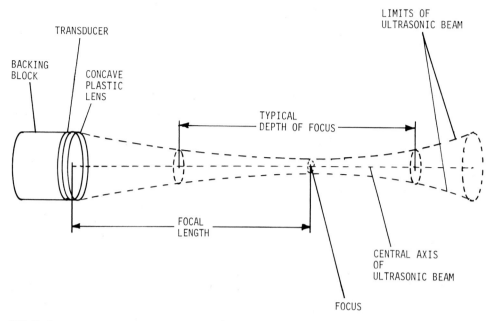

FIG. 7. Construction of the main components of a typical transducer probe for pulse-echo ultrasonic imaging, one of the type that can also be used for pulsed Doppler applications. The backing block improves the short-pulse performance (and, hence, the range resolution) of the transducer. The plastic lens focuses the ultrasonic beam to produce a narrow beam with optimal lateral and slice thickness resolutions over a limited depth of focus.

apply: only targets moving within the ultrasonic beam are capable of being detected. Notice that the effective beam shape is actually the product of the transmitting and receiving beams. If the same transducer is used as both transmitter and receiver, these two beams are identical. In any case, multiplying the two beams together results in an effective beam shape that is more sharply directional than either of the two beams alone.

When separate transducers are used for transmitting and for receiving, the situation is more complicated. First, it is necessary to arrange for the transmitting and receiving ultrasonic beams to overlap: obviously, the echo from a target in the transmitting beam can only be detected if it is also in the receiving beam. In the case of a specular reflector, even that may not be enough: the reflector also needs to be oriented so that it returns the ultrasonic pulse from the transmitting transducer to the receiving transducer. Since small scatterers reradiate spherical wavelets, however, small targets within the region of overlap are detected subject to the phenomenon of interference that has already been discussed.

From the point of view of the probe manufacturer, one of the simplest transducer arrangements for CW Doppler operation is provided by cutting a disk transducer along a diameter to form two D-shaped elements, one for transmitting and the other for receiving. This construction is illustrated in Fig. 8. Since the operation of the transducers depends on the transmitting and receiving beams overlapping, the two transducer elements are sometimes angled slightly so that the beams cross in the region where maximum sensitivity is required. The performance of the probe may

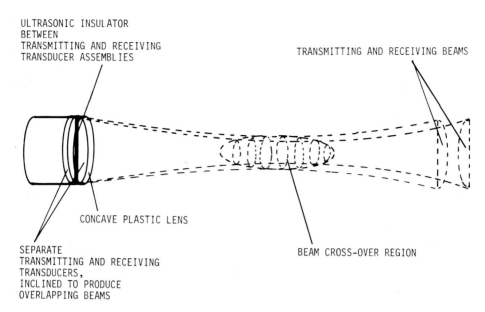

ULTRASONIC INSULATOR
BETWEEN
TRANSMITTING AND RECEIVING
TRANSDUCER ASSEMBLIES

TRANSMITTING AND RECEIVING BEAMS

CONCAVE PLASTIC LENS

SEPARATE
TRANSMITTING AND RECEIVING
TRANSDUCERS,
INCLINED TO PRODUCE
OVERLAPPING BEAMS

BEAM CROSS-OVER REGION

FIG. 8. Construction of a typical probe with separate transmitting and receiving transducers for CW Doppler operation. Note that in the diagram the beams are distinguished by their D shapes beyond the crossover region; real beams tend to be more circular in section as the distance from the transducer is increased.

be further improved by arranging for the two beams to be focused in the beam crossover region.

If the probe is required to operate at a relatively high ultrasonic frequency, above about 7 MHz, the individual transducer elements are usually quite small (about 1 or 2 mm in any dimension). The split-disk approach may then be more difficult to implement than the use of separate rectangular transducers mounted side by side.

The best shape for the sensitive region of the ultrasonic field depends on the particular clinical application. The two factors that are most important are the depth of the sensitive region beyond the probe and the dimensions of the sensitive region along and normal to the effective direction of the ultrasonic beam. When a single transducer is used for transmitting and receiving, the sensitive region extends along the entire beam length until the signals become too small to be detected as a result of attenuation in the intervening tissue. Single-transducer operation is generally limited to pulsed Doppler systems. When separate transducers are used for transmitting and receiving, the length of the sensitive region is limited to the overlapping parts of the two beams, and, in addition, attenuation in the intervening tissue is a further constraint.

An Analytical Approach to the Ultrasonic Field

The lateral dimensions of the sensitive region are determined by the dimensions of the ultrasonic beam, or beams, in the overlapping region. The mathematical analysis of the ultrasonic field is based on the application of Huygen's principle, in which the surface of the transducer is considered to be an array of separate elements each radiating spherical wavelets in the forward direction. The elements move in synchrony and with equal amplitudes (i.e., a disk transducer is considered to be a rigid oscillating piston). This is known as a "steady-state" condition. The method of analysis is illustrated in Fig. 9 by a simple example in which the source consists of an array of six small transducer elements. The wavelets interfere constructively in the regions where the maxima coincide (i.e., where the wavelets are in phase). In other places, there is a tendency for maxima and minima to coincide, so that destructive interference occurs and there is little or no net disturbance. Consequently, the ultrasonic field is concentrated within a beam that becomes more uniform (and eventually more divergent) with increasing distance from the array.

It is relatively easy to apply Huygen's principle to the simple case of the ultrasonic field produced by a linear array of a small number of transducer elements. The situation is much more complicated, however, if the source is in the form of, for example, a circular piston (i.e., a disk) transducer. The problem is one of three-dimensional geometry. The theoretical field for such a source is illustrated in Fig. 10. Moving along the central axis of the beam toward the source, the intensity increases until a maximum is reached at a distance of z'_{max} from the source given by

$$z'_{max} = a^2/\lambda \qquad [12]$$

where a is the radius of the source, and $a^2 \gg \lambda^2$ (as is usually the case in ultrasonic diagnosis). Increasingly closely spaced axial maxima and minima occur towards the source. At successive axial maxima and minima, starting at z'_{max} and moving toward the source, there are one, two, three, etc. principal maxima across the beam di-

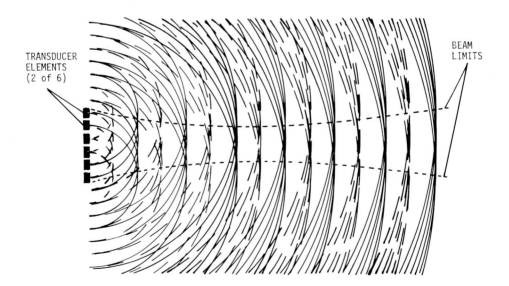

FIG. 9. Diagram illustrating the formation of an ultrasonic beam by interference among spherical wavelets emitted from (in this example) an array of six small transducer elements. Wavelet maxima are represented by *continuous lines,* and wavelet minima by *long-dashed lines.* The beam is the region in which the wavelets are in phase; outside the beam, destructive interference and divergence cause the intensity to be increasingly reduced.

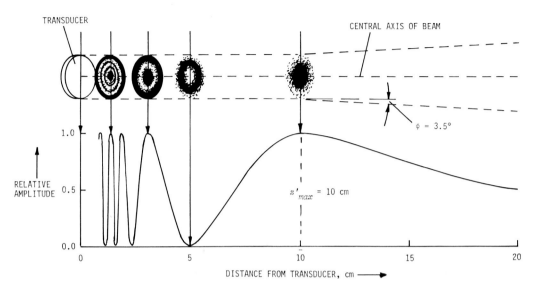

FIG. 10. The ultrasonic field. This example shows the distribution for a 1.5-MHz transducer with radius $a = 10$ mm. The ultrasonic beam normal to the central axis is circular in cross section; the elliptical diagrams represent such sections in the planes indicated on the graph, showing the variation in central axial amplitude with distance from the transducer.

ameter. The region between the source and the last axial maximum (at z'_{max}) is known as the "near field," and the region beyond this is the "far field." In the absence of focusing, the beam is roughly cylindrical in the near field. Deep in the far field, the beam diverges at angles $\pm\phi$ about the central axis, given by

$$\sin \phi \simeq 0.6\lambda/a \qquad [13]$$

Summarizing the results expressed in Eqs. 12 and 13, the length of the near field increases with increasing diameter of the transducer and with increasing frequency of the ultrasound (remember that $\lambda = c/f$), but the divergence in the far field decreases with increasing diameter and with increasing frequency.

This simple analysis corresponds to a single ultrasonic frequency, and consequently it applies to the situation with CW (steady-state) Doppler operation. When pulsed ultrasound is transmitted and received, however, the ultrasonic energy is spread over a spectrum of frequencies. With short pulses, and at the beginnings and ends of long pulses, the transient existence of a spectrum of ultrasonic wavelengths results in a smoothing out of the relatively well-defined inhomogeneities that exist at any particular single frequency.

Beam Forming: An Initial Discussion

Within the near field of an ultrasonic transducer, the beam profile can be modified by a variety of techniques, the most common of which is focusing. Focusing reduces the lateral dimensions of the ultrasonic beam within the focal zone and thereby greatly improves the resolution in azimuth and in elevation. In considering the phe-

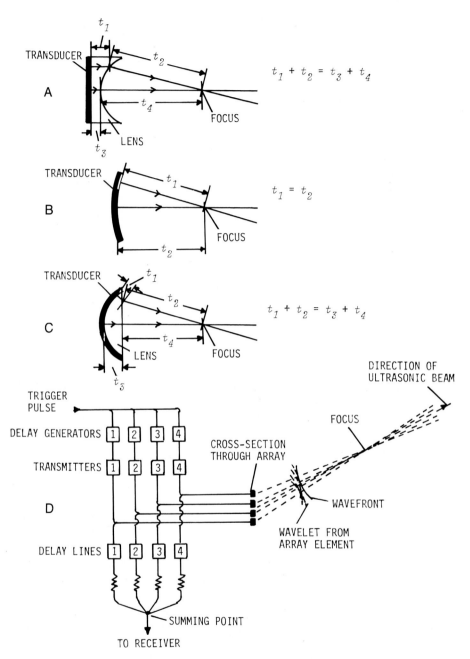

FIG. 11. Methods of focusing an ultrasonic beam. **A:** Concave lens. **B:** Concave transducer. **C:** Combined strongly focusing concave transducer and weaky defocusing convex lens. **D:** Electronic beam steering and focusing. The trigger pulse starts the delay generators 1 to 4, which introduce progressively longer delays in the excitation of the elements along the array. Consequently, the wavefront, which is the surface joining the cylindrical wavelets emitted by the transducer elements, has its normal (the direction of the ultrasonic beam) lying along a bearing that can be changed by changing the delay times. The beam can also be focused by fine adjustment of the delay times. Similarly, on reception the delay lines introduce time delays in the individual signal paths associated with each element in the array so that echoes from the focus arrive simultaneously at the summing point.

nomenon of focusing, a helpful concept is that the focus occurs at the point in the field at which the contributions from the entire surface of the transducer all arrive simultaneously, i.e., in phase. This is illustrated by the methods of focusing shown in Fig. 11. In Fig. 11A, a concave lens in which the speed of ultrasound is greater than that in the medium beyond the lens introduces appropriate thicknesses of lens material into ray paths of different lengths, so that the transit times along all ray paths from the transducer surface to the focus are equal. Focusing may also be achieved by means of a concave transducer giving equal-length ray paths from the transducer surface to the focus, as illustrated in Fig. 11B. Figure 11C shows how the combined effects of convergence by a concave transducer and divergence by a convex plastic lens can make it possible for a flat-faced probe to produce a focused ultrasonic beam. Finally, Fig. 11D shows how an array of small rectangular transducer elements can be used both to focus and to steer an ultrasonic beam by introducing appropriate time delays in the associated electronic circuits. With lenses and curved transducers, the focal length is fixed. With electronic focusing, the transmitting focal length can be chosen to be at any desired range, and, on reception, the focal length can be swept continuously along the beam to coincide within the echo-producing targets; this is called "dynamic focusing."

Effects of the Beam Shape on the Doppler Signal

The Doppler signals that are detected in any clinical situation may be quite dependent on the shape of the sensitive region of the ultrasonic beam. The directivity of the beam and its cross-sectional uniformity and, with pulsed Doppler operation, the sample length are particularly important.

In some situations, the diagnosis depends merely on the detection of a Doppler signal. This is often the case, for example, with the fetal heart detector. In this application, a probe of the type illustrated in Fig. 8 is often used. Ideally, the beam should have the minimum directivity (so that enclosing the fetal heart within the beam does not require careful directional adjustment) while maintaining adequate sensitivity to obtain a signal of detectable strength (obviously, the wider the beam, the more "dilute" is the signal from a moving structure within the beam). Toward the end of pregnancy, signals of adequate strength may be detected using a beam deliberately defocused to allow some degree of fetal movement to be tolerated. (The question of safety is discussed in Chapters 8 and 9; here it is sufficient to note that the use of excessive ultrasonic power cannot be justified if this is simply for operational convenience.) A probe designed for monitoring the fetal heart is illustrated in Fig. 12.

At the opposite extreme, ultrasonic beams optimized for pulse-echo imaging are designed to have the maximum directivity. Although such beams are also used for Doppler applications in many types of duplex scanners (see Chapter 2), they are often far from ideal because of the effect of the ultrasonic beam shape on the Doppler signal, particularly in the quantitative measurement of blood flow volume rate. Consider the situations illustrated in Fig. 13. The blood flow conditions are the same in all three of the situations shown, but the Doppler frequency spectra (discussed in

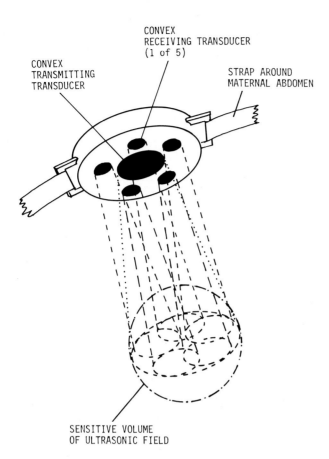

CONVEX
RECEIVING TRANSDUCER
(1 of 5)

CONVEX
TRANSMITTING
TRANSDUCER

STRAP AROUND
MATERNAL ABDOMEN

SENSITIVE VOLUME
OF ULTRASONIC FIELD

FIG. 12. Transducer assembly for monitoring fetal heart movements, especially during labor. The divergent transmitting and receiving beams overlap to produce an ultrasonic field with a relatively large sensitive volume, minimizing the loss of Doppler signal as a result of fetal movement.

the next section) are radically dependent on the relative dimensions of the blood vessel and the ultrasonic beam.

Some high-performance pulse-echo imaging systems employ annular array transducers (typically a central disk and two to five rings) to allow the depth of the focal region to be selected in the transmitting beam and to be swept dynamically in the receiving beam. When the same annular array transducer is used both for imaging and for Doppler studies in a duplex scanner (see Chapter 2), a pair of groupings of transducer elements can be used for CW Doppler operation, thus avoiding the dynamic range problem previously discussed. Recently, an instrument has become available that exploits the capability of an annular array, appropriately excited in phase and amplitude, to produce a wide, uniform ultrasonic beam ideal for quantitative measurement of blood flow volume rate from the attenuation-compensated frequency spectrum of the Doppler signal. This approach, which also depends on the ability of the annular array to produce a highly focused beam and thus to allow the spectrum to be corrected for attenuation in the overlying tissues, allows the blood flow volume rate to be measured without the need to estimate either the cross-sectional area of the blood vessel or the angle of attack of the ultrasonic beam relative to the orientation of the blood vessel. The instrument is described briefly in Chapter 2 and in more detail in Chapter 3.

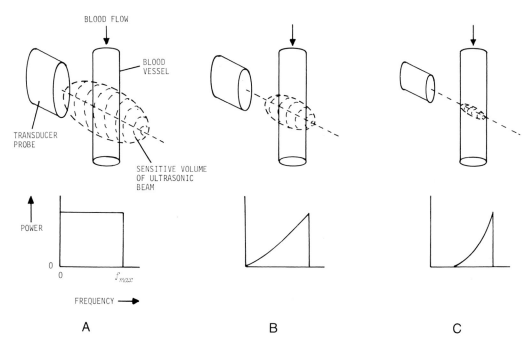

FIG. 13. The effect of the ultrasonic beam shape on the Doppler signal detected from flowing blood. In each diagram, the blood flow velocity profile is assumed to be parabolic, and the axes of the graph representing the frequency spectrum are the same. **A:** The ultrasonic beam is large enough to irradiate all the flowing blood uniformly, and the frequency spectrum has constant power from zero frequency to the frequency corresponding to the maximum blood flow velocity. **B:** The ultrasonic beam has the same diameter as the blood vessel, and, because the beam is nonuniform, the Doppler signals from the slowly moving blood at the edge of the vessel are at relatively low power. **C:** A narrow ultrasonic beam of the type used for imaging detects signals that mainly originate from the fastest flowing blood at the center of the vessel.

DOPPLER FREQUENCY SPECTRUM

Origin of the Spectrum

According to the Eq. 10, at any particular ultrasonic frequency, the Doppler shift frequency depends on the velocity of the reflecting target or ensemble of scatterers. If there is only one moving target in the sensitive region of the ultrasonic beam, there is obviously a single value of Doppler shift frequency at any instant, although of course this Doppler shift frequency does vary with time if the velocity of the target is changing. It is often the case, however, that there are many moving targets in the sensitive region, not all moving at the same velocity at any given moment. This is typically the case with blood flowing in a vessel: the blood at the center of the vessel has a higher velocity than that close to the vessel walls because of the effect of viscous drag. In this situation, signals covering a spectrum of Doppler shift frequencies occur simultaneously at any instant, and the spectral distribution changes if the velocities of the targets also change with time. This is illustrated in Fig. 14A.

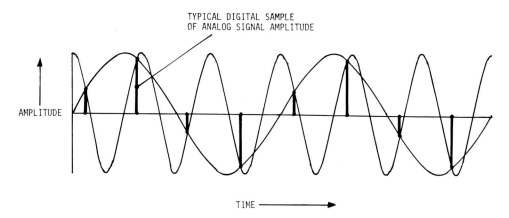

FIG. 15. Digital sampling of analog signals. In this diagram, the lower-frequency signal is adequately sampled at a rate of more than twice the signal frequency (i.e., within the Nyquist limit). The higher-frequency signal, however, is ambiguously represented when sampled at a rate below the Nyquist limit.

version of the analog signal into a time-varying series of digital data, which are subjected to fast Fourier transform (FFT) analysis in a specially built digital computer. There are two additional problems to be considered. The first problem relates to the process of digitizing the analog signal and, in particular, the rate at which digital samples are acquired. When a signal is digitized, the process is free from ambiguity only if the sampling rate is more than twice the maximum frequency present in the signal. This is known as the "Nyquist criterion"; it is illustrated in Fig. 15, which shows that a signal at a frequency below the Nyquist limit can be unambiguously represented by digital samples whereas one above is inadequately sampled because the digital samples derived from it could equally well have been derived from a lower-frequency signal. Incidentally, of course, the adequacy of digitization depends not only on the sampling rate but also on the resolution of the digitizing circuit: for example, a four-bit analog-to-digital converter has a resolution of one part in 16, five bits correspond to one part in 32, and so on. The second problem with digital techniques is concerned with the duration of the sample of signal that is digitized for frequency spectrum analysis. Fast Fourier transform analysis is subject to random statistical fluctuations, which increase with decreasing sampling time, so that the maximum sample duration should be used consistent with retaining the capability to follow changes in the spectral frequency distribution.

In summary, the time required to acquire a Doppler signal increases as the lowest frequency of interest decreases, and the noise in the displayed Doppler frequency spectrum increases as the duration of the sampling time is reduced. It is worth noting that, in many analyzers, the relationship between the ability to follow changes in the spectrum of the input signal and the variance of the spectral estimate are modified by "redundant" calculations in which several FFTs are calculated during the input record time, thus reducing variance and increasing the real-time bandwidth. For example, the input record time for 50-Hz address resolution is 20 msec, and the FFT might be calculated in 5 msec, allowing a redundancy of four.

PHYSICAL PRINCIPLES OF PULSED DOPPLER DETECTION

Range Measurement

As has already been noted, the output from a CW Doppler system is made up of Doppler frequency shift signals from all the targets moving within the sensitive region of the ultrasonic beam. The system is unable to discriminate between targets according to their ranges, or distances, from the probe containing the transmitting and receiving transducers.

In pulse-echo imaging, the ranges of the targets can be estimated from the corresponding time delays in the reception of echoes following the transmission of the ultrasonic pulse by assuming a value for the speed of ultrasound.

A pulsed Doppler system uses range-gated detection to apply the principle of pulse-echo range measurement to the selection of Doppler frequency shift signals from moving targets according to their distances from the ultrasonic probe. The principles are illustrated in Fig. 16. There are two essential steps in the process. First, the phases of the received echo signals are compared with that of a reference signal equal in frequency and having a fixed relationship in time to the transmitted ultrasonic pulses. The phase relationship between these two signals is constant in the case of stationary reflectors but shifted by the Doppler effect with echoes from moving reflectors. The second step involves the range gating of the output from the Doppler detector so the Doppler signals corresponding to the chosen depth along the ultrasonic beam can be selected according to the ultrasonic pulse-echo delay time. The range-gated samples are then fed to a sample-and-hold circuit so that the output from the system consists of the Doppler signal sequentially updated by each ultrasonic pulse.

Maximum Range Limitation

The maximum Doppler shift frequency that can be detected unambiguously by a pulsed Doppler system is set by the Nyquist limit. As has already been explained (see Fig. 15), an analog signal can only be unambiguously represented by samples if it is sampled at a rate that exceeds twice the highest frequency in the signal. This places a constraint on the operation of pulsed Doppler systems, best illustrated by means of an example. Imagine that it is desired to use a pulsed Doppler system to study blood flow at a maximum depth of 15 cm into the patient. The speed of ultrasound is about 1,500 m/sec, so the time delay between the transmission of an ultrasonic pulse and the reception of an echo from a depth of 15 cm is about 200 μsec (remember the round trip path length is 30 cm). The maximum pulse repetition frequency is limited by this time delay: following the transmission of an ultrasonic pulse, the echo from the deepest structure has to be detected before the next pulse is transmitted. In this example, a period of at least 200 μsec must be allowed to elapse between the transmission of consecutive pulses, so the maximum pulse repetition rate is 5,000 per second. Thus, the Nyquist limit to the maximum Doppler shift frequency that can be detected unambiguously is 2,500 Hz.

Now, the ultrasonic frequency for optimum Doppler sensitivity and resolution at

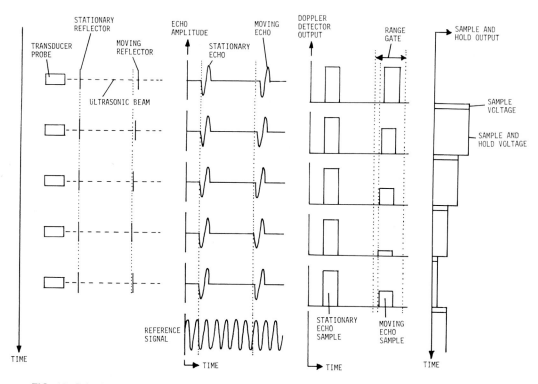

FIG. 16. Principles of pulsed Doppler detection. The diagrams on the left represent an ultrasonic transducer probe arranged to receive echoes from two reflectors in the ultrasonic beam, one stationary and the other in motion. (The *vertical dotted lines* are intended to help to appreciate position and time relationships.) The corresponding received echoes are shown in the adjacent group of diagrams, together with a reference signal at the frequency of the transmitted ultrasonic pulse and always having the same phase at the instant of transmission of each pulse. The echo signals from the stationary reflector have a constant phase relationship to the reference signal; those from the moving reflector vary in phase, however, as a result of the Doppler effect. The next diagrams show the output from the Doppler detector, which operates by comparing the phase of the received signal with that of the reference signal. The echoes from the stationary reflector produce constant detector outputs, but the outputs corresponding to the moving reflector vary in amplitude at the Doppler shift frequency corresponding to the reflector velocity. A gate can be adjusted to allow only the Doppler samples from the range interval of interest to be selected, by appropriate choice of time delay (i.e., target range) and duration (i.e., sample length). The sample output from the range gate can be fed to a sample-and-hold circuit so that the output from the system consists of the Doppler signal sequentially updated by each ultrasonic pulse; this is illustrated in the right-hand diagram.

a depth of 15 cm is about 2 MHz, as has already been explained in the discussion of Eq. 11. Consequently, the maximum vector velocity of blood flow along the effective direction of the ultrasonic beam (see Eq. 10) is just under 1 m/sec. Although it is thus a fortunate accident, structures and blood moving at physiological velocities can usually be detected with pulsed Doppler systems operating at ultrasonic frequencies and pulse repetition rates that are more or less optimum, but there are some clinical situations in which the velocities are so high that the corresponding Doppler shift frequencies exceed the Nyquist limit for unambiguous detection. This condition is known as ''aliasing'' because of the appearance of false signals on the display. In such situations, it is often possible to obtain satisfactory Doppler signals by increasing the pulse repetition rate above the ''limit'' set by the pulse-echo round-trip delay time because the additional spurious Doppler signals that may then si-multaneously occur are likely to be of lower frequency and smaller amplitude than the signals of interest.

BIBLIOGRAPHY

1. Atkinson, P., and Woodcock, J. P. (1982): *Doppler Ultrasound and Its Use in Clinical Measurement.* Academic Press, London.
2. Wells, P. N. T. (1977): *Biomedical Ultrasonics.* Academic Press, London.

2 / *Instrumentation Including Color Flow Mapping*

P. N. T. Wells

Department of Medical Physics, Bristol General Hospital, Bristol BS1 6SY, England

CONTINUOUS-WAVE DOPPLER SYSTEMS

The Basic System

A block diagram of a continuous-wave (CW) ultrasonic Doppler frequency shift detector is shown in Fig. 1. The transmitter operates continuously, providing an electrical output signal of constant frequency and amplitude. This signal is applied to the transmitting transducer mounted in the ultrasonic probe. The choice of frequency depends on the clinical application and is usually in the range from 2 MHz (for deep abdominal and obstetric studies) to 10 MHz (for peripheral vascular work). The factors that determine the geometry of the transducers are discussed in Chapter 1; the ultrasonic transmitting and receiving beams are designed to cross over to form a sensitive region appropriate to the particular clinical application.

The output from the receiving transducer consists of an ensemble of signals, some of a frequency equal to that of the transmitter (these are caused by reflections from stationary structures in the ultrasonic field and to direct electrical leakage from the transmitting circuit to the receiver) and some with frequencies shifted by the Doppler effect (these are caused by reflections from targets moving in the beam). When the transmitted "reference" signal and the amplified Doppler-shifted received signals are mixed, demodulated, and filtered, as shown in Fig. 2, the result is the extraction of the Doppler frequency shift signals corresponding to the moving targets in the ultrasonic beam. The process is called "noncoherent" detection because the echo signal provides its own source of phase and frequency reference. It has the advantage of simplicity and works well when only the magnitude of the Doppler shift frequency is required, but it cannot be used to provide directional information (i.e., it cannot distinguish between movements or flow toward and away from the ultrasonic probe). An audio frequency amplifier is usually arranged to follow the filter, and the operator can listen to the output from the amplifier (e.g., on headphones) or the output can be electronically recorded or analyzed.

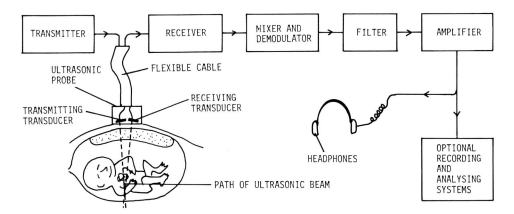

FIG. 1. Basic elements of the simplest type of continuous-wave Doppler frequency shift detector. This diagram shows the main components of a system designed to detect the movements of the fetal heart.

Directional Detection

It is often clinically useful to be able to separate Doppler signals according to whether they originate from targets moving toward or away from the ultrasonic probe. The essential difference between these two groups of signals is that those from approaching targets are shifted upward in frequency relative to the frequency

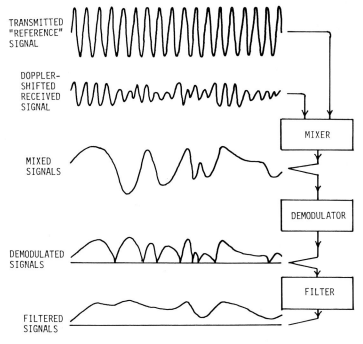

FIG. 2. Noncoherent detection of an ultrasonic Doppler signal. The "reference" signal is predominantly provided by echo signals from stationary structures and electrical leakage from the transmitter. The system does not provide directional information.

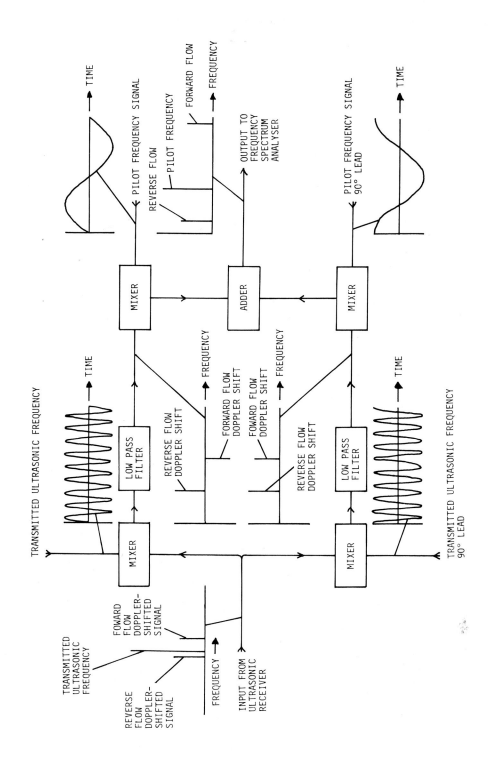

of the transmitter, whereas those from receding targets are shifted downward in frequency. Obviously, the most direct method of separating signals into those corresponding to forward and reverse flows (the term "flow" is often used in the remainder of this chapter, even in places where the argument applies equally to blood flow and to structure motion) is to use two sharply tuned filters, one accepting only signals with frequencies higher than that of the transmitted signal and the other, only lower-frequency signals. In this way, the signals can be separated into two channels and independently processed and displayed. This approach and variants of it, however, are expensive to implement because it is necessary to use a very stable oscillator and bulky high-performance filters.

The method that is now almost universally used for directional Doppler detection is the so-called "phase-quadrature" technique. Unfortunately, this method of signal processing is not amenable to explanation in terms of either simple concepts or illustrative analogy. The best that can be done here is to describe the circuit of a phase quadrature detector, and in the example shown in Fig. 3, the coherent detector is followed by a circuit employing frequency-domain processing to produce an output in which the forward and reverse flow signals are respectively represented by sidebands above and below a pilot frequency chosen to allow convenient display on a frequency spectrum analyzer. Thus, the pilot frequency corresponds to zero Doppler frequency shift (and thus to stationary targets) on the frequency spectral display; the displayed differences in frequency from the pilot frequency correspond to Doppler shift frequencies from moving targets, with forward and reverse flow appearing at higher and lower frequencies with respect to the pilot frequency. If complete separation of the signals corresponding to forward and reverse flow is required, an alternative technique, known as phase-domain processing, can be used after quadrature detection.

PRESENTATION AND DISPLAY OF DOPPLER SIGNALS

Listening to Doppler Signals

The analysis and interpretation of Doppler signals are discussed in Chapter 3. This section is concerned with the instrumentation for the presentation and display of Doppler signals, either as sounds for interpretation by ear or as waveforms or images for inspection and quantitative analysis.

Doppler signals obtained from moving structures and flowing blood are complicated, transient, and rather alien to diagnostic radiologists who are familiar with the

---

FIG. 3. Phase-quadrature detection of an ultrasonic Doppler signal followed by frequency domain processing. In this example, there is one forward and one reverse flow signal, the forward flow signal being at twice the frequency (i.e., originating from a target moving at twice the velocity) of the reverse flow signal. The first step is to divide the ultrasonic signals into two channels and to multiply the signals in each channel by a reference signal at the transmitted ultrasonic frequency; the reference signal for one channel is 90° out of phase with that for the other channel. Following mixing and low-pass filtering, the upper and lower Doppler sidebands are distinguished but not yet separated. The separation takes place when the signals in the two channels are first mixed with a signal at a conveniently chosen (i.e., within the audible frequency range) pilot frequency, again with 90° phase difference between the channels, and then added so that the output signal consists of forward and reverse flow signals in sidebands respectively above and below the pilot frequency.

more tangible art and science of image interpretation. In everyday life, however, the sense of hearing provides one of the most important channels for information transfer. The ear and brain are extraordinarily well adapted to selecting and inter-preting complex sound patterns immersed in a background of noise and irrelevant data.

Although the listener can learn to recognize clinically important sounds in Doppler signals, there are some sounds that are irrelevant and particularly distracting. Among these distracting sounds are the very strong low-frequency Doppler signals from the pulsating walls of blood vessels, known as "wall thump." Most Doppler systems incorporate high-pass filters that strongly attenuate signals with frequencies below around 200 Hz; some instruments have filters with adjustable cut-off frequencies, typically in the range 40 Hz to 1 kHz. The use of such filters can greatly facilitate the interpretation of the relevant higher-frequency sounds in Doppler signals, but it is important to be aware of the existence of the filter and the possibility that it may introduce errors, for example, in the measurement of flow volume rate in slowly moving blood.

When directional information is relevant to clinical diagnosis, this can be conveyed to the listener by providing separate channels for each ear, one corresponding to forward flow and the other, to reverse flow. Headphones or loudspeakers can be used, depending on the working environment and the preference of the listener.

Frequency Spectrum Analysis

The concept of frequency spectrum analysis is introduced in Chapter 1. Nowadays, most Doppler frequency spectrum analyzers employ digital techniques, usually based on the fast Fourier transform (FFT). The FFT has the advantage of easy software implementation on readily available hardware and avoids the need for expensive and bulky frequency-selective filters. The principal disadvantage is that the con-venience of the method, from the point of view of the user, may lead to forgetfulness and complacency concerning the physical limitations of frequency spectral analysis and the artifacts associated with it. Most important, it must not be forgotten that FFT analysis is subject to random statistical fluctuations, which are in addition to the other sources of noise tending to mask the true Doppler signals. These statistical fluctuations increase as either the frequency or the time resolution (or both) of the analyzer is increased.

Doppler signals entering an FFT analyzer are first converted into digital format. This process, and all the other processes within the instrument, are synchronized by a master clock. The digitized signals are stored in a buffer memory, and when this is full, the data are transferred to the processor memory. The processor then computes the FFT of these data and stores the results in an output buffer memory. Notice that the FFT analyzer operates on blocks of data that must be gathered in advance; the input and output buffer memories allow the process to proceed in real time. Suppose it takes the processor 7.5 msec to compute a 128-point transform on 256 words stored in the processor memory. This requires a sampling rate of 256/0.0075 Hz (i.e., approximately 34 kHz), which gives a Nyquist frequency limit of 17 kHz. After transformation, the 128 points are equally spaced from DC to 17 kHz, so the spectral frequency resolution is 17/128 kHz (i.e., approximately 133 Hz; notice that this is the reciprocal of 7.5 msec, the data input period). The range of frequencies in the displayed spectrum and the gain of the amplifier in the analyzer are usually under the control of the operator.

Although most modern Doppler frequency spectrum analyzers use FFT techniques, some machines are still in use that employ analog filters, and a few use zero-crossing counters. In principle, a zero-crossing counter determines the frequency at which amplitude of the analog Doppler signal waveform crosses the zero base line moving in either a positive-going or negative-going direction. (In practice, the counter actually operates on preset threshold levels slightly above and slightly below zero because this improves the reliability in the presence of noise.) The output from a zero-crossing counter can be presented on a spectral display in which time is plotted on one axis and the reciprocal of the time interval between zero crossings (i.e., a measure of the frequency of the signal) is plotted on the other axis; this form of display is called a "time interval histogram."

The power (or the amplitude) of the signal displayed by a frequency spectrum analyzer is usually presented as a gray scale; alternatively, color coding may be used. In addition to the complete frequency spectrum, there are several other quantities that can be used to represent the principal characteristics of the Doppler signal. The most important of these are the maximum frequency and the mean frequency time-varying waveforms, as illustrated in Fig. 4. Some FFT analyzers are able to compute these waveforms, and they may be displayed independently (or fed to waveform analyzers) or superimposed (sometimes in distinctive colors) on the frequency spectral display. It is worth noting that the output from a zero-crossing counter frequency meter is actually the root mean square of the instantaneous frequency spectral distribution; despite the fact that it is not a bad imitation of the mean fre-

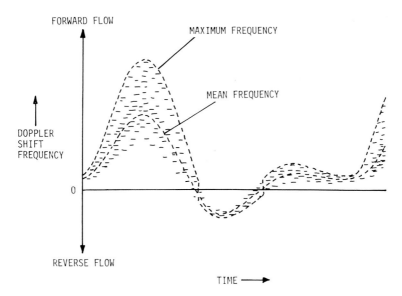

FIG. 4. Diagrammatic representation of a typical Doppler frequency spectrum. The maximum frequency waveform follows the instantaneous value of the frequency above which the power in the spectrum is below some small preset threshold. The mean frequency waveform follows the value of the instantaneous value of the frequency above and below which the powers in the spectrum are equal.

quency waveform and can be obtained inexpensively using simple analog circuitry, it is generally scorned by people with more elaborate equipment.

Hard Copy Devices

As described later in this chapter, Doppler signal frequency spectra and time-varying waveforms are often displayed simultaneously with other information, such as two-dimensional real-time ultrasonic pulse-echo images. In these situations, the Doppler data can be recorded on the same hard copy as the other images, for example, on a multiformat camera. Otherwise, Doppler data are conveniently recorded on any of the ordinary recording systems, including dry silver paper and even color ink-jet devices. Whatever the method of recording, it is frequently desirable to be able simultaneously to display time-varying physiological signals such as the electrocardiogram.

PULSED DOPPLER SYSTEMS

System Design

The physical principles of the pulsed Doppler system are introduced in Chapter 1. The basis of the method is the use of pulse-echo range measurement for the selection of Doppler frequency shift signals from moving targets according to their distances from the ultrasonic probe. Figure 5 is a block diagram showing the essential components of a pulsed Doppler system. In this system, the monostables controlling the sampling gates (adjustable by the operator) determine the duration of the Doppler sample and, hence, the length along the ultrasonic beam of the region sensitive to Doppler shift signals. The delay monostable (also adjustable by the operator) controls the depth from the transducer probe to the beginning of the sample. Notice that the delay monostable operates on the go-and-return path of the ultrasonic pulse (so 1 μsec corresponds to 0.75 mm), whereas the sample monostables actually control the duration of the pulse (and 1 μsec corresponds to 0.375 mm). Notice also that the system has to operate synchronously in order to ensure that successive Doppler samples are properly related to each other; in particular, the mixer and demodulator operate as a coherent detector. Moreover, the detector is normally of the phase-quadrature directional type already described.

System Limitations

The problem of aliasing that arises with Doppler systems when the Nyquist sampling limit is exceeded is discussed in Chapter 1. To recapitulate, the sampling frequency (which is equal to the pulse repetition rate) has to be more than twice the highest frequency in the Doppler frequency spectrum if ambiguities are completely to be avoided. Although this is not a perfect solution to this problem, satisfactory results can often be obtained simply by increasing the pulse repetition rate above the limit imposed by the pulse transit time from the transducer probe to the particular maximum depth from which echoes can be received. Although this leads to the avoidance of Doppler shift frequency ambiguity, range ambiguity is introduced be-

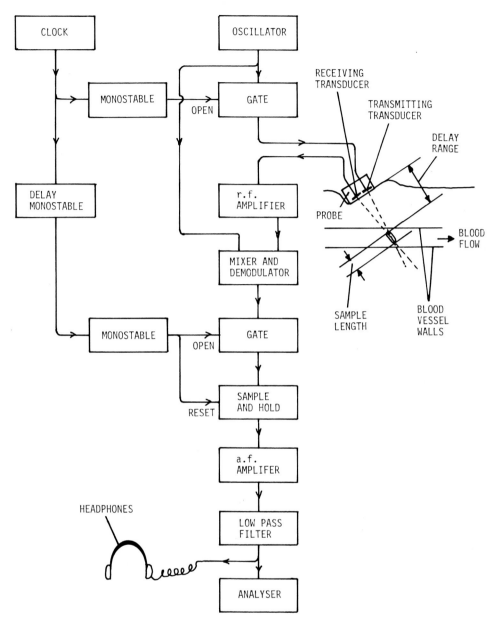

FIG. 5. Block diagram of simple pulsed Doppler system. The pulse repetition rate is determined by the clock; typically, it might be 5 kHz. Each time the clock emits a trigger pulse (in this example, once every 200 μsec), the monostable produces a pulse (say 5 μsec in duration) that opens the gate to allow a 5 μsec burst of the output from the oscillator (which runs continuously at the ultrasonic frequency, say 2 MHz) to excite the transmitting transducer in the probe to emit a 5 μsec pulse (corresponding to a length of 7.5 mm) of ultrasound into the patient. Echoes returning to the receiving transducer (including echoes from moving targets Doppler shifted in frequency) are amplified in the radio frequency (rf) amplifier before being mixed with a signal derived from the oscillator and coherently demodulated. The amplitude of the output from the demodulator thus depends on the velocity of moving targets in the ultrasonic beam, delayed in time according to their ranges, following the transmission of each ultrasonic pulse. The delay monostable is triggered by the clock at the instant that each pulse is transmitted, and it produces a trigger pulse (for example, for a delay of 100 μsec, the depth is 75 mm) to enable the associated monostable to open the gate (for 5 μsec) to allow the desired Doppler sample to be held by the sample-and-hold circuit until the process is repeated with the next pulse. The output from the sample-and-hold circuit (i.e., the range-gated Doppler signal) is amplified by the audio frequency (af) amplifier, filtered, and fed to the headphones and the analyzer.

cause echoes from more than one separately transmitted ultrasonic pulse are being received at the same time. The system can still be range gated to the depth of interest, but additional signals are collected simultaneously from what can be considered to be a second range-gated sample positioned somewhere else (exactly where depends on the actual pulse repetition rate) along the ultrasonic beam. It usually happens, however, that the desired range-gated sample is detecting signals from high-velocity targets and so has the highest Doppler shift frequencies; moreover, careful selection of the pulse repetition rate allows the other sample volume (or volumes) to be positioned where any Doppler signals that may originate are insignificant.

For the most effective Doppler operation, the ultrasonic waves traveling through the body need to have well-defined frequencies shifted only as the result of the Doppler effect. The condition is virtually completely satisfied with continuous-wave Doppler systems, but there are two phenomena that may lead to significant degradation with pulsed Doppler. First, any ultrasonic pulse is associated with a spectrum of ultrasonic frequencies rather than having a precisely defined single frequency, particularly at the beginning and end of the pulse. Consequently, very short pulses are unsatisfactory for Doppler operation because the method depends on comparison of the frequencies of transmitted and received signals for the detection of the relatively very small Doppler frequency shift. The main effect of this phenomenon is a broadening of the Doppler frequency spectrum that becomes more significant as the duration of the ultrasonic pulse is reduced. This limits the maximum range resolution of a pulsed Doppler system; in practice the transmitted pulse generally needs to be at least four complete cycles in length. The other phenomenon leading to reduced performance with pulsed Doppler systems is that of frequency dispersive attenuation in biological tissues. The attenuation is roughly proportional to the frequency of the ultrasound; consequently, the higher frequencies in the spectrum of a short ultrasonic pulse are preferentially attenuated, and the result is a downward shift in the frequency of the ultrasound as the pulse travels through tissue, leading to a change in Doppler shift frequency resulting from target motion at any particular velocity.

A pulsed Doppler system with a single range gate is capable of detecting Doppler signals from only one sample at a time. By providing parallel receiver channels, however, each fed through a gate controlled by a different time delay, Doppler signals can be received simultaneously from separate samples positioned sequentially along the ultrasonic beam. Multigated Doppler signals can be displayed in a variety of ways; for example, Doppler samples can be positioned across a blood vessel to measure the blood flow velocity profile at any instant, or the outputs from all the gates can be displayed as separate waveforms to show the variation with time in the velocity profile. Multigated systems typically have from six to 32 range gates and, if designed for studying superficial blood vessels, might operate at 5 MHz and have sample lengths of about 1 mm.

The Attenuation-Compensated Blood Flow Volume Ratemeter

The method commonly used for the ultrasonic measurement of blood flow volume rate depends on estimating the average blood flow velocity within the vessel of interest (which requires an ultrasonic beam with uniform sensitivity across the vessel and the measurement of the angle between the direction of blood flow and the ul-

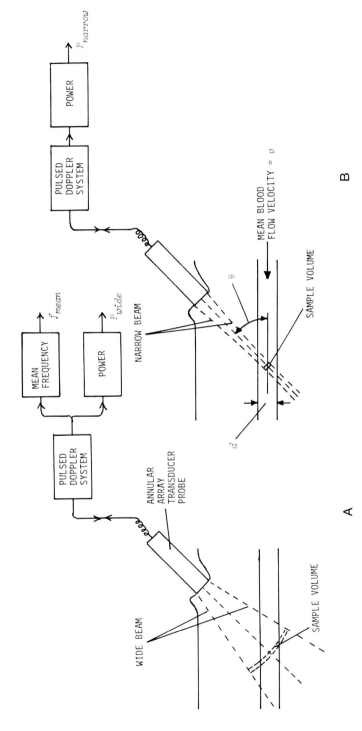

FIG. 6. The attenuation-compensated blood flow volume ratemeter. Wide and narrow beams are both produced by appropriate phasing and amplitude control of the signals associated with an annular array transducer. **A:** With the broad beam, $f_{mean} = v \cos \theta$ and $P_{wide} = kd^2/\cos \theta$. **B:** With the narrow beam, $P_{narrow} = kk'$, where k is an unknown constant (depending on the ultrasonic attenuation in the overlying tissue and the ultrasonic backscattering power of blood), and k' is a calibration constant. Now, $(v \cos \theta)(k d^2/\cos \theta) = k$ (volume flow rate); hence, (volume flow rate) $= (f_{mean})(P_{wide})(P_{narrow})k'$.

trasonic beam) and the cross-sectional area of the vessel (which usually requires the measurement of the diameter of the vessel and the assumption that it is cylindrical). This approach is discussed in Chapter 3.

A technique has recently been developed that can measure blood flow volume rate in vessels of appropriate size and anatomical position without the need to measure either the area or orientation of the vessel. It depends on the use of a pulsed Doppler system and two concentric ultrasonic beams, one wide and one narrow, as shown in Fig. 6. In essence, the wide beam provides the power spectrum of all the flowing blood, and the narrow beam allows this to be corrected for the attenuation in the overlying tissue so that the blood flow volume rate can be calculated. The necessary wide and narrow beams are obtained by appropriate phase and amplitude control of the signals associated with an annular array transducer; adequate performance can be obtained with accessible vessels using an array consisting of a central disk and one annulus. The signal-processing aspects of the instrument, known as the "attenuation-compensated blood flow volume ratemeter," are discussed in more detail in Chapter 3.

DUPLEX SYSTEMS

The Broad Concept

A duplex system is one that enables two-dimensional ultrasonic pulse-echo imaging to guide the placement of an ultrasonic Doppler beam and thus to allow the anatomical location of the origin of the Doppler signals to be identified. The imaging system may be static or real-time, and the Doppler system may be continuous wave or pulsed; the Doppler signals may be collected at the same time as the image information is being acquired, or a previously acquired image may be used for Doppler beam guidance. This very broad definition of the range of so-called "duplex" systems is given not because it is what the originators of the concept had strictly in mind but because many authors of papers on the subject have used the term loosely. What most people now consider to be a duplex scanner is one that has real-time imaging capability with either the imaging transducer or a separate transducer used to collect CW or pulsed Doppler signals, either simultaneously with imaging or sequentially. Instruments in this category are described in more detail here.

Typical Probe Arrangements

A convenient way to categorize transducer probe arrangements for duplex scanning is according to whether they use mechanical or electronic systems for real-time imaging. Figure 7 shows three probe designs typical of the numerous different arrangements possible for real-time mechanical scanning. As far as imaging is concerned, the image frame rate is limited by the depth of the scanned field and the number of image lines per frame. If the depth is, say, 15 cm, the go-and-return ultrasonic pulse-echo delay time is about 200 μsec per line. The corresponding maximum pulse repetition rate (equal to the number of image lines collected per second) is 5,000 Hz. This means that images made up of 100 lines per frame can be collected

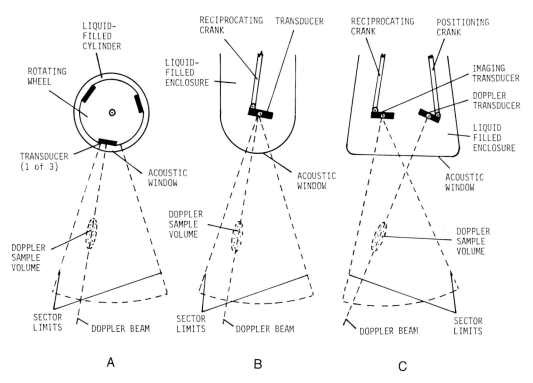

FIG. 7. Duplex transducer probe arrangements for mechanical real-time imaging. **A:** Rotating wheel with three transducers mounted on the rim, producing a sector scan; the wheel is servo controlled to the desired stationary position to allow an imaging transducer to be used for Doppler studies. **B:** Oscillating transducer, driven by a reciprocating crank, producing a sector scan; the transducer is servo controlled to the desired stationary position for Doppler studies. **C:** Oscillating transducer for imaging with separate offset Doppler transducer that can be directed (either manually or by servo control) to the desired orientation for Doppler studies.

at 50 frames per second, and so on; of course, the line density within the image depends on the sector angle of the scan.

In order to collect Doppler signals, it is necessary for the ultrasonic Doppler beam to be virtually stationary and to dwell in the desired direction sufficiently frequently and for a sufficiently long time during each acquisition period to allow adequate sampling of the moving targets. Generally, this excludes the use of a mechanically scanned imaging transducer for the collection of Doppler signals simultaneously with continuous real-time imaging (as in Fig. 7A,B); this is because the mechanical inertia of the moving parts prevents the necessary rapid stopping and starting of the scanning motion. The usual arrangement is for a line representing the desired eventual servocontrolled direction of the ultrasonic Doppler beam to be superimposed on the real-time image to allow appropriate orientation and positioning of the sample volume so that the operator can view the stationary image (as stored in a digital scan converter) when the system is actuated (perhaps by a footswitch) to collect Doppler signals. The system can be made to revert to real-time imaging (again with the footswitch) if it is desired to check the position of the Doppler sample, but, of course, Doppler signal acquisition is then again interrupted. This problem is avoided when separate transducers are used for imaging and Doppler operation (as in Fig.

7C). With this kind of arrangement, the timing of the Doppler pulses can be interpolated as desired among the pulse-echo imaging pulses so that the time is shared between the two modes of operation in the proportion and distribution that give the optimum compromise between Doppler and imaging performances. For CW Doppler operation, however, it is generally necessary to interrupt the pulse-echo imaging because the electrical timing and ultrasonic pulses interfere with the Doppler signals.

Two examples of duplex probe arrangements with electronically scanned linear and phased array transducers for real-time imaging are shown in Fig. 8. A linear imaging array with an end-mounted Doppler transducer (Fig. 8A) is often convenient from the point of view of obtaining a satisfactory Doppler angle, but it is not very versatile in terms of localization adjustment, and it may be difficult to ensure good coupling between the skin and the entire length of the probe. The problem of localization adjustment can be solved by arranging for the Doppler beam to be formed electronically at any desired angle, as in a phased array, from an appropriately chosen window of transducer elements on the linear transducer array. Pulsed Doppler operation can be interpolated among the imaging pulses, allowing simultaneous duplex

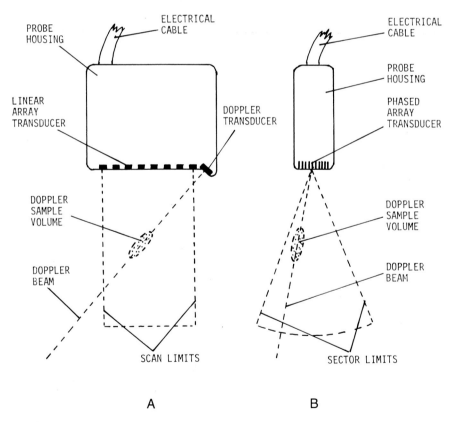

FIG. 8. Duplex transducer probe arrangements using electronically scanned arrays for real-time imaging. **A:** Linear array with end-mounted Doppler transducer; the Doppler beam angle may be fixed, as shown here, or adjustable. **B:** Phased array producing a sector scan. The phased array is also used for Doppler signal acquisition. The Doppler beam angle can be steerable within the sector with pulsed operation, but for CW operation, it is usually fixed in the direction normal to the surface of the array.

scanning. Figure 8B shows a phased array being used for duplex scanning. Again, simultaneous Doppler and imaging operation is possible because, unlike a mechanical real-time scanner, the direction of the beam can be changed instantaneously simply by electronic control of the time delays in the ultrasonic signal paths associated with each element in the array (the beam is said to be "agile").

Operating Frequencies

The choice of the optimum frequency for pulse-echo imaging is not affected by the fact that a system is designed for duplex scanning; for abdominal imaging, a frequency of about 3 MHz is likely to be chosen, and for peripheral vascular work, 7 MHz might be best. If the same transducer is to be used both for imaging and for Doppler operation, however, a compromise may be necessary. This is because a lower frequency may give better Doppler noise performance and, in any case, the range–velocity ambiguity problem is less likely to arise if the Doppler shift frequency for a given target velocity is lower. Some mechanical sector scanners employ two transducers, one for imaging and one for Doppler, the latter often operating at a lower ultrasonic frequency. Similarly, electronic array scanners whose transducers are capable of operating over a wide range of frequencies (i.e., they have a "broad" bandwidth) can work satisfactorily at relatively low ultrasonic Doppler frequencies and high ultrasonic imaging frequencies.

Data Display

The display of ultrasonic duplex real-time scans and Doppler signals affords opportunities for instrument designers to provide "user-friendly" systems based on ergonomic principles. Usually, the initial part of the clinical examination uses real-time imaging to allow the operator to survey the anatomy and to identify the site, or sites, for Doppler studies. The real-time images are displayed in the same way as in conventional scanning, and, superimposed on the scan, markers indicate the direction of the Doppler beam and (except when CW operation is involved) the position of the pulsed Doppler sample volume. Depending on the design of the instrument, simultaneous duplex imaging and Doppler operation may or may not be possible; if it is possible, the Doppler signals can be heard while the sample is being positioned, otherwise the Doppler signals can only be detected when the real-time image has been "frozen" in the frame store and the system has been changed over to Doppler operation. The Doppler signal analysis that is provided by the instrument may be limited to a simple frequency spectral display, or it may be quite comprehensive, providing FFT frequency analysis, maximum and mean frequency waveforms, and the computation of pulsatility and other indices describing blood flow waveforms. Frequency spectra are commonly on a "scrolling" display, continuously updated as new data are collected. Some instruments have electronic calipers that allow the diameters of blood vessels to be measured directly from the frozen image, and vector markers may be displayed at appropriate positions and orientations to permit automatic correction of the Doppler shift frequency for the vessel–beam angle. These latter two pieces of information can be used by the machine to compute the blood flow volume rate; it is important to remember, however, that the ultrasonic beam of a transducer optimized for high-resolution imaging is likely to be far from ideal for Doppler studies, which require uniform irradiation of, for example, a blood vessel. Moreover, single transducers cannot be used for CW Doppler studies; this problem can be avoided in duplex scanners using annular arrays because some transducers can be grouped together as transmitters and some, as receivers. Alternatively, a separate hand-held probe may be provided for CW Doppler studies.

Recordings of images and Doppler signals can be made using any of the methods familiar from nonduplex systems, and hard copies can be obtained on the recorders already in common use.

DOPPLER IMAGING SYSTEMS

Two- and Three-Dimensional Manual Doppler Scanning

The Doppler-shifted signals from flowing blood are sufficiently characteristic to allow them to be identified by electronic logic circuitry. This ability is exploited in a two-dimensional scanner designed to map out blood vessels. The position of the Doppler probe in space in a two-dimensional plane can be measured by means of resolvers mounted on a scanning frame, and this information can be used to control the horizontal and vertical deflection circuits of a cathode ray tube display, as illustrated in Fig. 9. The amplitude of the output from the Doppler detector controls the brightness of the display; in some instruments, the frequency controls the color, and, furthermore, the color coding may be extended to distinguish between forward and reverse flows. The probe is manually scanned systematically over the entire surface of the skin beneath which it is desired to map the blood vessels; only when the ultrasonic beam passes through moving blood is a signal registered on the display. Arterial and venous blood usually can be distinguished by their different flow directions.

The simpler two-dimensional Doppler scanners use continuous waves. More complicated three-dimensional scanners are based on pulsed multigated Doppler systems. They are capable of producing scans in any desired two-dimensional plane within the scanned three-dimensional volume.

Despite the fact that CW Doppler scanners are at least relatively inexpensive, their use has not gained widespread acceptance by radiologists although they remain popular with many vascular surgeons. There are two main reasons for this: satisfactory results depend on the skill of the operator, and the scanning time is rather long. Pulsed Doppler scanners have the added disadvantage of high cost and the problem of obsolescence as a result of the introduction of the technique of Doppler color flow mapping, described in the next section.

Doppler Color Flow Mapping

A conventional pulsed Doppler system can measure the Doppler shift frequency caused by motion in an isolated sample volume in about 10 msec; at a pulse repetition rate of 5,000 Hz, 50 Doppler samples can be collected in this time. The sample

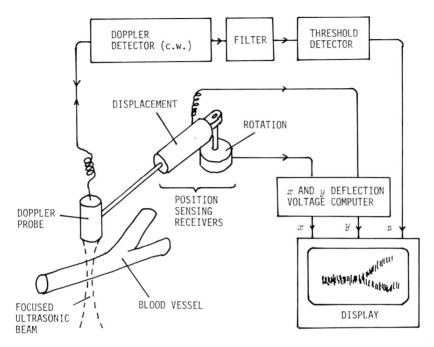

FIG. 9. Continuous-wave Doppler system for two-dimensional visualization of blood vessel distribution. The position of the probe is measured by a polar coordinate scanner, the resolvers of which control the *x* (horizontal) and *y* (vertical) deflection voltage computer driving the cathode ray tube display. The output from the Doppler detector is fed through a filter to remove low-frequency signals resulting mainly from skin contact changes and then goes to a threshold detector so that the *z* (brightness-controlling) signal is stored in the display system to form the two-dimensional image.

volume is typically a sphere with a diameter of 1 mm, although the length may be increased if it is desired to study blood flow in a larger vessel. A multigated pulsed Doppler system in which numerous independent receiver channels are time gated in sequence along the ultrasonic beam can measure the entire flow profile in the same time that a single channel can measure the point velocity, i.e., typically about 10 msec; the diameter of the beam line might optimally be as little as 1 mm. Until recently, the expense and complexity of a system with more than about 30 samples (i.e., capable of measuring the profile over more than about 3 cm) were usually prohibitive.

Single-sample or multigated pulsed Doppler systems, even when used in conjunction with real-time two-dimensional pulse-echo imaging, do not easily convey information about blood flow throughout the entire scan plane; the main application of duplex scanning is in the detailed study of precisely localized anatomical regions. Doppler color flow mapping, which is based on specialized types of pulsed Doppler systems, however, does produce real-time two-dimensional images color coded according to flow conditions and superimposed on real-time two-dimensional gray-scale pulse-echo images of anatomical structures. (The same technique can, of course, be used to color code M-mode recordings.) The principles of one realization of the method are illustrated in Fig. 10. For reasons that are explained later, best results are likely to be obtained using an electronically scanned linear or phased array. The key component of this particular type of system is the Doppler autocor-

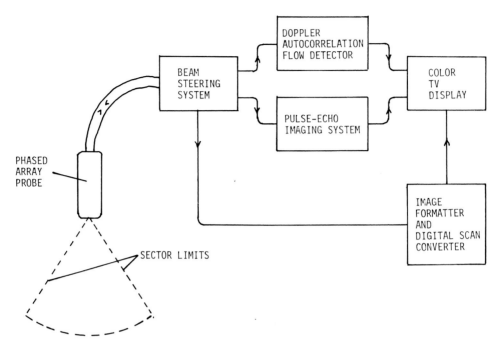

FIG. 10. Block diagram of typical Doppler color flow mapping system. The conventional phased array transducer probe produces a gray-scale real-time pulse-echo sector scan with electronic beam steering and digital scan conversion. Simultaneously, the Doppler autocorrelation flow detector color codes the two-dimensional image. Typically, flow toward the probe is coded in red, flow away from the probe is in blue, and turbulence (defined as the variance of the frequency spectrum) is in green; the brightness (luminance) of the color is controlled by the strength of the signal.

relation flow detector, the purpose of which is rapidly to extract Doppler signals line by line as the ultrasonic beam is scanned through the image plane. The Doppler signal processing and the real-time pulse-echo imaging proceed on a time-shared basis so that the displayed image is a combination of Doppler and anatomical information.

FIG. 11. Principle of Doppler autocorrelation flow detection based on pulse pair covariance. **A:** Input Doppler signal wave trains arrive sequentially (S_0, S_1, S_2, ...) from the phase quadrature detector. The multiplier accepts the wave trains directly and after being fed through the delay line; the delay line introduces a time delay exactly equal to the interval between consecutive ultrasonic pulses, so the multiplier processes pairs of consecutive wave trains ($S_0 \times S_1$, $S_1 \times S_2$, ...). If there is no movement of the echo-producing structures along the ultrasonic beam, the wave trains are identical; but if movements occur anywhere along the beam (in these diagrams, such movements are represented as occurring in the time between the pairs of *vertical dotted lines* drawn on the signal wave trains), corresponding phase changes occur in the echo wave trains of successive pulses, and these phase changes cause changes in the amplitudes of the multiplied pairs of wave trains ($S_0 \times S_1$, $S_1 \times S_2$, ...). Short-term variations in these multiplied waveforms are smoothed by the integrator [$\int(S_0 \times S_1)$, $\int(S_1 \times S_2)$, ...]. **B:** This graph shows the output signal consisting of successive integrated waveforms on the same time scale. At times when no movement has occurred along the ultrasonic beam, the instantaneous integrated amplitude of the output signal remains constant from pulse to pulse. When there is target motion, however, the integrated amplitude changes in correspondence with the Doppler frequency shift. In this example, target motion is represented at only one range interval, but the process is sensitive to motion at any velocity anywhere along the ultrasonic beam. The output signals are spatially identified in the digital scan converter (see Fig. 10), and the display is color coded according to the frequency (i.e., flow velocity) and frequency spectral variance (i.e., flow turbulence). Note that, for simplicity, only one channel of input signal is shown in this diagram; in a practical system, both channels from the phase quadrature detector are processed to provide directional information as well as velocity and turbulence signals.

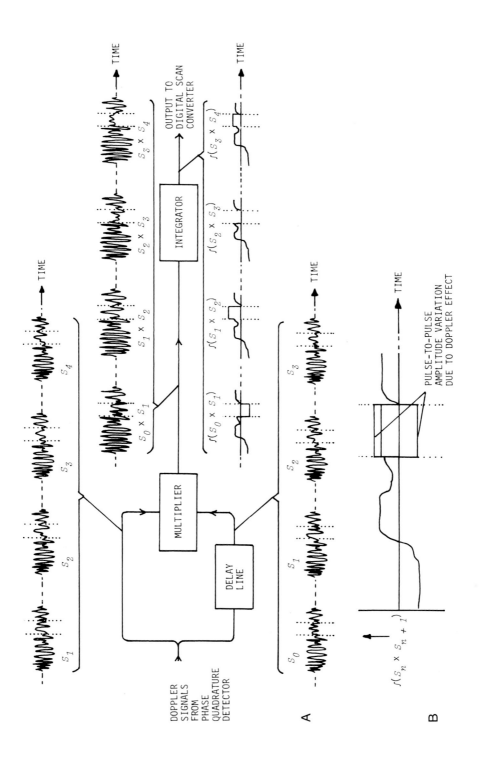

The Doppler autocorrelation flow detector is a kind of moving target indicator that avoids the need for a very large number of parallel receiver gates. Figure 11 shows how moving targets (such as flowing blood) can be identified by autocorrelation of the Doppler phase-quadrature-detected signals obtained with sequentially transmitted ultrasonic pulses. The autocorrelation function is defined as the product of the signal and a time-shifted version of itself. The function is obtained by multiplying the Doppler signal wave train with the signal wave train obtained from the immediately preceding ultrasonic pulse delayed (in a delay line) by a time exactly equal to the interval between pulses. Thus, a complete line of Doppler data can be obtained with a minimum of three ultrasonic pulses, so the method is up to about 20 times faster than the single-line multigated Doppler approach. (It is important to note, however, that satisfactory Doppler color flow mapping can be accomplished using a multigated system, since the spatial and frequency resolutions can be relaxed in comparison with the requirements for single sample volume studies. The multigated approach is demanding, however, in terms of hardware and software.)

Satisfactory operation of the autocorrelation method of flow detection depends on two important conditions. First, the echo wave trains from stationary structures must be identical from pulse to pulse. This means that the ultrasonic beam has to be stationary for at least three pulses. The minimum of three pulses is required because each pair of pulses gives a Doppler phase estimate; at least two phase measurements separated by a known time interval are needed to determine the target velocity. (In strict signal-processing parlance, the technique is known as "pulse pair covariance.") Generally, a completely stationary beam cannot be achieved if a mechanical real-time scanner is used, but this problem does not arise with electronic beam control, whether by linear or phased array. Secondly, so-called "clutter" signals have to be eliminated or they tend to mask the required Doppler signals. Although this can be done by a logic-controlled filter that passes low-amplitude high-velocity signals but not high-amplitude low-velocity signals, better results are obtained by a system known as a "delay-line canceler" that operates by subtracting stationary echoes in consecutive pairs of ultrasonic pulses.

The output from the autocorrelation detector consists of directional real-time velocity (i.e., Doppler frequency) signals. These are arranged to color code the two-dimensional real-time gray scale image; red is usually used to identify forward flow, and blue, reverse flow. In addition, the variance of the frequency spectrum is related to, among other things, the degree of turbulence in the blood flow, and this can be color-coded in green.

Doppler color flow mapping can be performed equally well with phased and linear array systems. With the sector of the phased array, it is usually easy to arrange for at least part of the vessel of interest to lie at a suitable Doppler angle of attack within the scan plane. This is not always the case with a linear array, however, and it is then necessary to use a wedge-shaped ultrasonic coupling device between the probe and the skin.

Doppler color flow maps contain a lot of information, and the acquisition of this ultimately limits the image frame rate. As with conventional pulsed Doppler systems, autocorrelation detection is subject to aliasing if the Nyquist limit is exceeded, and this causes color inversion. When imaging to a depth of 12 cm, a typical system uses an ultrasonic frequency of 3.5 MHz and produces a 50° sector at a frame rate of 30 per second. Similar considerations apply to the performance of linear array systems.

PLATE I

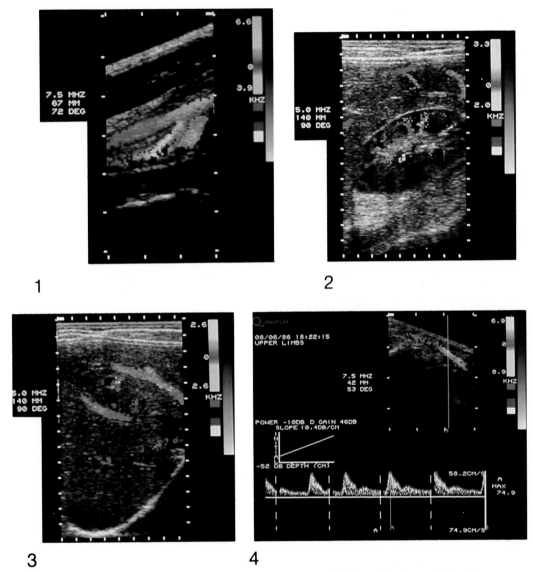

Plate I. 1: Normal carotid artery bifurcation; blood flow at the bifurcation demonstrates flow separation with reversal of flow in the bulb modulated in blue. **2:** Longitudinal section of liver and right kidney; the segmental and interlobar arteries appear in red, and the corresponding veins in blue. 3: Transverse scan of the liver shows the hepatic veins colored in blue or red, depending on the movement of blood away from the transducer or toward the transducer, respectively. **4:** Radial artery; spectral analysis and color Doppler display show the flow through a normal radial artery.

Some examples of Doppler color blood flow maps in various normal and pathological conditions are shown in Plate I.

FUTURE DEVELOPMENTS IN INSTRUMENTATION

It is a truism that the state of high-technology medicine is limited by the capability of the available technology. Thus, in medical Doppler ultrasound, the emergence and refinement of each new class of instrument has opened up new areas of clinical application. What will become clinically possible in the future will be determined by what new instruments become available and by what new methods of data analysis are developed.

Here are some ideas about prospects for innovation in ultrasonic Doppler instrumentation. Beginning with the transducer, improved efficiency (perhaps resulting from the use of plastic or composite piezoelectric materials) may allow the ultrasonic exposure to be reduced without loss of diagnostic information. Annular and two-dimensional arrays could be used to permit control of the lateral dimensions of the ultrasonic beam so that the sample volume, as opposed simply to the sample length, could be optimized for each particular clinical application. Improved Doppler transducer frequency bandwidth—or simply making use of what is already available—could allow several ultrasonic frequencies to be transmitted simultaneously, giving rise to uncorrelated Doppler frequency spectra that could be integrated to reduce fluctuations caused by random changes in backscattering from blood. Wideband operation might allow techniques to be adopted that could reduce the aliasing problem by providing distinctive pulse coding to avoid ambiguity. Several pulses could be transmitted simultaneously in different directions to increase the rate of data acquisition. Finally, specialized probes and catheter-mounted transducers could be developed for intraoperative, intravascular, and intracavitary investigations.

BIBLIOGRAPHY

1. Atkinson, P., and Woodcock, J. P. (1982): *Doppler Ultrasound and Its Use in Clinical Measurement.* Academic Press, London.

2. Kasai, C., Namekawa, K., Koyano, A., and Omoto, R. (1984): Real-time two-dimensional Doppler mapping using auto-correlation. In: *Acoustical Imaging, Vol. 13,* edited by M. Kaveh, R. K. Mueller, and J. F. Greenleaf, pp. 447–460. Plenum Press, New York.

3. Wells, P. N. T. (1977): *Biomedical Ultrasonics.* Academic Press, London.

4. Wells, P. N. T. (1980): Ultrasonic Doppler equipment. In: *Medical Physics of CT and Ultrasound,* edited by G. D. Fullerton, and J. A. Zagzebski, pp. 343–366. American Institute of Physics, New York.

3 / *Hemodynamics*

Peter N. Burns

Department of Diagnostic Radiology, Yale University School of Medicine, New Haven, Connecticut 06510

> *So much for the circulation! If it is either hindered or perverted or overstimulated, how many dangerous kinds of illness and surprising symptoms do not ensue?*
> —WILLIAM HARVEY, *De Motu Cordis et Sanguinis, 1628*

In clinical ultrasound studies, the Doppler signal is a consequence of the movement of the blood itself, with the Doppler shift frequency dependent on the velocity of this movement. Doppler information is, then, information concerning blood flow velocity. It is natural to ask how velocity might relate to other physiological variables, to pressure, flow rate, and peripheral resistance, for example. What velocity patterns should be considered normal for a given vessel and how might they change in the presence of a lesion that encroaches on the vessel lumen? What is the significance of the way in which velocity changes with time in arteries? In this chapter some of the concepts and relationships used to describe blood flow are introduced so as to form a background for the interpretation of Doppler signals obtained in clinical practice.

Although the laws governing the steady, organized flow of fluids, such as water in rigid pipes, have been understood for a long time, the study of pulsatile flow of blood in the elastic, branching, and rapidly tapering human arterial tree is still an area of active investigation. Indeed, the precise physiological significance of the pulsatile nature of arterial flow and pressure still remains somewhat obscure. Nonetheless, an acquaintance with the basic principles of fluid dynamics will serve as a constant aid in the application of the Doppler technique. Those readers who seek a complete discussion of the field of hemodynamics are referred immediately to the bibliography (1,5,6,9), to which for other readers it is hoped this chapter might provide a useful introduction.

STEADY FLOW

Basic Concepts: Velocity, Pressure, and Viscosity

Consider a tube that contains a steady flow of a liquid such as water (Fig. 1). The velocity v of flow of an element of fluid in the direction shown is then simply the distance s between any two points divided by the time t taken for the element to traverse them:

$$v = s/t \qquad [1]$$

In reality it is necessary to apply force to the liquid in order to maintain such steady flow. This force is required to overcome the tendency of the liquid to resist flow, a tendency that has its origin in the fluid itself and is a result of its "internal friction" or viscosity. The force may be transmitted to the liquid by means of a piston (Fig. 2) or equally through the fluid itself by contraction of a distant ventricle or even the action of gravity. If the force has a magnitude of F newtons (N) and is applied evenly to an area A of cross-sectional surface of a liquid, there is a pressure of F/A [measured in newtons per square meter (N/m^2), or pascals (Pa)] exerted on the fluid.

As long as the flow is steady, the pipe itself plays relatively little role in the origin of the fluid friction. Intramolecular forces cause the fluid in immediate contact with the internal surface of the pipe to adhere to it; this infinitesimally thin cylindrical element of fluid is stationary and is referred to as the boundary layer. It is helpful to think of the flow bounded by this layer as comprising a series of thin, cylindrical laminae sharing a common axis with the tube. Neighboring laminae of blood slide over each other with progressively higher speed as the diameter of the laminae becomes smaller, much in the same way that cylindrical leaves can be forced out of a rolled up newspaper (Fig. 3). The fastest flowing elements are then towards the center of the vessel, with a decreasing velocity towards the edge.

The rate of change of velocity of flow as one moves from the outer edge of the vessel toward its center is known as the velocity gradient. Neighboring molecular elements between laminae are attracted to each other by the same binding forces that are responsible for the cohesion of the liquid, which consequently resists such deformation. The force required to overcome this resistance increases with the viscosity of the liquid. It is greater for thick, sticky fluids such as treacle and less for thin, volatile fluids such as alcohol. Blood, as might be expected from its composition as a suspension of particles in a liquid plasma, has rather complicated viscous properties. These can change according to the size of the velocity gradient,

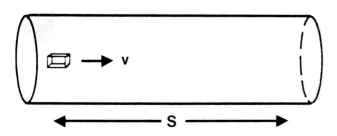

FIG. 1. An element of fluid in steady flow at velocity v takes a time t to traverse a distance s.

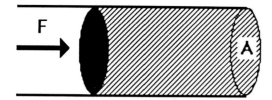

FIG. 2. A force *F* is applied to a fluid to maintain flow against viscous resistance.

but for blood vessels above a millimeter or two in diameter, blood behaves approximately as a constant-viscosity or Newtonian, fluid. In such a fluid the larger the
velocity gradient, the larger the force (called the shear stress) that opposes the sliding
of adjacent laminae. The constant of proportionality is the coefficient of viscosity,
measured in poise after the French physician and physicist Jean Louis Poiseuille.
The Pascal-second is the SI (Système International) unit of viscosity, 10 of which
are equal to 1 poise (P). The viscosity of blood is about 3.5×10^{-2} P, or 3.5×10^{-3} Pa sec.

It was Poiseuille who first described how the steady flow of a fluid is influenced
by its viscosity, showing that for a pressure difference $P_2 - P_1$ along a length of
vessel l, the pressure is related to the flow Q in the following way (Fig. 4)

$$P_2 - P_1 = \frac{8l\eta Q}{\pi r^4} \qquad [2]$$

where η is the viscosity and r the radius of the vessel lumen. If we write this equation
in a simpler form, we may see a parallel with the familiar Ohm's law, which relates
a steady electrical current I to the potential difference E

$$E = RI \qquad [3]$$

where R is, of course, the electrical resistance. Pursuing the analogy we could denote

$$R = \frac{8l\eta}{\pi r^4} \qquad [4]$$

the fluid resistance. Notice how the resistance increases with the fourth power of
decreasing radius. Thus, halving the radius means that a 16-fold increase in pressure
is required to maintain the same flow. The human vascular tree is a rapidly dividing,
narrowing network of vessels. The total resistance of many parallel paths is clearly
less than that of each individual path. In fact, if the resistance of a number of parallel

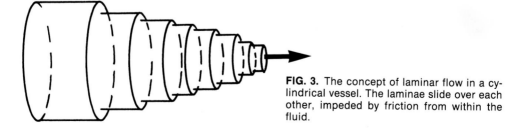

FIG. 3. The concept of laminar flow in a cylindrical vessel. The laminae slide over each
other, impeded by friction from within the
fluid.

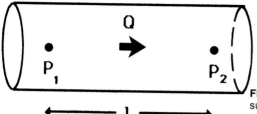

FIG. 4. Poiseuille's law. Steady flow rate Q is sustained in a long rigid tube. The pressure drop over a length I is $P_2 - P_1$.

vessels is R_1, R_2, R_3, and so on, then the total resistance R_{TOT} to flow is smaller than each of the individual values and is given by

$$\frac{1}{R_{TOT}} = \frac{1}{R_1} + \frac{1}{R_2} + \frac{1}{R_3} + \cdots \qquad [5]$$

This raises the interesting question of which part of the vascular tree makes the greatest contribution to the overall resistance to steady flow. Thus, although there is one aorta of considerable length and with a cross-sectional area of about 3 cm², there are more than a thousand million parallel capillaries, each with a cross-sectional area of less than one millionth that of the aorta. Which offers the greatest resistance to flow? Using Poiseuille's law and ignoring, for the moment, the anomalous viscous properties of blood in small vessels, Burton (1) has tabulated the anticipated size and length of vessels on the basis that each level of the circulation must support the same volume flow, and calculated from Poiseuille's law that the greatest contribution to resistance must occur at the arteriolar level (Table 1; Fig. 5). This is, of course, the portion of the circulation in which vasomotor tone acts to control tissue perfusion, a significant fact for Doppler measurements because it illustrates one way in which the state of vessels of physiological interest—but in which flow velocity is too low to measure—influences flow in the much larger vessels from which we obtain most Doppler signals.

Laminar Flow

Another consequence of Poiseuille's law is that the variation of velocity across the lumen of a long rigid vessel with steady viscous flow is smooth and can be predicted: it has the form of a parabola or, to be precise for the case of the cylindrical

TABLE 1. *Geometry of mesenteric arterial bed of the dog*

Vessel	Diameter (mm)	Number	Total cross-sectional area (cm²)	Length (cm)
Aorta	10	1	0.8	40
Large arteries	3	40	3	20
Main branches	1	600	5	10
Terminal branches	0.6	1,800	5	1
Arterioles	0.02	40,000,000	125	0.2
Capillaries	0.008	1,200,000,000	600	0.1

Adapted from Burton (1).

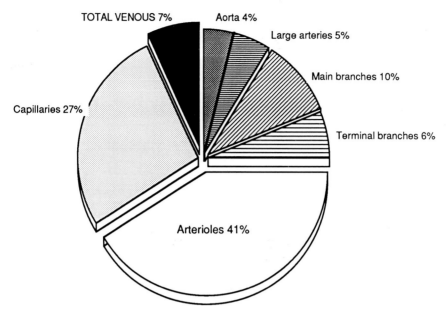

FIG. 5. Relative resistance to flow in portions of the arterial bed calculated from Poiseuille's law and the data of Table 1. After Burton, ref. 1.

pipe, a paraboloid of rotation (Fig. 6). Such a parabolic velocity profile is characteristic of flow in these idealized conditions and is actually observed in some smaller vessels of the abdomen. Flow is said to be laminar when the velocity gradient is smooth and continuous and the streamlines of flow are linear and aligned. Of course, real vessels bend, turn, and branch; their flow velocity is not constant with time, and their walls are not rigid. Velocity profiles deviate from a parabolic form in most of the major arteries (they are generally flattened in the middle) and are themselves a changing function of time. This is an important consideration in the quantitative interpretation of Doppler shift spectra, especially in the measurement of volumetric flow rate.

Geometric Influences on Velocity Profile

As no blood vessel in the body conforms to the conditions for Poiseuille's law, it is not surprising that the velocity profiles, especially in large vessels, are rarely parabolic. Geometry plays an important role among the factors influencing velocity profile and therefore should be considered carefully when one interprets Doppler shift spectra.

Tapering

The arterial system tapers steadily. A converging tube has the effect of stabilizing laminar flow and flattening its velocity profile (Fig. 7). A diverging tube, on the other hand, tends to destabilize flow and elongate the profile, at the same time lowering

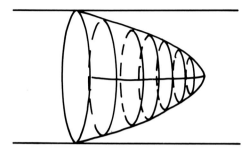

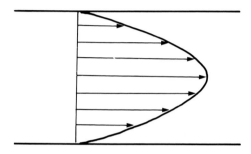

FIG. 6. Parabolic velocity profile in a vessel.

the critical Reynolds number and thus making flow disturbance and turbulence more likely (9).

Entrance Effects

If a small branch has its origin in a large vessel, the profile is flat at the beginning and gradually reverts to a parabolic shape along the new branch. The distance required for this to occur is related to the Reynolds number and the radius of the branch. For the human iliac artery, it is about 100 cm for a velocity of 10 cm/sec, indicating that parabolic flow is never established in this vessel. In practice, then, the velocity profile bears a heavy dependence on the point of measurement along the artery.

Exit Effects

When a vessel widens suddenly (for example, after a constriction), the profile elongates and again eventually reestablishes itself as parabolic. At the outlet itself, the inertia of the flowing blood may cause the boundary layer to separate from the vessel wall, leaving a region of fluid that is stagnant or has a slight retrograde movement toward the region of lower pressure (Fig. 8) (see the following discussion of stenotic flow). This flow separation is known to occur at the origin of the normal internal carotid artery in the area of the bulb. The confusion between the Doppler detection of this normal reverse flow and the turbulent eddies associated with stenosis has been responsible for some false positive Doppler diagnoses of carotid lesions

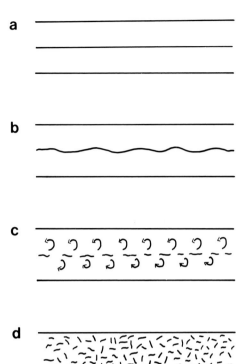

FIG. 11. The transition from laminar flow (**A**) through disturbed flow (**B** and **C**) to turbulence (**D**), illustrated by the course of a streamline of imaginary dye.

which small instabilities gradually formed into circular rotating vortices and then finally broke up into chaotic, disorganized motion, filling the entire pipe (Fig. 11).

In turbulent flow, the velocity of the fluid elements changes rapidly with time, with chaotic movement superimposed on smooth flow. These random movements are similar to the swirling eddies that are swept along a shallow stream flowing over rocks. Such vortices have several effects. First, they increase the resistance to flow: this is known as Reynolds stress. Second, the rotating elements produce flow vectors in the transverse or radial direction as well as in the opposite direction to the overall flow. Finally, the presence of irregular velocity gradients produces forces that tend to upset the homogeneous distribution of red blood cells in a region of turbulence. Superimposed on the turbulence is the overall steady flow along the axis of the pipe. The velocity profile is no longer parabolic but relatively flat (Fig. 12). This means that the velocity gradient and hence the shear stress near to the wall of a vessel in which the flow is turbulent can be very great.

Reynolds showed that the critical velocity at which the transition from laminar to disturbed and then turbulent flow occurs depends on the viscosity and density of

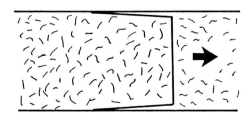

FIG. 12. Velocity profile in turbulent flow.

the liquid as well as on the diameter of the tube. In fact,

$$v_c = \frac{R_c \eta}{d\rho} \qquad [6]$$

is the critical velocity, where η is the viscosity; d is the diameter of the tube; ρ is the mass density of the fluid; and R_c is a constant for critical flow. This constant has led to the definition of what has become known as the Reynolds number for a given "free stream" velocity v of flow:

$$R = \frac{dv\rho}{\eta} \qquad [7]$$

Reynolds found that the critical value of his number for water in a pipe was about 2,000. However, under carefully controlled conditions he found it possible to maintain laminar flow up to Reynolds numbers of 12,000 or much greater. Experiments have shown that the critical value of the Reynolds number for flowing blood is also about 2,000, with vortex formation occurring at around 1,600. In the presence of other factors that disturb the flow, however, the transition to turbulence can occur at much lower Reynolds numbers. In reality, where lengths of blood vessels are much smaller and where a stenosis responsible for the increase in flow velocity may be highly localized, critical values of less than 500 have been observed.

Downsteam from a narrowing of the vessel flow velocity decreases and laminar flow is gradually restored. This occurs at a somewhat lower Reynolds number than that at which turbulence was established. As the cause of turbulence in major arteries is often a local stenosis, the turbulence may occur only in the region immediately downstream to the constricting lesion and may take place only over the systolic portion of the cardiac cycle, at which the critical value of the Reynolds number is attained. This underlines the need for Doppler systems with both spatial and temporal resolution to assess velocity patterns associated with arterial stenosis.

FLUID ENERGY: WHY BLOOD FLOWS

It is a common misconception that the impetus for the flow of a fluid is a difference in pressure and that consequently flow is always from a point of high pressure to one of low pressure. Although it is often true that flow occurs down a pressure gradient, this only represents part of the picture. In fact, it is a difference in fluid energy that determines the direction and character of flow. A mechanical analogy could be that of a bicycle free-wheeling down a hill: any cyclist knows that it is possible to free-wheel up a hill if enough speed has been built up at the foot of the hill. Similarly, fluid with sufficient kinetic energy is capable of flowing up a pressure gradient. The property of a fluid that determines the direction and speed of flow is its total fluid energy; this is the real "driving force" for flow.

Fluid energy can take several forms, which are generally combined in real situations:

1. *Pressure energy (P)*. Pressure in a fluid may be thought of as the ability to do work (to overcome viscous resistance, for example) and is hence a form of potential energy.
2. *Kinetic energy*. Each volume of moving fluid has energy by virtue of its mass and motion, determined by $\frac{1}{2}\rho v^2$, where ρ is the density and v the velocity of flow.

3. *Gravitational potential energy.* Fluid at a higher level than an arbitrary point is also capable of doing work; its weight imparts a potential energy equal to ρgh, where h is height, ρ the density, and g the acceleration of gravity. This gravitational energy may be transformed into kinetic energy by, for example, allowing the fluid to flow downhill.
4. *Viscous energy.* Flow against a viscous resistance described above may also be seen as a form of energy loss, in which kinetic or potential energy of the fluid is transferred to heat. With laminar flow the magnitude of this loss depends on vessel geometry.

Considering a single streamline of flow, the principle of conservation of energy holds that the sum of these individual energies, the total fluid energy E, must remain constant at each point along the path of flow. Thus,

$$E = P + \rho gh + \tfrac{1}{2}\rho v^2 + R_L = \text{constant} \qquad [8]$$

where R_L is the viscous loss. This is a form of the Bernouilli equation, an embodiment of Newton's classical laws of mechanics applied to a fluid. Application of this fundamental principle of fluid mechanics is of great help in understanding situations encountered clinically, such as the flow of blood through a stenosis.

HEMODYNAMICS OF STENOSIS: BERNOUILLI'S PRINCIPLE

By analyzing the total energy of a fluid passing through a stenosis and applying Bernouilli's principle, it is possible to predict the patterns of velocity change and hence the Doppler characteristics that form the clinical basis of, among other things, the carotid Doppler examination. It also explains why criteria based on velocity are likely to be far more sensitive to the presence of mild stenosis than, for example, measurements of pressure or flow rate. Furthermore, it gives an indication of how noninvasive velocity measurements can be used to determine the point at which pressure and flow are reduced to a significant extent and hence threaten the perfusion of the downsteam tissue bed.

Flow and Velocity

It is a trivial observation that the flow of a fluid speeds up through a narrowing of its passage. However, this is the starting point for the interpretation of Doppler signals in stenosis (Fig. 13). The quantity of fluid Q flowing per second is simply the product of the average velocity and the cross-sectional area:

$$Q = v_1 A_1 \qquad [9]$$

Since the volume flow remains constant through the region of the narrowing,

$$Q = v_1 A_1 = v_2 A_2 \qquad [10]$$

Thus,

$$\frac{v_2}{v_1} = \frac{A_1}{A_2} = \frac{d_1^2}{d_2^2} \qquad [11]$$

Halving the diameter of a circular vessel (i.e., a 50% diameter stenosis) therefore results in a fourfold increase in average velocity (Fig. 14).

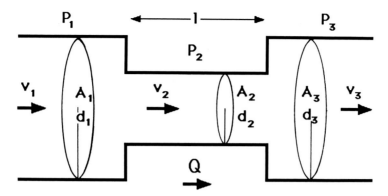

FIG. 13. Schematic depiction of a stenosis: *v* is velocity; *l* is length; *P* is pressure; *A* is cross-sectional area; *d* is diameter; and *Q* is flow rate.

Fluid Energy Without Losses

If there is no energy loss and the system is horizontal so that we can ignore the action of gravity, the total fluid energy is simply the sum of the pressure and kinetic energy:

$$E_1 = P_1 + \tfrac{1}{2}\rho v_1{}^2 \qquad\qquad [12]$$

$$E_2 = P_2 + \tfrac{1}{2}\rho v_2{}^2 \qquad\qquad [13]$$

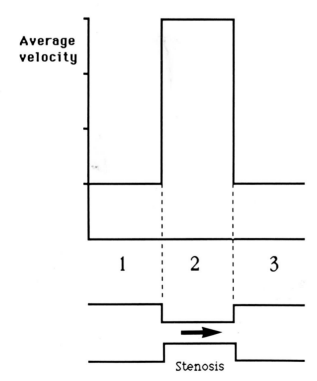

Average velocity

1   2   3

Stenosis

FIG. 14. A 50% stenosis producing a fourfold increase in velocity.

According to Bernouilli's principle,

$$E_2 = E_1 \qquad [14]$$

or

$$P_1 + \tfrac{1}{2}\rho v_1^2 = P_2 + \tfrac{1}{2}\rho v_2^2 \qquad [15]$$

So that

$$P_1 - P_2 = \frac{\rho}{2}(v_2^2 - v_1^2) \qquad [16]$$

Thus, in our example of 50% diameter stenosis,

$$P_1 - P_2 = \frac{\rho}{2} v_1^2 (4^2 - 1^2) = \frac{\rho}{2} 15 v_1^2 \qquad [17]$$

In other words, the 50% diameter stenosis has resulted in a 15-fold increase in kinetic energy of the fluid. This energy is derived from the pressure energy, which consequently falls in the region of the narrowing. This is the well-known "Bernouilli effect," in which the pressure is reduced in a region in which the flow is speeded up. If there are no energy losses, the flow slows down again in the poststenotic area, and the pressure returns to its original value (Fig. 15).

Energy Losses

In real stenoses, energy is lost; indeed, the loss of potential energy (pressure) may have catastrophic consequences on flow downstream. In the brain, for example, autoregulation of perfusion fails at pressures below about 50 mm Hg. Poiseuille's law indicates that the viscous energy loss in the stenotic portion is proportional to its length and inversely proportional to the fourth power of the radius. This tells us

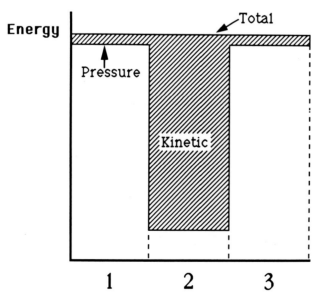

FIG. 15. Pressure change in a hypothetical stenosis without energy loss. The pressure is reduced in the region of the narrowing as kinetic energy increases.

immediately that the radius of the lumen is the most important factor in determining viscous energy loss. Because of the fourth-power dependence, the resistance to flow in our 50% diameter stenosis is 16 times that of the unstenosed segment. This energy is dissipated in the form of heat as blood flows through the narrowing. Additional energy is lost as the blood is forced to flow faster in the stenosis and the conditions for steady flow are breached. Just how much energy is associated with the acceleration of blood into the narrowing stenosis depends on how abrupt the narrowing is and on the mass, or inertia, of the blood itself. This inertial loss is less for smoothly tapering stenosis than for sharp, well-defined lesions. Inertial loss at the entrance to the stenosis is also transformed into heat (Fig. 16). Note that the inclusion of

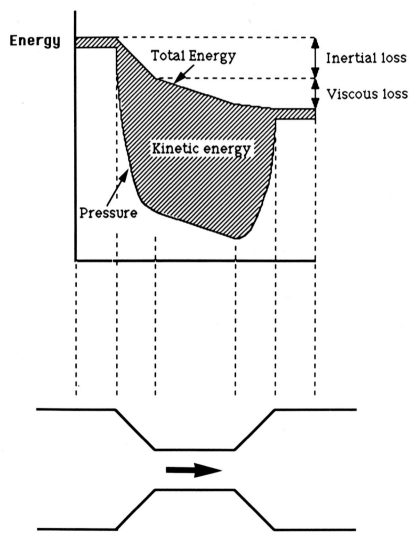

FIG. 16. Viscous and inertial losses in a stenosis with laminar flow. The size of the inertial loss depends on the geometry of the narrowing.

energy losses shows that there is now a pressure drop ΔP across the stenosis, equal to the sum of the viscous and inertial losses.

Turbulence

As the residual lumen diameter decreases, the velocity of blood flow v_2 increases. As an example, consider a 1-cm diameter internal carotid artery at peak systole, with a normal velocity of 50 cm/sec. If there is a 70% diameter reduction (Fig. 17),

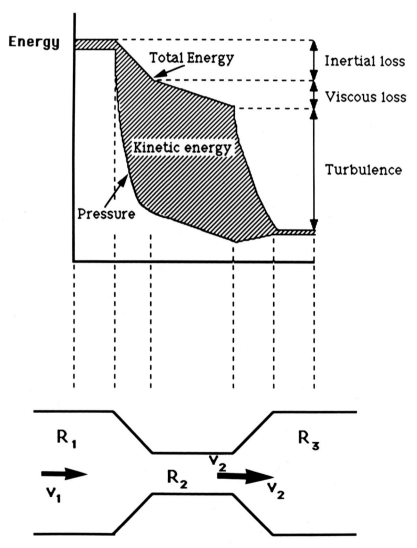

FIG. 17. Losses in a stenosis with turbulence. The Reynolds number R increases as the lumen diverges, creating turbulence. This dominates the energy losses, the combined effect of which is to cause a drop in pressure.

the velocity in the stenosis is

$$\frac{50}{(0.3)^2} = 556 \text{ cm/sec} \tag{18}$$

The Reynolds number in the proximal segment is

$$R_1 = \frac{\rho}{\eta} d_1 v_1 = 1,250 \tag{19}$$

($\eta = 0.04P$, $\rho = 1$ g/cm^3)
In the stenosis,

$$R_2 = \frac{\rho}{\eta} d_2 v_2 = 4,170 \tag{20}$$

indicating that there is likely to be flow instability. As the rapidly moving blood emerges into the poststenotic region at velocity v_2, the Reynolds number is given by

$$R_3 = \frac{\rho}{\eta} d_3 v_2 = 13,900 \tag{21}$$

Thus, there is tubulence. The inertia of the jet overcomes the cohesive forces between laminae of blood as it enters the widened section of vessel. The flow then "separates," with fluid near the edge of the vessel moving slowly or even backward toward the region of lower pressure in the stenosis. Notice that in this region the pressure gradient is in the opposite direction to flow.

Rotating eddies, or vortices, are established, and at higher velocities these can propagate downstream. Such vortices passing through the stationary sensitive volume of a Doppler system placed downstream to the lesion give rise to one of the characteristic Doppler features of turbulent flow. At higher Reynolds numbers the eddies give way to completely random, disorganized flow. Viscous losses for turbulent flow are much greater than those for laminar flow, with additional kinetic energy of the blood being dissipated as heat. The flattened velocity profile gives rise to high velocity gradients near the vessel wall, which can produce oscillatory patterns of shear stress, affecting the elastic properties of arterial walls and giving rise to "poststenotic" dilatation of the vessel. This energy can also result in mechanical damage to endothelial tissue and to low-frequency vibrations in the wall of the vessel itself. The transmission of these vibrations to the horn of the physician's stethoscope is the origin of the stenotic murmur, or bruit. Figure 17 shows how the losses caused by inertial entrance effects, viscous resistance within the stenosis, and turbulence combine to create the pressure drop across the stenosis.

Pressure and Flow: The "Critical Stenosis"

Although a stenosis of a major vessel contributes a resistance in series with that of the distal vascular bed, it has been assumed to this point that this resistance is small compared to the overall resistance, so the flow rate remains relatively unaffected. As the residual lumen diameter decreases, however, Poiseuille's law predicts a rapid increase in resistance. Inevitably, a point is reached at which this resistance constitutes a significant proportion of the resistance of the total vascular circuit. Overall flow diminishes, and a large pressure is dropped across the stenosis. High flow velocities in the stenosis cause additional losses because of turbulence, exacerbating the drop in pressure. As already discussed, both the pressure drop caused by viscous resistance and that caused by kinetic energy loss in turbulence increase with the fourth power of decreasing radius. The sum of these two effects is therefore a steeply changing function of lumen diameter. We might expect there to be a certain residual lumen diameter below which a small increase in the degree of stenosis would result in such a large pressure drop that flow would be affected significantly. Beyond this point we would expect flow to drop rapidly further until the point is reached at which the vessel has been occluded. This prediction seems to be borne out by observation. There does indeed appear to be a critical degree of narrowing beyond which flow is reduced and appreciable pressure drops are seen: this is often referred to as "critical" or "hemodynamically significant" stenosis.

At the same time as flow decreases, so, of course, does velocity. Thus, Doppler measurement shows an increase of velocity up to a maximum near the point of critical

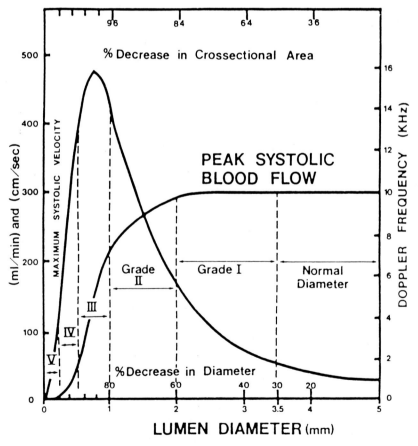

FIG. 18. Flow, diameter, and velocity in a graded stenosis predicted by a simplified theoretical model. The stenosis is assumed to be smooth and axisymmetric, and the effects of turbulence are not considered. Collateral and distal resistance are in the normal clinical range. (From Spencer and Reid, ref. 8, with permission.)

stenosis, followed by steady decline down to zero velocity at occlusion. For more minor encroachments into the vessel lumen, though, velocity increases with the inverse square of lumen size, so that velocity changes are apparent long before pressure and flow drop at the point of critical stenosis. Figure 18 summarizes the situation based on this very simple model. Velocity begins to increase noticeably at about a 30% diameter stenosis, then increasing rapidly above 50%. Flow remains substantially unaffected until about 75 to 80% diameter reduction. After about 85%, the critical point has been exceeded, and both flow and velocity drop. It is worth noting that this theoretical prediction assumes a particular value for downstream resistance; if distal resistance were to decrease, the critical point could be reached with a less severe lesion. Peripheral vasodilation after exercise of the lower limb, for example, can cause a nonsignificant stenosis upstream to become critical and thus produce symptoms.

In applying Poiseuille's law to arterial stenosis, the assumption of idealized flow conditions has been stretched to its limit. We are now far from the original caveat that flow should be steady and the vessel long, symmetric, and rigid. Stenoses are often abrupt and axially asymmetric, and the inner wall of the artery far from smooth. Furthermore, flow is pulsatile, and vessel walls are elastic. The result is that velocity profiles in such vessels are parabolic and irrotational only in the most exceptional circumstances, and flow disturbance and turbulence are time-dependent phenomena. Although qualitative aspects of stenotic flow can be described using the simple fluid models discussed above, it should be stressed that diagnostic criteria for the classification of velocity patterns in disease must rely ultimately on clinical experience.

PULSATILE FLOW

Real arteries are viscoelastic, curved, and branching, and the flow in them is pulsatile. This presents a truly daunting problem of the analysis of flow, one that has yet to succumb completely to the repeated onslaughts of theoreticians. Those interested are referred to the seminal work of Womersley, described in detail by McDonald (5). Here, a few of the aspects of pulsatile flow that may help in the interpretation of Doppler signals are presented.

Basic Concepts: Acceleration, Inertia, Compliance

Let us return to the pipe with flowing fluid (Fig. 19) and suppose now that the velocity of flow is changing with time. Flow may, for example, be low at first, speed up, and finally slow down again. A fluid element's position might change with time

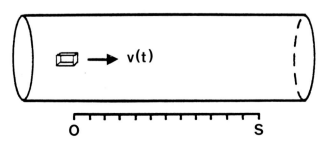

FIG. 19. An element of unsteady flow in a rigid pipe. The velocity *v* now varies and is thus a function of time *t*.

in the way shown in Fig. 20A. The velocity of the element would then look like Fig. 20B, rising to a maximum value and then declining to zero. Finally, the acceleration of the element (that is, the rate of change of the velocity with time) would be represented by Fig. 20C, in which deceleration is denoted by a negative acceleration. These three graphs are related in a fundamental way. The steepness or gradient of the position at any time gives the velocity at that point in the journey:

$$v(t) = \lim_{\delta t \to 0} \frac{\delta s}{\delta t} = \frac{ds}{dt} \qquad [22]$$

where ds/dt is the derivative of position with respect to time. Similarly, the derivative of velocity (that is, the rate of change of velocity with time) is the acceleration,

$$a(t) = dv/dt \qquad [23]$$

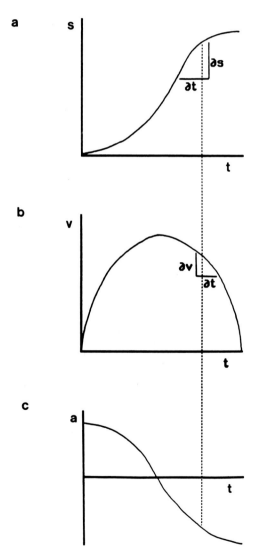

FIG. 20. A: The distance covered s varies with time t. The rate of change of distance ds/dt at any point is the velocity. **B:** The velocity v also varies with time. The rate of change of velocity dv/dt at any point is the acceleration. **C:** The acceleration (a) as a function of time.

Now, the total distance s divided by the total time T is seen to be the average velocity. In fact, we can deduce the total distance from the area under the velocity curve (Fig. 20b). This is given by the integral

$$s = \int_0^T v(t)\, dt \qquad [24]$$

Thus, if we only know the velocity (as is the case with Doppler studies), we can deduce the distance traveled in a given time period during which there is acceleration by simply integrating the instantaneous velocity. In the next chapter it can be seen that this forms the basis of Doppler methods for the measurement of volumetric flow rate.

Of course, in order to change the velocity of flow, we must apply force to the fluid. We may use a piston (Fig. 21), in which case for a mass of fluid (m) Newton's law of inertia states that the force required to produce an acceleration is proportional to its mass or inertia, m:

$$F = ma = m\frac{dv}{dt} \qquad [25]$$

In order for velocity to change, then, pressure energy must be expended.

Suppose now that we consider the walls of the pipe to exhibit elasticity, as do the walls of a blood vessel. As fluid enters a segment, the pressure rises and flow rate is increased at the same time as blood is leaving the segment. In Fig. 22, $Q_2 < Q_1$. In this segment, the pressure P rises to $P + \delta P$, the radius r to $r + \delta r$, and the volume V to $V + \delta V$. The rate of change of volume with pressure is

$$dV/dP = C \qquad [26]$$

where C is known as the volume compliance. It is related to the vessel radius and wall properties such as thickness and modulus of elasticity. The modulus of elasticity is approximately constant in arteries undergoing small deformations (6).

Laws of Motion for Pulsatile Flow

Using these relationships, we can extend and qualify Poiseuille's law for varying flow in much the same way as alternating current theory extends Ohm's law:

1. Poiseuille's law: $\qquad P_2 - P_1 = RQ \qquad$ R: resistance $\qquad [27]$

2. Continuity equation: $\qquad Q_2 - Q_1 = C\,\dfrac{dP}{dt} \qquad$ C: compliance $\qquad [28]$

3. Navier equation: $\qquad P_2 - P_1 = L\,\dfrac{dQ}{dt} \qquad$ L: inertia $\qquad [29]$

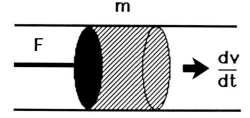

FIG. 21. Inertia. In order to accelerate a mass of fluid m, a force F must be applied.

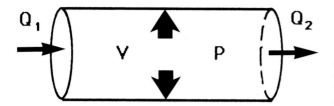

FIG. 22. Compliance. An increase in pressure *P* in an elastic vessel results in an increase in volume *V*. The volume increases, and the vessel wall stores energy.

Here, R, C, and L can be compared to electrical resistance, capacitance, and inductance, respectively. One simple (but incomplete) approach is to apply these laws individually to situations in which one of these properties dominates. Thus, for example, the peripheral bed offers mainly viscous resistance, so that L and C are negligible and Poiseuille's law is appropriate for its description. For steady flow, Eqs. 28 and 29 are zero, and we are left with Poiseuille's law. For pulsatile flow, Poiseuille's law gives only the minimum energy loss that will be sustained.

Propagation of Arterial Pulses

These concepts provide tools that can help describe patterns of flow velocity seen using the Doppler technique at different points of the arterial tree. For example, flow in the ascending aorta is highly pulsatile, reaching a peak velocity in systole and dropping rapidly to zero, as might be expected from the behavior of the left ventricle. Figure 23 shows that by the time the flow pulse has reached the descending thoracic aorta, there is already some flow in diastole. The major branches of the aorta that supply organs of the upper abdomen are all seen to carry appreciable flow in diastole (Chapter 6). This flow has its origin in the ability of a compliant vessel to store energy. A simple visualization of this effect is provided by the "Windkessel" Model (6) (Fig. 24). In this model, the great vessels act as a compliant reservoir, storing the pulsatile energy from the heart and issuing a more steady outflow, which passes into a Poiseuillian peripheral resistance. Inflow to the reservoir is then the sum of the compliant and resistive flows (Eqs. 27 and 28 above):

$$Q(t) = C \frac{dP}{dt} + \frac{1}{R} P \qquad [30]$$

This model predicts flow that rises to a peak and then decays exponentially throughout diastole (Fig. 25).

Although this waveform does not look much different from that of the renal vessel illustrated in Fig. 26, it bears little resemblance to those encountered in the lower reaches of the aorta. The Doppler waveforms of Fig. 23 show a marked reverse flow component in diastole, which becomes more pronounced as one progresses downstream, with a clear oscillatory form visible in the velocity envelope of the common femoral artery. Such a development of the velocity pulse requires a "transmission" theory for its description, one that is capable of describing the evolving relationship between pressure and flow along the arterial paths. In such a model the inertia of

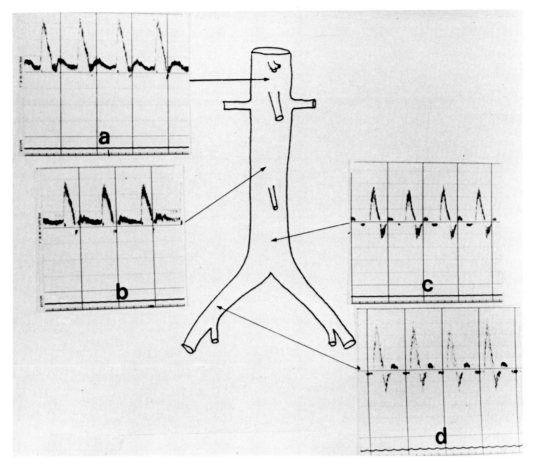

FIG. 23. Doppler signals from the aorta. Note the development of a reverse flow component as the pulse progresses distally.

blood and the compliance of the vessel combine to propagate the pressure pulse down the arterial tree at a predictable speed. In the major arteries this is about 6 m/sec; in small branches it is much lower.

By considering pressure waveforms at successive points in the circulation, we can see how the reverse flow observed with the Doppler technique is capable of appearing. Suppose that points *A* and *B* are separated by a few centimeters. Then the pressure waveforms at the two points changes with time as shown in Fig. 27A. Now the flow direction and magnitude are determined by the difference in pressure between the two points. If we subtract curve *A* from curve *B*, we obtain Fig. 27B, which shows that in this example the pressure gradient reverses twice during the cardiac cycle, thus creating two periods of reverse flow. Whether such flow reversal is actually seen on Doppler examination depends on whether there is a superimposed steady flow, raising the negative excursions above the zero velocity axis, and also on the precise form of the pressure wave itself. In fact, both of these factors are influenced by the condition of the distal vascular bed. Because this may be the actual object of the Doppler examination itself, we shall consider it further.

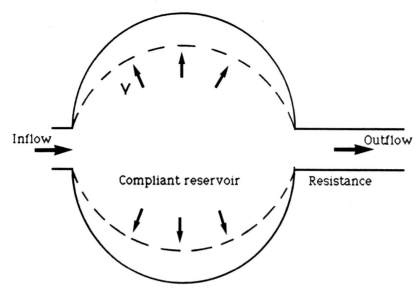

FIG. 24. The Windkessel concept. The aorta acts as a reservoir of fluid with a pulsatile input and less pulsatile output.

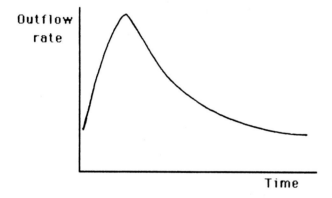

FIG. 25. Flow predicted by the Windkessel model. The decay is exponential.

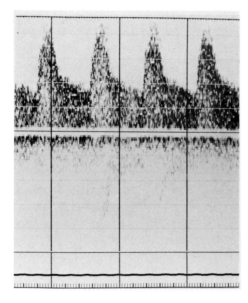

FIG. 26. Doppler signal from a renal artery.

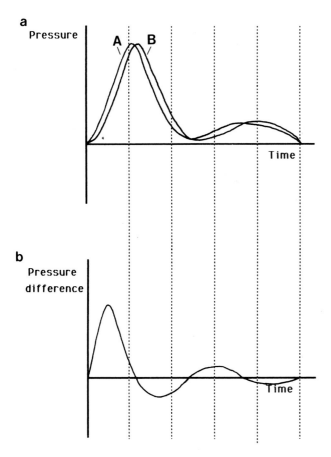

a
Pressure

A B

Time

b
Pressure
difference

Time

FIG. 27. The direction of flow between two adjacent points A and B is determined by the direction of the instantaneous pressure difference. (Adapted from McDonald, ref. 5.)

Wave Reflection: Impedance

The difference between peak systolic and diastolic pressure—the pulse pressure—is observed to increase as the pulse travels distally. Peak-to-peak flow velocity, however, decreases steadily (Fig. 28). The explanation is that reflections of the pressure wave occur at various points in the distal vascular bed; the superposition of the reflected pressure waves on the forward wave has the effect of increasing the pulse pressure. The transmission model predicts such reflections and describes them using another concept borrowed from electrical theory: impedance. With steady flow, the relationship between pressure and flow is described by resistance. With dynamic flow, in the presence of compliance and inductance, this relationship is described by impedance. More specifically, any periodic waveform (such as that of the pressure and flow pulses) can be decomposed into a series of sinusoidal components, each a multiple of a single frequency. In a linear system, the pulse will behave as the sum of these Fourier components. Considering a single point in the arterial system, the input fluid impedance to the distal circulation is then defined as the ratio of pressure to flow for each of these components and hence is a function of frequency. The impedance at zero frequency (i.e., steady flow) is simply the resistance. Transmission theory predicts that reflection will take place whenever there is a discontinuity in impedance, as usually occurs at a site of arterial branching.

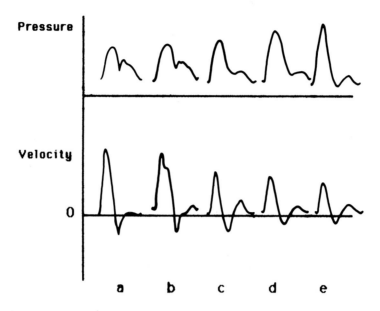

FIG. 28. The peak-to-peak pressure increases as the pulse travels distally. Peak-to-peak flow velocity decreases, but the waveform becomes more pulsatile. a, ascending aorta; b, thoracic aorta; c, middle abdominal aorta; d, distal abdominal aorta; e, common femoral artery. (Drawn from McDonald, ref. 5.)

At the bifurcation of the canine aorta, for example, a reflection of about 14% of the pressure wave occurs (5). Large reflections also occur at the periphery of the circulation. These reflections combine with each other and with the forward-going pulse to modify the pressure pulse waveform. Although the reflections are quite large, their path backwards through arterial branches results in considerable attenuation in amplitude, especially of the high-frequency components.

Investigations have shown that vessels of less than 1 mm diameter contribute most to arterial reflections, and of these, arterioles appear to be especially significant (7). If vasoconstriction or vasodilation is induced in these vessels, the impedance and hence the reflection coefficient at a range of frequencies is seen to change. Phase measurements further suggest that the site of reflection remains constant. Thus, we may conclude that a significant portion of the reflections that give rise to the pulsatile form of the distal pressure wave have their origin at the arteriolar level of the circulation. This is a crucial observation for the burgeoning number of Doppler techniques that rely on changes in the shape of the velocity pulse upstream to assess relative impedance of an arteriolar bed. Thus, if vasoconstriction occurs, for example, the reflection coefficient increases, and a more pulsatile velocity (and pressure) pulse is observed upstream. At the same time, vasoconstriction increases viscous resistance, reducing the mean, or steady, component of flow. These two factors combine to produce the familiar distinction between time-velocity waveforms associated with low and high distal impedances (Fig. 29). Indices for the quantitative classification of this difference are described in Chapter 4.

The Effect of Pulsatile Flow on Velocity Profile

Several aspects of pulsatile flow conspire so as to preclude the formation of a parabolic flow profile. First, acceleration in systole flattens the profile, especially

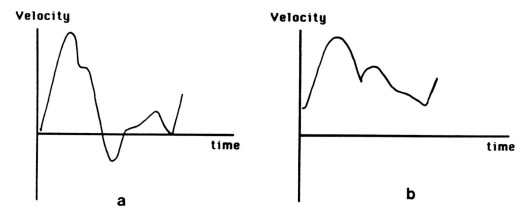

FIG. 29. Typical flow waveforms when the distal impedance is (**A**) high and (**B**) low.

in large vessels. In diastole, flow begins to revert to a parabolic form, but the next cardiac cycle begins before this process can be completed. During diastole there may be reversals in the pressure gradient; the effect of these on flow depends on the fluid energy. Fluid energy in turn depends on position within the vessel lumen; blood near the edge has less kinetic energy than that in the center, so it tends to reverse flow direction after a smaller change in pressure gradient. The result is that arteries commonly support reverse flow near their edge with forward flow simultaneously in the center of the lumen (Fig. 30).

The tendency for large arteries to have a blunt flow profile suggests the concept of "plug" flow, in which the central portion of the fluid moves as a single mass with very little shear and with inertia as its dominant fluid property. Near the wall, on the other hand, viscous forces reign, and a high velocity gradient exists. Thus, aortic flow has been seen experimentally to be inertia dominated with a large unsheared core and relatively thin boundary layers accompanied by high wall shear stresses (2).

Bernouilli Equation for Varying Flow: Estimation of Pressure Difference from Velocity

Since the Bernouilli equation is simply a statement of conservation of energy, it must hold for unsteady as well as steady flows. Now, however, the flow variables along a streamline are changing functions of time. Just as in the case of velocity, we may integrate the expressions for fluid energy along a streamline **s**. A new term is introduced that corresponds to the inertial energy required to accelerate or decelerate a volume of blood. Thus, the Bernouilli equation becomes

$$E = P + \rho g h + \tfrac{1}{2}\rho v^2 + \rho \int_s \frac{d\mathbf{v}}{dt}\, d\mathbf{s} + R_{\mathrm{L}}(\mathbf{v}) \qquad [31]$$

| total fluid energy | pressure energy | gravitational potential energy | kinetic energy | inertial energy | viscous energy |

As before, the total fluid energy is constant for a given streamline.

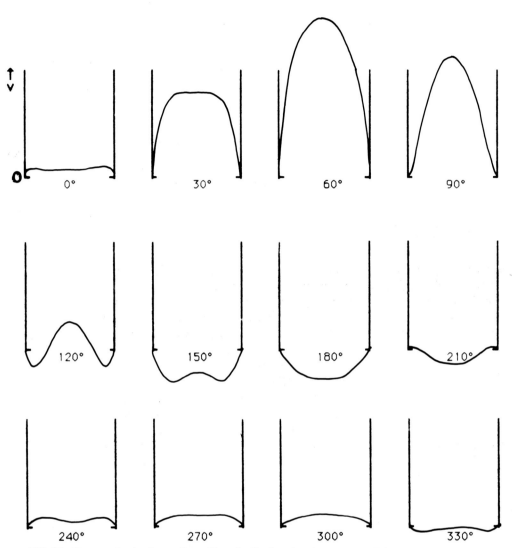

FIG. 30. Measured velocity profiles with pulsatile flow in a large artery. The cardiac cycle has been divided into 360°. (Adapted from McDonald, ref. 5.)

In general, this expression is as intractable as it looks: the estimation of each of the individual terms for a given situation is virtually impossible. In certain cases, though, an intelligent guess can be made that some terms in the equation are so small as to be of negligible importance. One such situation is that of aortic stenosis during late systole. Here, flow has been accelerated through a relatively large orifice and has a plug profile. The shear within the moving plug is low, so that viscous resistance is insignificant in relation to the high kinetic energy of the moving plug. In late systole there is little acceleration, so that the effects of inertial energy on pressure also may be ignored. If we concentrate on a region sufficiently small that the gravitational potential (or hydrostatic) energy is constant, then between two adjacent points 1 and 2 (Fig. 31),

$$P_1 + \tfrac{1}{2}\rho v_1{}^2 = P_2 + \tfrac{1}{2}\rho v_2{}^2 \tag{32}$$

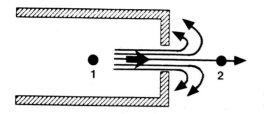

FIG. 31. Estimation of pressure drop across an abrupt stenosis using a simplified Bernouilli equation.

which implies that

$$P_1 - P_2 = \frac{\rho}{2} (v_2{}^2 - v_1{}^2)$$ [33]

allowing an estimate of pressure drop across the stenosis to be made on the basis of a velocity measurement alone. The velocity may be measured, of course, using Doppler techniques. Equation 33 is expressed in compatible (for example, SI) units. But if we use meters per second for velocity, millimeters of mercury for pressure, and substitute a value for the density of blood, we obtain

$$P_1 - P_2 \approx 4(v_2{}^2 - v_1{}^2)$$ [34]

an expression familiar to the Doppler echocardiographer.

Could this technique allow one to estimate pressure drop across a smaller stenosis by measuring velocity alone? The answer is probably not. Holen and colleagues (3) have shown that the assumptions explained above are only valid for orifices larger than about 3.5 mm in diameter and for pressure drops of more than about 70 mm Hg. Below this, viscous energy losses become significant, and actual pressure drops exceed those predicted by Eq. 33. This probably rules out the technique for estimation of pressure difference associated with stenosis outside the heart.

Turbulence in Unsteady Flow

Pulsatile flow renders more elusive the already vague distinction between flow disturbance and turbulence. Since Reynolds numbers increase during systole, disturbed flow can be detected in normal major vessels such as the aorta, explaining the "innocent" murmurs often associated with high cardiac output. Turbulence caused by stenosis, on the other hand, might be equally short-lived because deceleration in diastole can have the effect of stabilizing the flow and reestablishing laminar conditions. (An example of such periodic turbulence is shown in Fig. 19 of Chapter 4.) Acceleration, as it flattens the flow profile, also has the effect of stabilizing flow, so that the onset of turbulence is often seen to take place around the peak of systole and to be sustained into diastole.

When time-varying flow passes through a stenosis, its pulsatility is affected. Resistance of the stenosis and compliance of downstream arteries combine to absorb high-frequency components of the pressure pulse, resulting in less pulsatile flow downstream from a stenotic lesion. This introduces a potential ambiguity in the interpretation of time velocity waveforms in arteries: an unusually dampened waveform in, say, the popliteal artery could be produced either by the lowering of peripheral impedance or by the presence of an upstream stenosis.

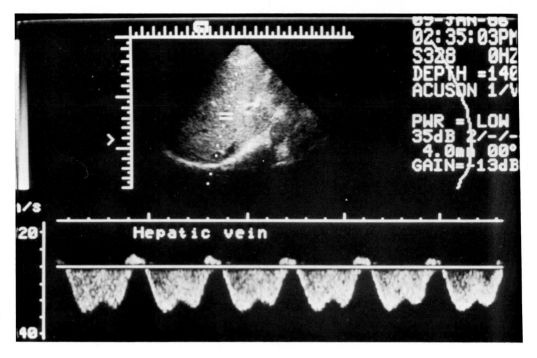

FIG. 32. Doppler signal from a hepatic vein.

FLOW IN VEINS

The venous system is isolated from the pulsatile pressure in arteries by the vascular beds themselves. Venous pressure is lower, and flow more continuous. Energy to return blood to the heart is derived from gravity, the muscle pump, and changes in abdominal and thoracic cavity pressures. Flow velocities are low, so that disturbed flow is unusual. Acceleration in venous flow is mild, so that parabolic flow profiles can be seen in many medium-sized veins. Because of the low pressure and multiplicity of collateral paths, venous flow in general reflects to a greater extent pressure changes in surrounding tissue rather than conditions in distant downstream branches. Two exceptions are the upper inferior vena cava and the main hepatic veins, which, because of their proximity to the right atrium and the absence of a valve in their path, experience pulsatile flow variation under the transmitted influence of fluctuating right atrial pressure (Fig. 32).

SUMMARY

1. Difference in total fluid energy is the impetus for flow. Fluid energy can take the form of pressure, weight, or inertia of moving blood.
2. The principal source of resistance to flow in blood vessels is the blood itself. Blood viscosity remains relatively constant in large vessels.
3. Poiseuille's law holds that for steady flow in a long rigid tube, flow rate is proportional to pressure, with the constant of proportionality related to the

inverse fourth power of vessel radius. In idealized conditions, the flow velocity profile is parabolic.

4. Energy dissipated in a stenosis through the production of turbulence results in a loss of pressure. Whereas this loss begins to become significant around a critical degree of stenosis, raised velocity and disturbed flow occur at milder degrees of stenosis.

5. In a pulsatile system, the relationship between pressure and flow is more complex. The total opposition to flow is represented by the fluid impedance; losses are greater than for steady flow. The velocity profile changes with time and can contain multidirectional flow.

6. Discontinuities in fluid impedance give rise to wave reflections. These reflections combine with the traveling velocity pulse to influence its shape.

REFERENCES

1. Burton, A. C. (1972): *Physiology and Biophysics of the Circulation,* ed. 2. Yearbook Medical Publishers, Chicago.

2. Clark, C., and Schultz, D. L. (1973): Velocity distribution in aortic flow. *Cardiovasc. Res.* 7:601–613.

3. Holen, J., Aaslid, R., Landmark, K., Simonsen, S., and Ostrem, T. (1977): Determination of effective orifice area in mitral stenosis from noninvasive Doppler data and mitral flow rate. *Acta Med. Scand.,* 201:83–88.

4. Ku, D. N, Giddens, D. P., Phillips, D. J., and Strandness, D. E. (1985): Hemodynamics of the normal human carotid bifurcation: *In vitro* and *in vivo* studies. *Ultrasound. Med. Biol.,* 11(1):13–26.

5. McDonald, D. A. (1974): *Blood Flow in Arteries,* ed. 2. Edward Arnold, London.

6. Noordergraaf, A. (1978): *Circulatory System Dynamics.* Academic Press, New York.

7. O'Rourke, M. F., and Taylor, M. G. (1966): Vascular impedance in the femoral bed. *Circ. Res.,* 18:126.

8. Spencer, M. P., and Reid, J. M. (1979): Quantitation of carotid stenosis with continuous wave (CW) Doppler ultrasound. *Stroke,* 10(3):326–330.

9. Strandness, D. E., and Sumner, D. S. (1975): *Hemodynamics for Surgeons.* Grune & Stratton, New York.

4 / Interpretation and Analysis of Doppler Signals

Peter N. Burns

Department of Diagnostic Radiology, Yale University School of Medicine, New Haven, Connecticut 06510

That Doppler ultrasound signals from moving blood produce audible sounds is a purely fortuitous consequence of the combination of the ultrasonic and physiological parameters together with the Doppler equation itself. Ultimately, the content of a Doppler signal is a reflection of the interaction between the sound beam and a series of targets in a moving medium. In clinical diagnosis, it is the properties of the moving medium that are of interest, so the interpretation of Doppler signals must concentrate on extracting this information from the sound. The ear is capable of quite subtle discrimination of this Doppler noise; indeed, for many years clinical diagnoses using Doppler techniques were made entirely through the ears of trained operators. Today, with a variety of signal-processing techniques and visual displays incorporated routinely in commercial equipment, it is worth noting that the seasoned Doppler practitioner still derives benefit from listening carefully to the sounds themselves. In many contexts, however, the use of spectral analysis not only is helpful in understanding the variety of factors that may contribute to an individual Doppler signal but is useful as a means of documenting an examination and essential for quantitative analysis.

In its simplest, most qualitative application, duplex pulsed Doppler techniques may be thought of as offering a "directional stethoscope" for the user. Doppler signals from a specific site may be used to infer the presence and direction of flow, whether the flow is laminar or turbulent, whether there is a jet, the approximate distribution of flow velocities within the sample volume, and whether distal arterial impedance is high or low.

In using Doppler ultrasound as a tool for the evaluation of hemodynamics, one may also contemplate the direct measurement of physiological quantities. If it is possible to obtain Doppler signals in a particular vessel, is it practicable to estimate velocity, volume flow rate, or pressure? In this chapter some of the factors contributing to the content of the Doppler signal are discussed, and the use of simple signal processing in the interpretation of the signals is explained. In addition, some of the techniques available for quantitative measurement are reviewed together with their known sources of error.

SCATTERING OF ULTRASOUND BY BLOOD

The composition of blood is responsible for some important aspects of the Doppler signal. Blood consists of a suspension of erythrocytes (red blood cells), leukocytes (white blood cells), and platelets in a liquid plasma. Because of the relatively low numbers of leukocytes and small size of platelets, it is generally assumed that the erythrocytes are responsible for the scattering of ultrasound by blood. The mean diameter of an erythrocyte is 7 μm, much less than the wavelength of the ultrasound. which is about 0.2 to 0.5 mm. Individual erythrocytes therefore act as point scatterers, whose combined effect is referred to as Rayleigh–Tyndall scattering. The size of the echo from blood is small compared to that produced by specular reflection from solid tissue interfaces, as is apparent from the echo-free appearance of blood-filled structures on ultrasound images. One consequence of the Rayleigh–Tyndall process is that the intensity I of the scattered wave increases with the fourth power of frequency f ($I \propto f^4$). Thus, doubling the ultrasonic frequency results in an echo from blood that is 16 times stronger. This is partly responsible for a dramatic difference in performance between Doppler instruments detecting blood flow using different ultrasonic frequencies. Of course, attenuation in soft tissue also rises with frequency, tending to offset the advantage of the increased efficiency of scattering at higher frequencies. The choice of the optimum ultrasonic frequency with which to perform a Doppler examination is thus an inevitable compromise.

Another effect of the scattering of ultrasound from many small moving targets is that the intensity of the echo fluctuates with small displacements in space and over small periods of time. This accounts for the distinctive noise-like character of Doppler blood flow signals. It also allows a prediction to be made about the average strength of the signal. Atkinson and Berry (1) developed a statistical diffraction theory that accounted for the fluctuations. The theory gave a mean value of the acoustic pressure Π of the returning ultrasonic echo as

$$\Pi = k[n(1 - \alpha n)]^{1/2} \qquad [1]$$

where n is the number density of erythrocytes, and α is the effective volume of the erythrocyte, and k is a constant; α is approximately 90 μm^3 (29), and if n is small, then $\alpha n \ll 1$. Neglecting the small amount of attenuation in blood, the backscattered intensity I is then simply proportional to the number of red blood cells in the beam:

$$I \propto \Pi^2 \propto n \qquad [2]$$

Thus, the intensity of the Doppler signal is related to the quantity of blood lying within the sensitive volume of the Doppler beam. This forms the basis of the most common method for volume flow measurement with Doppler ultrasound.

CHOICE OF INSTRUMENTATION

The various types of Doppler instruments available are described in Chapter 2. In practice, the choice is narrowed considerably by the specific application being considered. Continuous-wave systems, for instance, use two (usually adjacent) transducers, one to transmit, the other to receive. Their beams overlap to form a sensitive volume defined by their spatial product (Fig. 1). The Doppler system is then sensitive to any moving target lying within this volume. Should the volume contain moving solid structures as well as moving blood, strong low-frequency "clutter" signals are superimposed on those of the blood flow. This may be more than an inconvenience: if the dynamic range of the receiver is limited, overloading of the demodulator can occur with the result that part of the blood flow signal itself is lost.

Even where clutter is not a problem, the presence of several vessels within the sensitive volume gives rise to a superposition of several Doppler signals. If these are simply an artery–vein pair (say the carotid artery and jugular vein), the directional resolution of the spectral display and the distinct characteristics of arterial and venous flow allow their identification. In the upper abdomen, however, there are usually too many vessels present to allow continuous-wave systems to be very helpful. The usual solution is to confine continuous-wave techniques to the examination of superficial structures and to employ a sufficiently high ultrasound frequency that attenuation limits the penetration of the beam and hence the extent of the sensitive volume. Thus, 7 to 10 MHz systems are often used without imaging for the examination of the carotid and superficial vessels of the limbs. Many configurations of the continuous-wave transducer assembly have been made, allowing, for example, probes to be clipped onto vessels at surgery. The continuous-wave method is also capable of quite high sensitivity to weak signals, so that it is preferred for the examination of smaller vessels such as the ophthalmic and supraorbital arteries and those supplying the female breast (4). One exceptional application to deep-lying structures is in obstetrics, where some workers use continuous waves at 3 MHz to obtain signals from the fetal and uterine vessels (see Chapter 9).

The pulsed Doppler technique overcomes the principal disadvantages of the continuous-wave system by providing axial localization of the sensitive volume. By

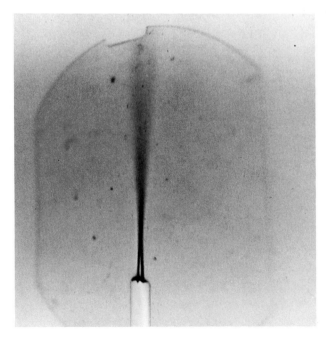

FIG. 1. Schlieren visualization of the acoustic field from a continuous wave transducer. The sensitive volume is defined by the region of overlap of the two beams (courtesy D. H. Follett).

transmitting short bursts of ultrasound and timing the return of echoes, the pulsed Doppler technique combines the range resolution of pulse-echo imaging with Doppler flow detection (Chapter 2). This gives some control over the location and extent of the sensitive volume. Changing the timing of the electronic gate in the receiver controls the depth of the sensitive volume, whereas altering the time for which the gate is open determines its effective axial length. The lateral dimensions of the sensitive volume are determined by the lateral beam width, both within and orthogonal to the scan plane. For single-transducer systems, this is fixed by the transducer geometry and therefore varies with depth. The result is a volume with an approximately teardrop shape of a length of between 1 and 15 mm, which is positioned at an axial depth controlled by the operator.

Such control is clearly required for abdominal scanning and is preferred for examination of carotid vessels. It is, however, of little practical use without some form of visual guidance. In a duplex scanner, this is provided by the real-time ultrasound image. Some duplex scanners use the same transducers for imaging and Doppler measurement; other mechanical sector scanners are able to use different transducers and possibly different frequencies for the two functions. These might exploit the superior performance of a swept-focus annular array for imaging and a single disk or dual element (for continuous waves) transducer for Doppler mode. Typical combinations might be 7 to 10 MHz for imaging and 5 MHz for Doppler studies in the carotid, or 5 MHz imaging together with 3 MHz for Doppler studies in the abdomen. Electronic sector scanners are capable of switching between imaging and Doppler modes at a sufficiently high rate to permit real-time "duplex" imaging at a somewhat reduced frame rate. Although this is sometimes at the expense of signal-to-noise performance of the Doppler system, the facility of simultaneous imaging and Doppler scanning is useful where there are slow movements (such as those of respiration or of a fetus) that can make the positioning of the Doppler volume difficult. Electronic arrays may also address the problem of the different optimum imaging and Doppler frequencies by employing sufficiently broadband transducers that the two functions can be served by the same array operating at different frequencies. The agility of the beam produced by such arrays is capable of providing imaging, Doppler frequencies, and M-mode functions at such rapid alternation as to allow real-time examination of the heart. Using an array for the pulsed Doppler system allows electronic control of the lateral extent of the beam in the direction of the array elements but places quite heavy demands on the performance of the beam-forming electronics. High-performance Doppler systems using such arrays have only become available relatively recently.

The pulsed Doppler duplex scanner has become the standard instrument on which most examinations described here are based. It does, of course, have some limitations, which are important to appreciate. The problem of aliasing described in Chapter 1 sets an effective limit on the maximum Doppler shift frequency that it is possible to detect unambiguously at a given pulse repetition frequency: the Nyquist limit is one-half the pulse repetition frequency. Thus, high velocity flow requires a high pulse repetition frequency for its detection. However, increasing the Doppler angle or decreasing the ultrasound frequency has the effect of reducing the Doppler shift for a given target and so are two ways of surmounting the problem of aliasing. Another is to increase the pulse repetition frequency itself, but this reduces the maximum depth from which signals can be obtained (more frequent pulses imply

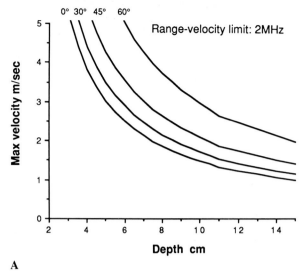

A

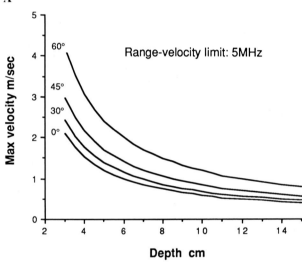

B

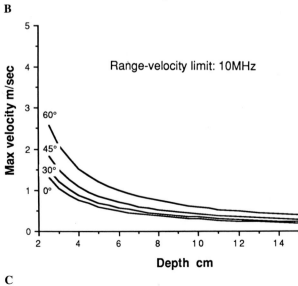

FIG. 2. The Doppler range–velocity limit at various angles and ultrasound frequencies. This represents the highest velocity it is possible to measure unambiguously with a conventional pulsed Doppler system. (**A**) 2 MHz; (**B**) 5 MHz; (**C**) 10 MHz.

C

less time to wait for echoes to return to the transducer before the next pulse is emitted: echoes from deeper structures take longer to return). Thus, the maximum velocity it is possible to detect unambiguously is determined by the ultrasound frequency, the Doppler angle, and the depth of the target (Fig. 2). Continuous-wave Doppler devices do not suffer from such a limitation.

Less obviously, pulsed Doppler instruments tend to emit pulses of a higher average intensity than their continuous-wave counterparts. The signal-to-noise ratio of a pulsed system is inherently poorer than that of a continuous-wave system because of its higher bandwidth; that is, the pulses transmitted contain wider range of ultrasound frequencies. Narrowing this range improves signal-to-noise performance but degrades spatial resolution. At comparable intensities, then, pulsed Doppler systems generally offer a poorer signal-to-noise ratio. Manufacturers often address this problem by increasing the power of the transmitted pulse. Some practical implications of the resulting acoustic exposure levels are discussed in Chapter 9.

Finally, it is now possible to extend the multigate pulsed Doppler system into a duplex scanner, which can provide color flow mapping by the same technique of rapid alternation of beam function combined with fast signal processing (Chapter 2). The superposition of flow information as colors on a gray-scale real-time image presents the Doppler formation in a novel and appealing way. These systems are clearly well suited to identifying the location of high velocity flow (such as in a stenosis) or of mapping the extent of flow in a certain region (24). However, the Doppler information presented is that of the single parameter encoded in color, a parameter whose value is changing rapidly and is derived from, but does not describe, the full Doppler frequency spectrum. It therefore seems likely that spectral analysis should remain an essential component of most Doppler examinations, whether or not color flow mapping is included. Indeed, present color instruments offer the flow-mapping facility as an addition to, rather than a replacement for, conventional duplex scanning and spectral analysis (24) (see Plate I).

TECHNIQUE

The results of the Doppler ultrasound examination are very much dependent on the operator. Doppler sonographers cultivate a coordination of hand, eye, and ear that is best acquired by experience. Although clinical technique depends on the precise application, a few notes concerning physical aspects of the Doppler examination may be helpful as a guide.

Ultrasound Frequency

The optimum Doppler frequency is generally the one that gives the best signal-to-noise ratio in a given situation. Higher frequencies can provide small sample volume sizes and greater sensitivity to flow but suffer greater loss by attenuation in tissue; lower frequencies give better penetration but at a cost of spatial resolution and detectability of flow. In general, the optimum frequency for Doppler examination is below that for imaging the same structure (for example, 5 MHz for a carotid artery being imaged at 10 MHz). When a machine in which the image and Doppler systems share a transducer and are at the same frequency, it may be better to perform the imaging examination separately so that the Doppler portion can be carried out using a different, lower-frequency transducer.

Beam–Vessel Angle

In ultrasound imaging, the operator seeks to display specular reflections that show the boundaries of structures most clearly. Thus, a blood vessel is best imaged with the beam perpendicular to the vessel axis. If flow is aligned with the axis of the vessel, this is the worst angle of approach for Doppler examination. It is indeed only rarely that the best image is likely to produce the best Doppler signal. Some duplex systems offer Doppler transducers offset from the imaging system (see Figs. 7 and 8 of Chapter 2). For others, the field of the scan must be altered for the Doppler examination in order to reduce the beam vessel angle. Smaller angles, below 60°, are best (Fig. 3).

Pulse Repetition Frequency

In most instruments, the Doppler pulse repetition frequency (PRF) is linked to the frequency scale of the spectrum analyzer, so that a high PRF increases the range of Doppler shift frequencies that can be displayed. The PRF should be set high enough that aliasing does not take place but not so high that the spectral trace of the signal only occupies a small part of the display. When searching for signals it is best to start with a relatively low PRF and increase it when the signal has been

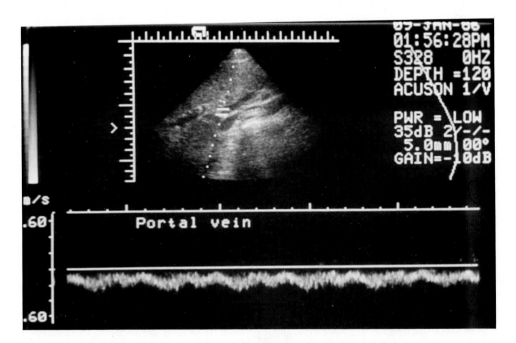

FIG. 3. Duplex Doppler scan showing flow in the portal vein of an adult liver. The real-time image is above, the real-time sonogram display of the Doppler signal below.

located. A low PRF also means a narrower bandwidth and less electrical noise from the Doppler receiver, thus making the search easier. Pulse repetition frequency is often labeled "frequency scale" or "maximum depth" on the control panel of an instrument.

Aliasing

The effect of aliasing on a spectral display is shown in Fig. 4A. Aliasing occurs at velocities corresponding to Doppler shifts above the Nyquist frequency, so when this velocity is attained (here in systole), the signal "folds over" into the reverse-flow portion of the display. Aliasing ceases as soon as the velocity drops back below the same point. It is important to note that the Doppler sound itself, and not just the display, suffers artifactual distortion when aliasing is present. Increasing the PRF has the effect of Fig. 4B. However, if depth does not permit the PRF to be increased and the flow is in one direction only, most instruments will permit the time axis of the display to be shifted down (Fig. 4C), so devoting the entire range of frequencies on the display to one flow direction. This signal-processing trick alleviates the visual artifact associated with an aliased signal but does not generally change its sound. In some newer instruments, though, further processing is introduced automatically that synthesizes the signal and remedies the distortion of the sound as well. Without such a facility, this "base-line shift" should be used only when essential. If aliasing persists, the Doppler shift frequency may be reduced by adjusting the beam vessel angle or by using a lower ultrasound frequency. Finally, at the expense of range ambiguity, it is possible to use "extended" or "multiple" PRF systems, or, by sacrificing axial resolution altogether, one can always eliminate aliasing by using continuous-wave Doppler.

Doppler Transmit Power

The prudent use of ultrasound dictates that acoustic exposure should be maintained at the minimum level consistent with obtaining satisfactory diagnostic information. Thus, the transmit power should be set at its minimum and increased only when there is no other way to rescue a Doppler signal that is buried in noise. Many pulsed Doppler instruments function at spatial peak temporal average (SPTA) acoustic exposure levels 10 to 100 times greater than those of imaging systems, and some clinical protocols (for the Doppler examination of the fetus, for example) may not permit the transmit power to be raised beyond a certain level (see Chapter 9).

Doppler Receiver Gain

When searching for a Doppler signal it is often best to have the overall system performance at its most sensitive. This can be achieved by increasing the receiver gain to the point that receiver noise is heard and seen on the display and the signal occupies an adequate range of gray levels. Once a signal is obtained, the gain is reduced so that noise is not present on the display. Gain settings that are too high can result in an overloaded receiver and loss of directional resolution, seen as a

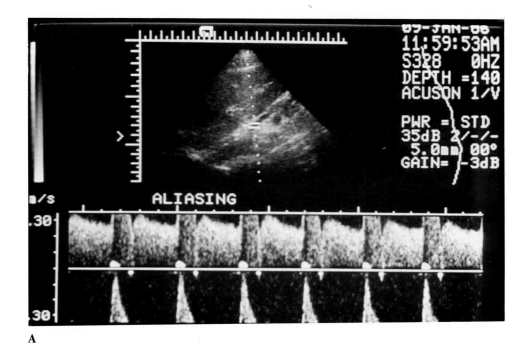

A

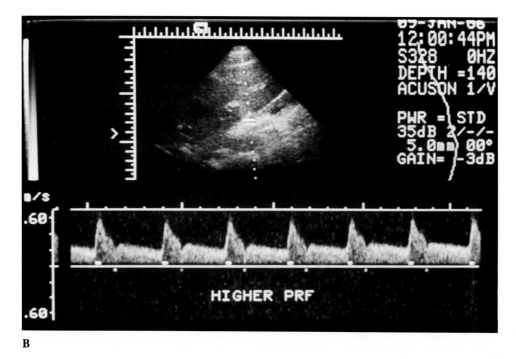

B

FIG. 4. Aliasing of a pulsed Doppler signal from the celiac trunk. **A:** Note the folding over of forward flow in systole into the reverse flow channel. **B:** The effect of raising of the pulse repetition frequency.

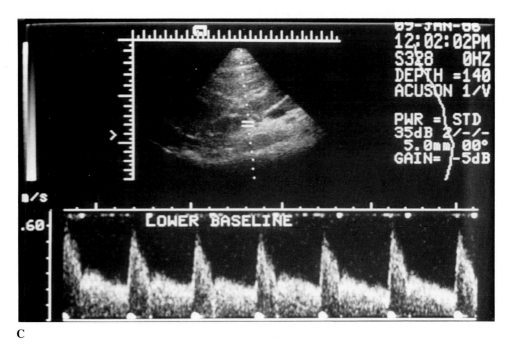

C

FIG. 4. (*continued*). **C:** The effect of lowering the base line.

"mirror-image" artifact of the spectral display about its horizontal axis. Gain settings that are too low can result in undetected flow.

Sample Volume Size

The axial length of the sample volume is its only dimension under the control of the operator. Long sample volumes help in locating the desired signal, whereas shorter sample volumes are used to exclude unwanted contributions from the signal. These may be from flow in a neighboring vessel, from flow at the edge of the same vessel, or from movements of the vessel wall. This last source of interference produces the low-frequency, high-amplitude signals referred to as clutter. An example of how a signal (from an aorta) can be overwhelmed by the effects of clutter is shown in Fig. 5. The first move to improve such a signal should be to reduce the sample volume size. Note that the narrower beam of a higher-frequency ultrasound transducer usually creates a smaller overall sample volume size.

Filters

Every Doppler instrument has a high-pass filter used to eliminate the lowest Doppler shifts from the display; the frequency at which this filter operates is usually variable. Its most useful function to the operator is to eliminate clutter that cannot otherwise be avoided (for example, from moving solid structures in the heart). However, it also has the effect of eliminating signals from low-velocity blood flow, which

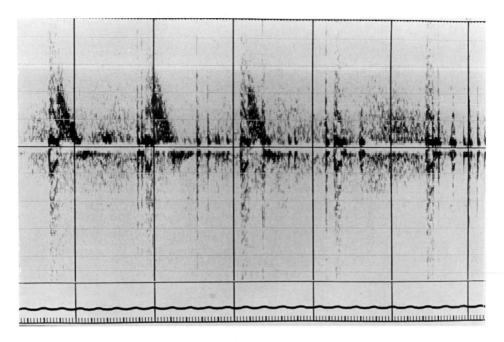

FIG. 5. A signal badly affected by clutter, mainly at the beginning of systole. Note that the resulting artifact in the display can mask the blood flow signal.

can cause serious misrepresentation of the real velocity spectrum. This is of particular significance when diastolic flow, often at low velocity, is being assessed in abdominal vessels. The filter should therefore be kept at its lowest setting (50–100 Hz) unless it is necessary to increase it.

Doppler Display Dynamic Range

In exactly the same way that the wide range of amplitude of echoes constituting the ultrasound image is mapped or "compressed" into the range of gray shades available on the video display, so the amplitude of output of the spectrum analyzer (corresponding to the amplitudes of the Fourier components of successive samples of the Doppler signal) is mapped onto the gray scale of the Doppler display. The operator can often limit the range of amplitudes displayed (the dynamic range) or alter the mapping characteristic itself (the postprocessing). Both can be used to enhance contrast between adjacent gray levels in the display or to eliminate the display of noise. It should be noted that both these controls and the receiver gain can have the effect of increasing the apparent width of the spectral display, hence introducing an artifact in the assessment of spectral broadening. A consistent approach should be used: one is to leave the dynamic range fixed at a high enough level to be able to display the full range of amplitude levels present in a typical signal as well as some background noise and to use the receiver gain control to adjust for stronger signals. Many instruments are equipped with some form of mean power level meter, which can be used to achieve a standard display level, thus helping in the visual assessment of spectral content. The widespread tendency of echocardiographers to reduce the dynamic range to produce a "cleaner" display should be avoided when using Doppler display outside the heart, as it causes the weaker signals to be lost from the display.

Image Update

Whether or not the facility to update the B-scan image is used, and at what rate, is largely a matter of preference for the operator. Only electronically controlled arrays allow image updates at a rapid rate. In many instruments there is a discernible loss in signal-to-noise quality of the Doppler signal when the image update is used. In others the Doppler pulse repetition frequency is reduced, thereby increasing the risk of aliasing. Many mechanical sector systems, which require an appreciable time to switch between functions, leave a gap in the Doppler signal. Others are able to synthesize the missing portion of the signal so that the display appears unaffected. Increasingly, the trade-offs implicit in sharing time between the two functions are being reduced; however, for weak Doppler signals, it is still probably good practice to sacrifice the image update altogether and thus obtain optimum performance from the Doppler system.

Angle Correction

Doppler shift frequency depends on some factors in addition to the velocity of flow (Eq. 10 of Chapter 1). These are the velocity of sound, the ultrasound frequency, and the angle between the ultrasound beam and the direction of flow. Many Doppler systems are equipped to calculate velocity from Doppler shift frequency and hence allow for these factors. The first two are known and may be programmed into the machine. The Doppler angle, however, must be measured. Assuming that flow is parallel to the wall of the vessel (that there are not, for example, substantial helical components to flow), this angle may be measured from the ultrasound image. Inevitably, errors are associated with the measurement: the vessel axis may not lie within the scan plane, the vessel may be curved, or the flow may not be aligned with the axis of the vessel. As is discussed below, the error in velocity estimation resulting from such an inaccuracy is strongly dependent on the beam vessel angle itself. Velocity should not be estimated when this angle is above about 60°. In correcting for the operating frequency of the Doppler system, velocity estimates eliminate one factor that may vary between individual duplex instruments. Thus, even if a constant angle of insonation is used in the examination, estimated velocity is a better parameter to report than Doppler shift frequency.

ANALYSIS OF THE DOPPLER SPECTRUM

Spectral Display

Although the movement of the single target gives rise to a Doppler shift signal of one frequency whose pitch is proportional to the target velocity, the same volume

INTERPRETATION OF DOPPLER SIGNALS

of a pulsed Doppler signal (or the sensitive region of a continuous wave Doppler signal) usually insonates blood cells moving at a large number of differing velocities, sometimes even in opposite directions within the same vessel (Fig. 6). The Doppler signal is therefore perceived by the operator as a complex and changing set of sounds. The successful application of quantitative techniques in a clinical setting relies to a great extent on the appropriate choice of subsequent processing and measurement

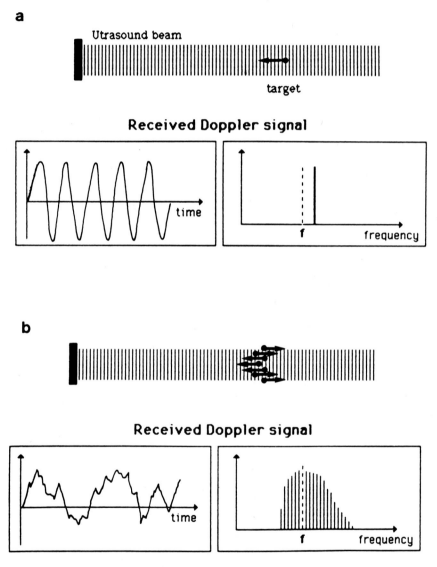

FIG. 6. A: A single scatterer moving towards the transducer gives rise to a Doppler signal of a single frequency, Doppler shifted by an amount proportional to its velocity. **B:** The Doppler signal from a number of scatterers moving both toward and away from the transducer is a sum of Doppler shift frequencies, represented by the Doppler spectrum (**right**).

made on this signal. To this end a variety of signal-processing methods are available, some of which are now incorporated routinely in commercial instruments.

Because the basis of information contained within the signal lies in the combination of different Doppler shift frequencies of which it is composed, it is natural that the fundamental tool of the processing of Doppler signals should be the frequency (or spectrum) analyzer. This instrument is capable of determining the relative powers of the various frequency components that are present in the signal at a given time. Although there are several methods for implementing spectral analysis, the most common uses the digital fast Fourier transform (FFT). Short periods of the signal (from 1 to 10 msec) are digitized and analyzed mathematically for their frequency components. Dedicated arithmetic processors can perform the necessary calculations at sufficient speed to be able to accept the next period for analysis as it arrives, thus producing a series of spectra in real time. These spectra are simply graphs showing the relative amplitude of each of the frequency components constituting the Doppler signal.

If the target is blood flowing in a single vessel that is uniformly insonated by the ultrasound beam, the power at a given frequency relates to the quantity of blood flowing at the corresponding velocity. The spectrum is usually displayed as a sonogram, in which a single spectrum is depicted as a vertical line on whose axis lies frequency, brightness modulated at each point to represent amplitude. Subsequent spectra are displayed as vertical lines at a fixed distance apart, creating an image that scrolls from left to right with time. The three variables—time, frequency, and amplitude—are thus shown in real time as the signal is heard. Figures 7 and 8 illustrate this process for a phantom target consisting of a fine jet of microspheres directed into a tank of water. The final sonogram display of Fig. 8 illustrates the same data as the spectrum of Fig. 7B. With *in vivo* signals the power spectrum changes with time, and the sonogram becomes the most useful display format. Figure 3 shows a typical duplex Doppler scan, here of the portal vein of the adult abdomen, along with the sonogram spectral display. An example of an alternative form of display is shown in Fig. 9. Here the three variables are plotted in an isometric display generated by a computer. The amplitude of the Doppler signal is now the vertical axis, with Doppler shift and time on the horizontal axes. This form of display can be useful for more detailed assessment of the distribution of signal amplitude in the Doppler spectrum.

Factors Affecting Content of the Spectrum

The relationship of the three signal variables—time, frequency, and power—to the actual velocity of blood flowing in a vessel is complicated by a variety of physical factors that it is essential to understand when interpreting Doppler signals. The spectrum illustrated in Figs. 7 and 8, for example, contains a range of Doppler shift frequencies. Do these correspond to a range of real velocities in the target? In this particular case it was possible to determine with a high degree of confidence that the actual velocity profile of the experimental jet was very nearly flat, so that all the targets could be regarded as moving at a single velocity. Why then does the illustrated spectrum of Figs. 7B and 8 show a definite range of frequencies, and why

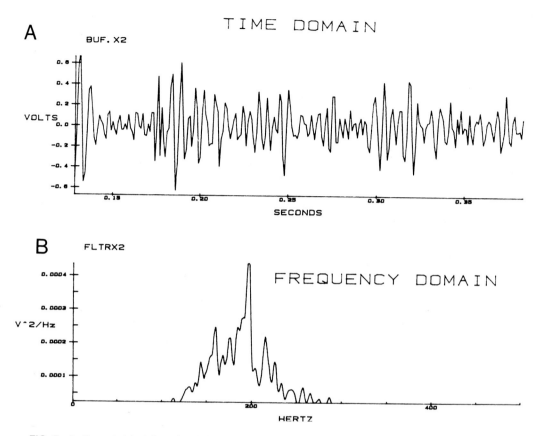

FIG. 7. A: Demodulated Doppler shift signal obtained from a fine jet of microspheres moving at nearly uniform velocity. This is the signal that is fed to the loudspeaker and perceived to contain a mixture of frequencies. **B:** The frequency domain representation (obtained from the Fourier transform of **A**) displays this mixture of frequencies. The Doppler shift is seen to center around 200 Hz.

does it contain gross fluctuations of power with frequency? First, the Doppler shift obtained from a single target moving at a steady velocity is only a single frequency in the idealized situation of an infinite plane target in an equally infinite acoustic field (Fig. 10A). In practice, a moving target enters and leaves a beam of finite width, and as it does so the backscattered echo received by the transducer rises and then fades (Fig. 10B). Even if the target is moving at a steady velocity, this amplitude modulation of the received echo causes a similar modulation of the Doppler difference signal. This modulation is equivalent to the introduction of additional frequencies above and below the main Doppler shift frequency. The consequent broadening of the spectrum is known as transit-time broadening and is one manifestation of a fundamental ambiguity inherent in simultaneous measurements of a moving target's position and velocity using sound. Thus, for example, narrowing the beam (and therefore localizing the target) results in a more rapid modulation of the Doppler shift frequency and a broader spectrum (and therefore greater uncertainty in the target's velocity).

With pulsed Doppler beams, the transit-time broadening effect arising from the beam geometry is additionally affected by the receiver gate length. For a single moving scatterer and a short sample volume, which may contain as few as three cycles of ultrasound, it is possible to experience a transit-time broadening of as much as 33% (16). It is not possible to determine from the Doppler spectrum alone whether such broadening is the result of many scatters moving at different velocities (as is the case, for example, with disturbed flow in a large vessel) or an artifact of the transit-time effect on scatterers that are really moving at one velocity. Such uncertainty inevitably affects the ability of any pulsed system to measure flow velocity with a high degree of spatial resolution. For this reason, long sample volumes or continuous-wave systems provide a more reliable means of measuring the velocity of highly localized jets.

Because most vessels contain blood flowing at a range of velocities across the lumen diameter, the effect of transit-time broadening in practice is to smear the Doppler shift power spectrum in relation to the velocity profile (Fig. 11).

Another important influence on the Doppler spectrum is the form of the acoustic beam itself. The sample volume is often smaller than the vessel, in which case the spectrum changes according to the velocity of those flow laminae that lie within the beam. This in turn depends on the velocity profile (6). This is the explanation of the disquieting ability of the operator to increase or decrease the spectral width of the Doppler display from a vessel with a blunted flow profile by manipulation of the beam position (Fig. 12). Furthermore, the beam in reality is not uniform across its lateral dimensions. Thus, unless the vessel is small compared to the beam width, it

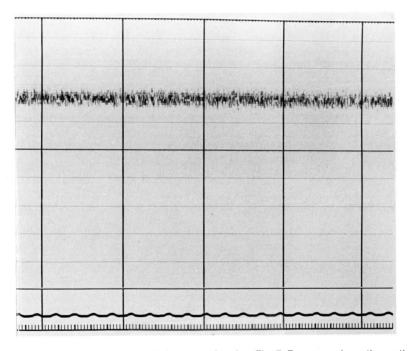

FIG. 8. The sonogram representation of the same signal as Fig. 7. Frequency is on the vertical axis, time on the horizontal, with the gray scale corresponding to the power of the Doppler shift at that frequency. The horizontal markers represent 1 sec, and the vertical markers 100 Hz.

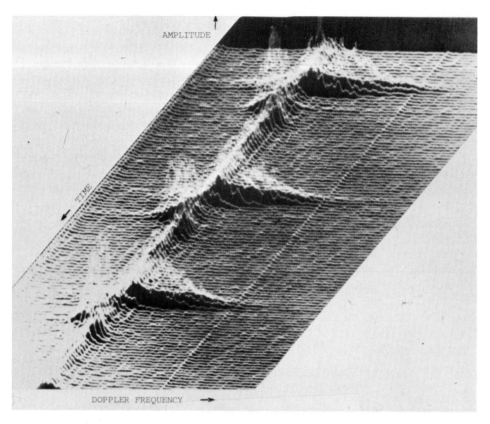

FIG. 9. Isometric display from a posterior tibial artery signal showing the three spectral variables: time, amplitude, and Doppler shift frequency. Each line of the display is a Doppler amplitude spectrum.

is unlikely that each of the flow elements contributes equally to the Doppler signal. A beam plot of a typical 2 MHz Doppler transducer is shown in Fig. 13. The −3dB (that is, half-amplitude) width of the beam near its focus is only 3 mm, indicating that it is not possible to interrogate equally all the blood flowing in a large vessel using such a device.

Examples taken from three vessels with different velocity profiles, insonated in a manner to minimize the effects of transit-time broadening, are shown in Fig. 14. Here, if the Doppler sample volume has a uniform sensitivity and embraces the entire vessel lumen evenly, the relative power of different frequencies reflects the relative volumes of blood moving at the corresponding velocities. Where there is a plug flow profile, that is, one in which the entire cross section of blood is moving at one velocity, there is one Doppler shift corresponding to that velocity, and we would expect a signal that appears similar to that obtained in the abdominal aorta in early systole (Fig. 14A). In other smaller arteries, such as in the celiac trunk, a blunted parabolic flow profile develops in diastole, and the power spectrum shows a broader band of Doppler shift frequencies during diastole (Fig. 14B). In the case of a parabolic flow profile in a smaller vessel, theory predicts a flat distribution of power with frequency up to the Doppler shift corresponding to the center-stream

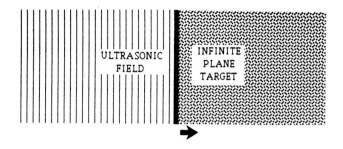

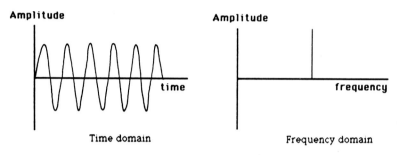

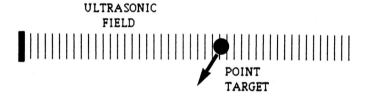

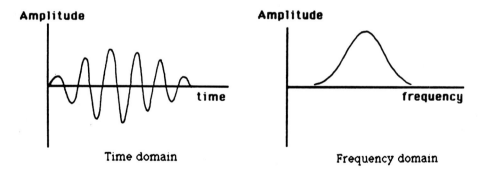

FIG. 10. A: Only an infinite plane target moving in an ultrasonic field gives rise to a Doppler shift of one frequency (**bottom right**). **B:** Transit-time broadening in the CW flowmeter. A point target moves across an ultrasound beam of finite width. The range of amplitudes of the Doppler shift signal (**bottom left**) is equivalent to a range of Doppler shift frequencies, causing a broadening of the spectrum.

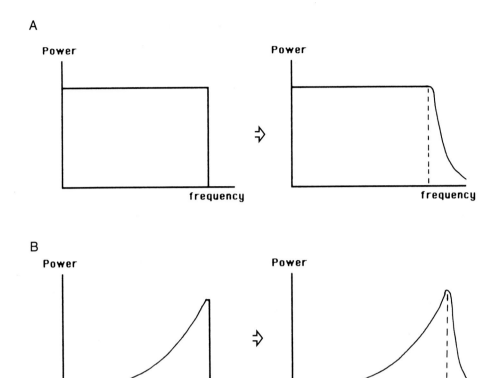

FIG. 11. Effect of transit-time broadening on the theoretical Doppler shift spectrum from a distribution of scatters moving in a vessel with (**A**) a parabolic flow profile and (**B**) a blunted flow profile.

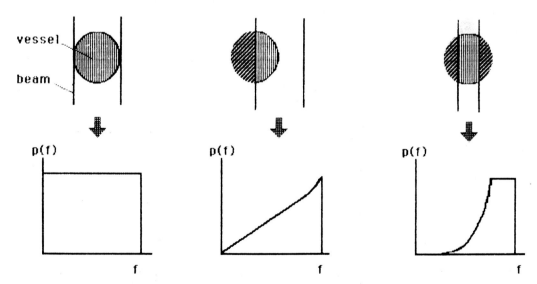

FIG. 12. Illustration of how a single vessel with a parabolic flow velocity profile can give different Doppler shift spectra according to the position and size of the beam in relation to the vessel lumen. *f* is frequency; *p(f)* is the power of the Doppler signal at frequency *f*.

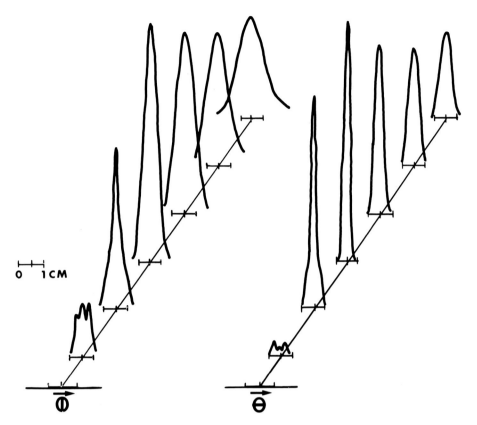

FIG. 13. Beam plot of typical 2-MHz continuous-wave Doppler transducer (13-mm diameter, focused) used for cardiac applications. The two graphs correspond to the amplitude perpendicular (**left**) and parallel (**right**) to the line between the D-shaped elements.

velocity. The uniform gray of the resulting sonogram is illustrated in Fig. 14C, which is from an ovarian artery. Note the low Doppler shift frequencies from this small vessel.

Finally, and as explained in Chapter 1, it should be noted that the process of spectral analysis provides only an estimate of the true power spectrum of the Doppler signal and is itself responsible for certain artifacts in the resulting display. The FFT algorithm examines discrete lengths of the Doppler signal (the input records) and analyzes them for their frequency content. The process of dividing the continuous Doppler signal in this way itself causes artifacts in the calculated spectrum; these, however, can partly be overcome by the use of a weighting function (such as a Hamming window) and probably do not contribute any noticeable effect to real Doppler signals (2). Of more significance is the choice of the length (corresponding to the duration of analyzed segment) of the input signal record. The more records obtained in each second, the more FFT calculations on new data can be performed, and the greater will be the time resolution of the spectral display. However, the length of time over which the signal is sampled for each analysis also determines the frequency resolution of the spectrum. Decreasing the input record time improves the time resolution of the spectrum at the expense of poorer frequency resolution.

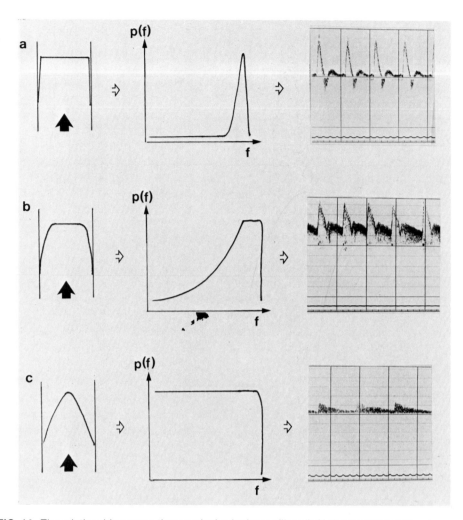

FIG. 14. The relationship among three typical velocity profiles: (**left**) the Doppler shift power spectrum (**center**) and the resultant spectral display (**right**). **A:** Plug flow (the aorta). **B:** Blunted parabolic flow in diastole (the celiac trunk). **C:** Parabolic flow (an ovarian artery).

In general, input record lengths of 5 to 50 msec are used, giving a maximum resolution of 20 to 200 Hz. The amplitude of each of these discrete frequency components is then subject to additional random inaccuracies associated with the sampling of a changing waveform. This variance may be reduced by performing the FFT calculation in a shorter time than the input record length. The next calculation may then begin immediately using data in the record that has not yet been completely replaced. Thus, some data are analyzed two or more times. This redundancy has the effect of averaging the final spectrum produced and reducing its variance. Increasing the redundancy also improves the ability of the spectrum analyzer to respond to rapid changes in the input signal (the system's "real-time bandwidth") and is generally desirable in the analysis of Doppler signals. These factors explain the rather wide variation in the visual appearance of different displays on different instruments. In practice, it is hard to make allowance for such factors in judging a spectrum, but one should certainly be aware of its reliance on the characteristics of the particular signal-processing method used.

Processing the Doppler Spectrum

It is often useful to derive waveforms that help to describe the form of the Doppler spectrum. As the spectrum changes with time, so do the shapes of these waveforms, creating a trace that may be submitted to further analysis. The two most commonly used waveforms are simply the maximum and mean Doppler shift frequencies. Various digital and analog signal-processing techniques are available for the automatic derivation of these waveforms, and some are to be found in modern instruments.

Maximum Frequency

The maximum Doppler shift frequency at a given moment corresponds to the velocity of the fastest moving lamina of blood within the sample volume. In an artery this quantity is likely to attain its maximum value at peak systole. In grading a stenosis or in estimating pressure difference from the velocity of the jet, this is the quantity used. The variation of the maximum Doppler shift frequency with time creates a time velocity trace, which is also used to assess downstream vascular impedance (see below).

An example of an individual Doppler spectrum corresponding to a short period of time might look like that of Fig. 15. Because of the presence of noise, the high

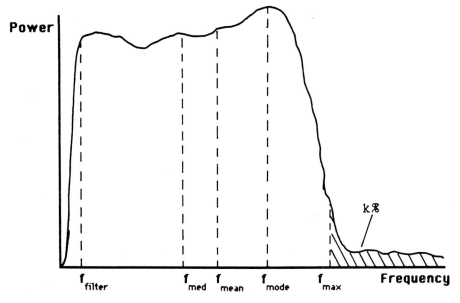

FIG. 15. Definition of parameters obtained from the Doppler spectrum. f_{filter} is the frequency of the high-pass filter; f_{med} is the frequency above which 50% of the power lies; f_{max} is defined here as the frequency above which k% of the power lies (k is chosen to lie between about 1 and 5); f_{mean} is the mean frequency; and f_{mode} is the frequency with the greatest signal power.

frequency of the blood flow signal may be difficult for the machine to identify reliably. One method is to define the maximum frequency as that frequency below which 95% (or 98% or 99%) of the power of the Doppler signal lies. The frequency can be calculated easily by measuring the areas under the curve of Fig. 15: it is the point at which 95% of the area lies below and 5% lies above. Mathematically, this may be described by

$$\int_0^{f_{max}} p(f)\,df = \frac{100 - k}{100} \int_0^{\infty} p(f)\,df \qquad [3]$$

where k is the centile; f_{max} is the maximum Doppler shift frequency; and $p(f)$ is the power of the signal at frequency f. As long as the signal has a relatively steep falloff of power with frequency, this estimated maximum frequency lies close to the real one. A threshold filter, which eliminates all signals below a certain amplitude, improves the performance of such a device. Problems can occur, however, during periods in which the flow velocities are low and the Doppler signal-to-noise ratio is consequently reduced. Figure 16A shows an example of a signal from a descending aorta in the adult obtained using the suprasternal notch approach. Note that there is flow throughout diastole. Figure 16B illustrates the performance of a maximum-frequency estimator on this signal. On the first half of the trace a high-pass filter has been used to eliminate the low Doppler shift frequencies depicting diastolic flow; the waveform "envelope" is well traced by the estimator. Halfway through the trace (arrow), the filter was removed, and diastolic flow appears in the spectral display. On this unexpurgated signal the estimator gives a more erratic trace, latching on to higher-frequency noise during portions of the cycle in which the flow velocities are low.

Mean Frequency

The mean Doppler frequency is the average Doppler shift in a given spectrum, calculated from the weighted sum of the amplitude elements. In Fig. 15 this corresponds to the normalized area under the spectral curve:

$$f_{mean} = \frac{\int_0^{\infty} fp(f)\,df}{\int_0^{\infty} p(f)\,df} \qquad [4]$$

Again, this may be derived using digital or analog (12) techniques. If the sample volume is sufficiently large compared to the vessel and is uniform in sensitivity, the mean Doppler shift frequency corresponds to the average flow velocity in the vessel. This is an important parameter which is necessary for the most commonly used method of volume flow measurement with the Doppler technique. For a parabolic flow profile, geometry predicts that the maximum velocity at the center stream is exactly double that of the mean velocity across the entire vessel lumen.

Figure 17 shows a signal processed from the anterior cerebral artery of the neonatal brain. Here the flow profile is nearly parabolic, and the sample volume of the Doppler system is large compared to the dimensions of the vessel. The maximum frequency has been estimated from the 97th centile of the power spectrum. Figure 17C shows

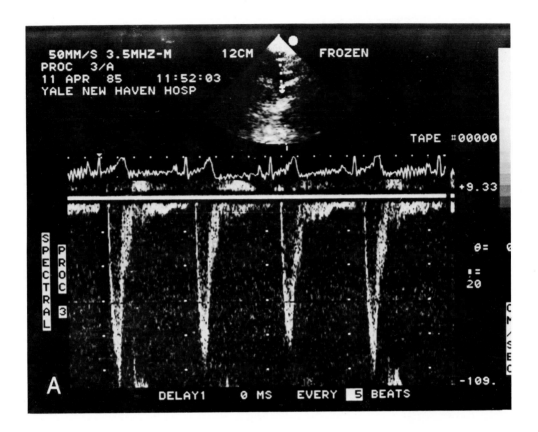

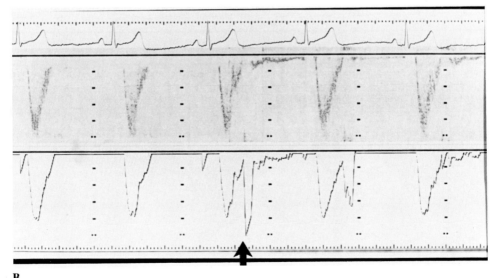

FIG. 16. A: Duplex scan of descending aorta using suprasternal notch approach. Note the low-velocity flow in diastole. **B:** Maximum frequency estimator's performance on the Doppler signal. Half way through the scan (*arrow*), the high-pass filter was removed, revealing the diastolic flow component.

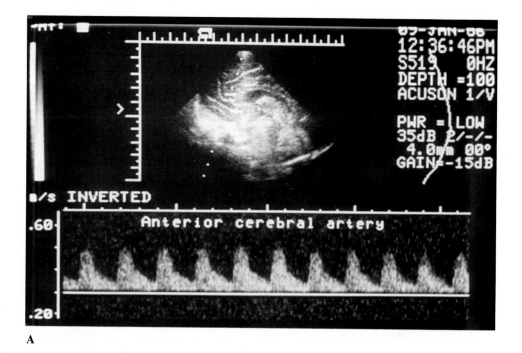

A

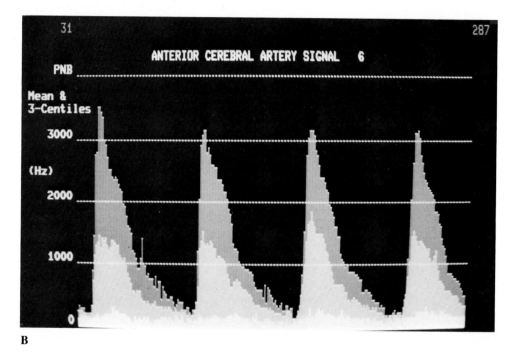

B

FIG. 17. Analysis of a signal from a vessel with a near-parabolic velocity profile (the anterior cerebral artery of a neonate). **A:** The duplex scan. **B:** Maximum and mean frequency Doppler waveforms. **C:** Calculation of the average ratio f_{max}/f_{mean} gives a value of 1.7. With perfect estimation and a true parabolic profile, this ratio would be 2.

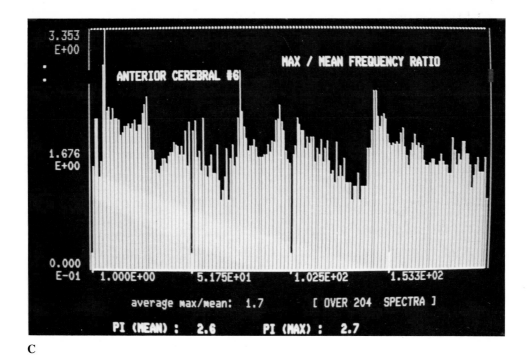

C

FIG. 17. (*continued*).

that the average ratio of the maximum to mean frequency over 200 spectra is approximately 1.7. Note that this method of measuring the maximum Doppler shift frequency is likely to err on the side of underestimation.

Modal Frequency

The mode of the frequency spectrum is that frequency with the highest amplitude value. Some digital systems use the variation of this parameter with time as a method of tracing the shape of the time velocity waveform. Fluctuations in spectral content add a random component to this variation.

Median Frequency

The median frequency is the frequency below which one-half of the total power in the Doppler spectrum lies. It is, therefore, defined by Eq. 3, where $k = 50$. As an expression of an "average" value for the spectrum, the median is less influenced by the presence of low-frequency (clutter) or high-frequency (noise) interference than is the mean.

Root Mean Square Frequency

The root mean square frequency (rms) is the normalized second moment of the power spectrum. In practice, this is a reasonable approximation to the mean value.

It is encountered most commonly as the output of some analog devices such as the zero-crossing detector. Though simple, this latter method is particularly susceptible to error in the presence of a broad spectrum of frequencies and is probably best avoided in favor of methods based on Fourier analysis (22).

INTERPRETATION OF THE DOPPLER SPECTRUM

Qualitative Methods

Presence of Flow

Determining whether flow is present is one of the simplest but perhaps most useful applications of Doppler ultrasound. It may be used to exclude occlusion by thrombosis, for example, or to determine the point of occlusion of a limb vessel during a pressure measurement. Confirming the absence of flow is, by its nature, a little more difficult. It is necessary to be certain that the lack of Doppler signal is a consequence of lack of flow rather than of the acoustical or electrical parameters of the system. It is prudent to check that normal flow signals can be detected with the same machine settings from comparable structures at comparable depths before concluding that flow is absent at a particular location.

Direction of Flow

The directional resolution of the Doppler system is best when the beam–vessel angle is relatively low and the signal lies in the middle of the dynamic range of the receiver. If a mirror image of the signal is seen in the reverse flow sideband of the display, care should be taken with the adjustment of angle and receiver gain so as to obtain a trace showing an unambiguous direction.

Identification of Characteristic Flow

It is apparent that normal flow in various parts of the arterial circulation shows distinct characteristics according to its precise location (Chapter 6). Those characteristics of waveform shape and spectral distribution are mostly consequences of the hemodynamic factors discussed in Chapter 3. These often allow the identification of the origin of a flow signal from spectral display (and the aural quality of the sound) alone and are particularly useful in circumstances in which the image may be ambivalent.

Semiquantitative Methods

Disturbed Flow

The characteristics that distinguish disturbed and turbulent flow from laminar flow are reflected in the content of their respective Doppler signals.

In a vessel with a flat velocity profile, the spectral display shows a narrow range of Doppler shift, especially in systole (Fig. 18A). This is the origin of the "window" below the spectral trace in systole—a Doppler sign of laminar flow with a blunt profile. More slowly moving laminae are found toward the edge of the vessel, so the size of the window (and with it the contrast between laminar and disturbed flow signals) can be increased by employing a small sample volume situated toward the center of the vessel. Flow disturbance produces velocity vectors whose direction varies. This means that the components of velocity along the direction of the Doppler beam change with time. The combination of many such components results in a wide range of Doppler shifts, seen as a broadening of the spectral display and a reduction in the size of the window (Fig. 18B). As the Reynolds number nears its critical value, vortices form, and the Doppler sample volume includes rotating flow elements. Velocities, and hence Doppler shifts, are noticeably higher. The vortices contain simultaneous and forward and reverse flows at a range of velocities. Vortex formation is time dependent in arteries; Fig. 19 shows their appearance on a Doppler trace in which the critical number is attained in the upstroke of systole. Suddenly, laminar flow gives way to rotating flow, and the Doppler spectrum shows simultaneous forward and reverse velocities together with a broad range of Doppler shifts. Note that laminar flow reappears in diastole at a slightly lower velocity: this is the hysteresis effect described in Chapter 3.

As flow velocities increase, vortices are shed and travel downstream. As they move through a Doppler sample volume, they are responsible for fluctuation of Doppler shift frequency with time. These rotational components can also have their origin in geometry: Fig. 20 shows a signal from a quite normal but tortuous splenic artery, showing dramatic variation in the maximum frequency.

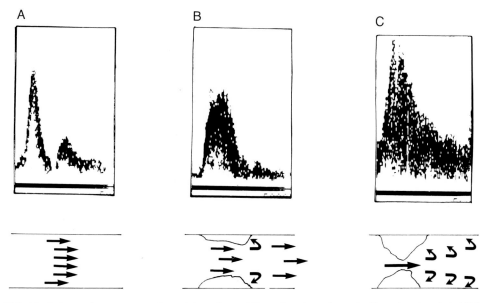

FIG. 18. Schematic representation of the effect of flow disturbance on the Doppler signal. **A:** With normal flow and a blunt velocity profile, there is a "window" below systole. **B:** Flow disturbance causes spectral broadening. **C:** Critical stenosis results in high Doppler shifts, large spectral width, and a damped waveform shape.

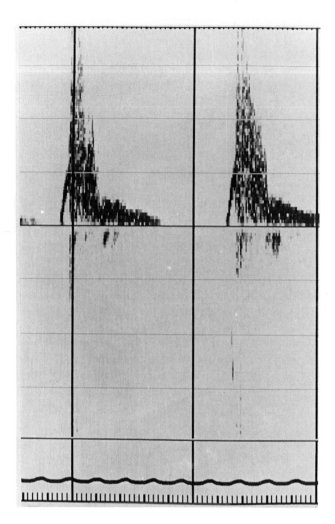

FIG. 19. Periodic turbulence in a renal artery. Note how laminar flow suddenly gives way to simultaneous forward and reverse velocities. During the turbulent period the peak Doppler shifts are high, and there is a wide range of frequencies. Here, laminar flow is reestablished in diastole.

At high Reynolds numbers, turbulence ensues and is sustained throughout the cardiac cycle. The cardiac waveform produced by a tight stenosis is very much less pulsatile than its normal counterpart. Simultaneous disorganized forward and reverse Doppler shifts are seen, and velocities remain high throughout the cardiac cycle (Figs. 18C and 21).

These are, then, four particular Doppler features of disturbed flow: increased velocity, spectral broadening, simultaneous forward and reverse flow, and fluctuations of flow velocity with time. Criteria for the clinical classification of these findings in the context of carotid diagnosis are discussed in Chapter 5.

There are many methods for the objective identification of Doppler spectra associated with disturbed flow. In general, the mean, median, and mode frequencies decrease relative to the maximum frequency as the spectrum broadens. Of course, the ratio of any two of these frequencies derived from the same spectrum is independent of Doppler angle. A variety of indices based on such ratios have been proposed. These include f_{max}/f_{mean} (27); $(f_{max} - f_{mean})/f_{mean}$ (3); and various measures of spectral "bandwidth" based on the mode frequency (26). Figure 22 shows

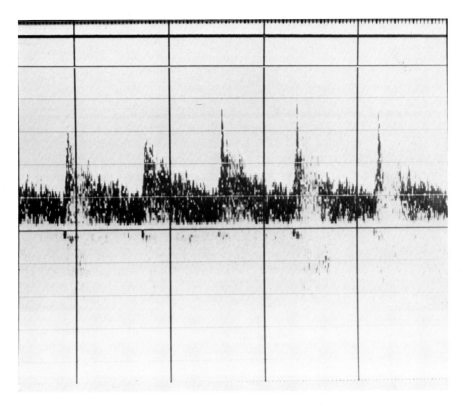

FIG. 20. Normal signal from the splenic artery showing flow disturbance. Here, the origin is probably geometric, associated with tortuousity of the vessel's path.

how f_{max}, f_{mean}, and f_{min} (defined as the third centile of the power spectrum) change with increasing degrees of stenosis of the internal carotid artery. Note that in the normal vessel, f_{mean} and f_{max} are very close to each other, especially in systole. With a critical stenosis (75% diameter reduction), f_{max} may be more than double f_{mean}, which now shows much less pulsatile variation.

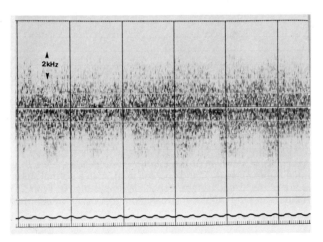

2kHz

FIG. 21. Severe turbulence distal to critical stenosis. Note the high Doppler shifts, simultaneous forward and reverse flow, and greatly reduced pulsatility.

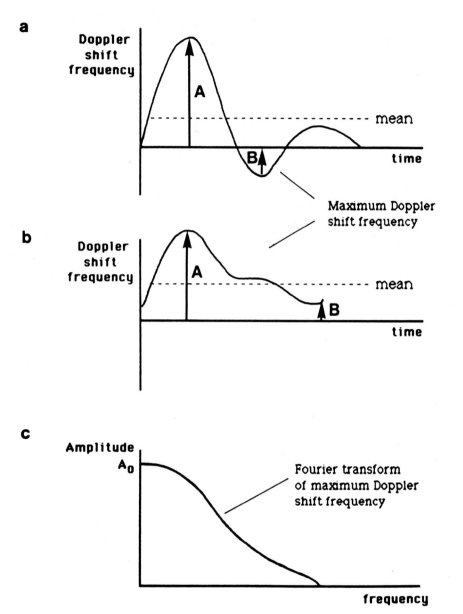

FIG. 23. Typical time velocity waveforms when the distal impedance is (**A**) high and (**B**) low. **C:** The Fourier transform of the time velocity waveform.

is unity, the pulsatility index (PI_F) is the area under the curve,

$$PI_F = \frac{1}{A_0^2} \sum_{i=1}^{n} A_i^2 \qquad [5]$$

where A_i is the amplitude of the ith Fourier component. The PI is higher for pulsatile waveforms and lower for damped waveforms.

Although this index has certain advantages (such as its relative insensitivity to heart rate), it is cumbersome to calculate in a practical setting. Therefore, it has been largely replaced by a number of indices calculated in the time domain, directly from the Doppler trace. Each of these indices is a ratio of Doppler shift frequencies and so independent of Doppler angle. One of the most commonly used is the pulsatility index (PI) defined as

$$PI = \frac{A - B}{mean} \qquad [6]$$

where A is the maximum, B is the minimum, and "mean" is the time average of the maximum Doppler shift frequency over the cardiac cycle. The mean and A_0 are identical. Again, high PIs describe pulsatile waveforms. Note that a slower heart rate in Fig. 23B would also result in a high PI because B and the mean would be reduced. Table 1 shows a variety of other indices that have been suggested as ways of describing the time velocity waveform shape. It should be noted that some of the more arbitrarily conceived of these ratios behave in a particularly extravagant fashion as B becomes small. In vessels in which end-diastolic flow is zero, for example, A/B is infinite.

Because it is not necessary to know the Doppler angle when calculating one of these indices, pulsatility can be assessed in vessels that are too small or tortuous to be imaged (e.g., the arcuate vessels of the kidney). For any measurement reflecting the shape or spectral content of the Doppler waveform, the index should be calculated for each of several cardiac cycles and an average value taken. Beat-to-beat variation in the adult suggests that about five heartbeats are adequate for a measurement of pulsatility.

Quantitative Methods

Local Pressure Difference

By using the modified Bernouilli equation and taking careful note of the limitations described in Chapter 3, it is possible to estimate the pressure drop across a wide orifice carrying a fast jet of blood by measuring the jet velocity using Doppler techniques.

TABLE 1. *Some indices used to describe the shape of the time velocity waveform*

Index	Expression
"Full" pulsatility index (PI$_F$)	$\frac{1}{A_0^2} \sum\limits_{i=1}^{n} A_i^2$
Pulsatility index (PI)	$(A - B)/mean$
Resistance index (RI)	$(A - B)/A$
S–D ratio	A/B
B/A ratio	$B(100\%)/A$

[a] A is the maximum value over the cardiac cycle, B the minimum, "mean" the average value, and A_i the amplitude of the ith component of the Fourier transform of the waveform.

The practical technique for this method of estimating the pressure drop across, for example, a stenotic aortic valve requires insonation of the fastest moving stream of blood. If a jet is present, its orientation must first be ascertained because its axis may not be aligned with that of the vessel. The maximum Doppler shift frequency at peak systole is then measured, and the corresponding velocity deduced. In many circumstances the velocity before the orifice is so small compared to that of the jet that it may be ignored (16). If the angle between the jet and the Doppler beam is less than 20°, a maximum error of only 6% is obtained by assuming it to be zero (Fig. 24). With pulsed Doppler systems, aliasing at the high Doppler shifts obtained is often a problem, and care should be exercised in choice of the pulse repetition frequency and interpretation of the spectral display. Finally, it should be borne in mind that underestimation of pressure drop because of ignorance of the viscous term is the most likely source of error with this method and that the risk of such error increases with progressively smaller orifice sizes. Comparison with invasive pressure measurements (17) suggests that accuracy is reasonable when the orifice diameter is above about 3.5 mm and the velocity is greater than about 3 m/sec.

Measurement of Velocity and Acceleration

In estimating velocity using the Doppler angle and Doppler shift frequency, the size of potential errors induced by an uncertainty in the angle measurement should be borne in mind. Figure 24 shows that these increase rapidly with increasing angle. At 45°, for example, a 5° uncertainty in angle measurement results in a 9% error in velocity. At 70° the same uncertainty results in a 25% error in velocity. At angles less than 20°, on the other hand, these errors are reduced to insignificance.

If velocity is to be measured from the maximum Doppler shift frequency, it is generally more reliable to assess the location of the maximum frequency by eye from the spectral display rather than to rely on the output of the maximum frequency processor, which is generally more prone to the effects of noise.

Flow acceleration may also be measured from the gradient of the velocity–time

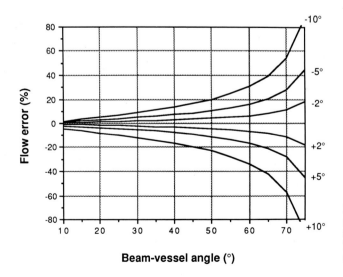

FIG. 24. Graph showing effect of various errors in the measurement of the angle between the beam and the flow direction on the estimate of flow velocity.

waveform; facilities for this procedure are frequently incorporated into the scanner's own analysis software. Clearly the precision of an acceleration measurement during the upstroke of systole in the aorta, for example, is enhanced by choosing a fast sweep rate of the Doppler spectral display.

VOLUME FLOW MEASUREMENT

Noninvasive measurements of volume flow rate using Doppler ultrasound have attracted a great deal of attention in recent years, mainly in relation to cardiac output and transvalvular flow in the heart, to umbilical venous flow in the fetus, and to portal flow in the adult abdomen. As techniques improve and specialized instrumentation becomes more widely available, the variety of clinical applications for volume flow determination is likely to increase.

A number of methods are available, based on somewhat diverse principles. All have in common the use of Doppler ultrasound to determine an average velocity in the vessel lumen and hence a mean flux of blood across a section of vessel. This is then integrated over time to yield the volume flow rate.

Velocity Profile Method

In this method, the velocity profile is measured at successive intervals throughout the cardiac cycle and integrated to give a volume flow rate. A pulsed Doppler system with a sample volume much smaller than the vessel lumen cross section is required. The sample volume is moved slowly across the vessel lumen or a multigated system is used, and the velocity is calculated using a beam–vessel angle derived from the real-time image. Angle may also be deduced from a series of Doppler measurements a known angle apart (10). Assuming circular symmetry of the profile, each velocity is multiplied by the corresponding semiannular area, and the resulting flow components are summed. Multigate or "infinite" gate systems that are capable of interrogating an entire vessel at one time have the advantage that they can acquire the necessary data in a single heart beat and therefore are less prey to problems of beat-to-beat variation (10). This method is particularly suited to applications in which the transducer may be placed directly on the vessel of interest and a high ultrasonic frequency used. This permits a small sample volume and high precision (9). For transcutaneous applications the method seems to remain at present only suitable for large and accessible vessels such as the aorta and common carotid arteries.

Uniform Insonation Method

The principle of the uniform insonation method is shown in Fig. 25. The entire volume of blood whose flow rate is to be assessed is exposed to a uniform ultrasonic beam. The mean Doppler shift is then calculated. If each element of blood contributes equally to the Doppler shift signal and the angle between the beam and flow direction is constant over the entire volume, the mean Doppler shift frequency corresponds to the mean flow velocity in the vessel. Simply multiplying this velocity by the cross-sectional area of the vessel or orifice gives the instantaneous flow rate. This product

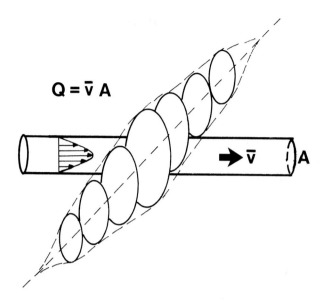

Q = v̄ A

FIG. 25. Principle of even insonation method for the estimation
of volume flow rate Q. The instantaneous mean velocity v̄ is
calculated from the mean Doppler shift frequency and multiplied by the cross-sectional area
A of the vessel.

is then integrated over the cardiac cycle to yield the time average flow rate. For
arterial flow both the cross-sectional area and the velocity change with time, so that
ideally one would form the product of the instantaneous mean velocity and the cross-
sectional area at the same time,

$$Q(t) = \bar{v}(t)A(t) \tag{7}$$

where $\bar{v}$ is the mean velocity and A the cross-sectional area at time t. Time-averaged
volume flow rate Q is then given by

$$Q = \frac{1}{T}\int_0^T \bar{v}(t)A(t)\,dA\,dt \tag{8}$$

where $\bar{v}(t)$ is calculated using a mean frequency processor from the first moment of
the Doppler power spectrum (Eq. 4).

In practice, the goal of simultaneous diameter and flow velocity measurement is
not attainable using this approach. The optimum ultrasonic approach for the former
is perpendicular to the vessel or orifice, whereas for the latter an acute angle of
approach to the direction of flow is best. Because it is difficult to arrange for two
noninterfering beams to be used at the same time, it is usual to measure the mean
velocity and mean area separately and take their product after, rather than before,
temporal integration. The error so introduced depends on the rate of change of both
the cross-sectional area and the flow velocity over the cardiac cycle. It is mitigated
by the fact that most flow takes place during one portion of the cardiac cycle. For
the highly distensible fetal aorta, it has been estimated (5) that by taking the area
from the mean of ten diameter measurements on a real-time scan, an error of approximately 10% is introduced. Most workers, then, take an average area $\overline{A}$ and
multiply it by the time-averaged mean velocity:

$$Q = \overline{A}\int_0^T \bar{v}(t)\,dt \tag{9}$$

For the uniform insonation method, then, it is necessary to measure the beam vessel angle and a cross-sectional area of the lumen and to establish that the assumption that the mean Doppler shift corresponds to the mean spatial velocity (the uniform insonation assumption) is as nearly as possible valid.

The beam vessel angle is easily measured using the duplex scanner, but as already discussed (Fig. 24) the cosine dependence of velocity on angle means that this angle should be less than about 55° if substantial errors are to be avoided. This creates a difficulty when using a single-transducer sector duplex scanner to measure flow in a vessel parallel to the skin surface; low angles are easiest to achieve with a system using a separate Doppler transducer offset from the imaging assembly. Some practical implementations are described in Chapter 9. The vessel axis must lie within the scan plane for the image to give the correct angle. Gill (13) has estimated that it is necessary to visualize at least 2 cm of the vessel lumen, thus rendering flow measurement impractical for tortuous vessels. If two Doppler transducers aligned at a fixed angle are arranged to insonate the same volume of blood, the Doppler angle can be calculated from the signals themselves. Again, the two beams must lie within the plane of the axis of flow—a 90° angle between the two transducers gives the most reliable results. One such system (30) has been made for use on superficial vessels: it consists of two receiving elements inclined at a fixed angle to each other and to a central transmitting transducer, which is also used to measure the vessel diameter.

Measurement of the cross-sectional area of the lumen presents a more challenging problem. One approach is simply to measure the apparent internal diameter of the vessel from the ultrasound image and assume that its section is circular. This measurement is best carried out at right angles to the vessel, where reflections are specular and the axial resolution of the scanner determines precision. This is, of course, an impossible approach for Doppler ultrasound. Considering the ambiguity introduced by multiple echoes from a vessel wall and the axial resolution of the image, the precision of diameter measurement is unlikely to be better than 1 mm in all but the most superficial vessels. Figure 26 shows the error resulting from such

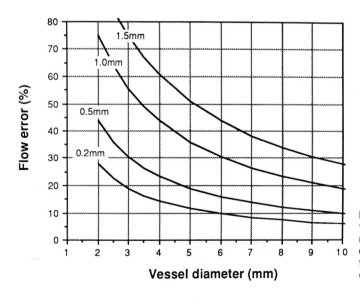

FIG. 26. Graph showing the effect of precision of diameter measurement on the error in the estimation of area (and hence flow) when the cross section is circular.

a margin in the diameter measurement and indicates that the method is best reserved for use on large vessels. Clearly, most vessels (especially veins) are not circular in section. If, for example, the section is an ellipse with a major axis 50% longer than the minor axis, a 50% error can result from assuming circularity. In this case imaging must be used to estimate the area, forcing reliance on the lateral resolution of the scanner. Additional errors accrue from the distensibility of the vessels, especially arteries, some of which are capable of changing their cross-sectional areas by up to 40% over the cardiac cycle (Chapter 9).

Uniform insonation itself requires that the sensitivity of the sample volume be essentially smooth over the volume occupied by the moving blood. By controlling the receiver gate, the axial length of the sample volume may be extended to include the entire vessel. It should be ensured that the receiver electronics are such that the amplitude and frequency response of the system are uniform along the axial extent of the sample volume. The lateral beam width is more difficult to control, especially if the transducer is used for imaging as well, in which case this width is designed to be as small as possible. Even low-frequency, poorly focused Doppler transducers do not have a uniform sensitivity over the dimensions of the typical large vessel (Fig. 13). If the beam and vessel axes are aligned, the less sensitive portion of the beam insonates the more slowly moving blood near the vessel walls, and the result is a weighting of the mean toward the high Doppler shifts and an overestimation of mean velocity (6). It appears, however (13), that for small beam–vessel angles, the sample volume whose length exceeds the width of the vessel partially compensates for inadequacy of the beam width. In practice, most beams are inhomogeneous over their width, and although mathematical techniques to compensate for this effect do exist, they are difficult to apply to a beam in tissue.

Additional difficulties may arise from more subtle aspects of the interaction of sound with tissue. The process of absorption by tissue is strongly frequency dependent, so with pulsed systems the center frequency of the received signal is lower than that of the transmitted signal. This results in a downward shift of the mean Doppler frequency, whose severity depends on the length of the ultrasonic path but can be as great as 15% (18) (Fig. 27).

For small angles of insonation such as those likely to be used in estimating cardiac output from the suprasternal notch, it is also possible that refractive differences between the vessel wall and the blood itself can result in total internal reflection in which some or all of the acoustic energy of the beam does not reach the moving blood but is refracted outside the vessel. Acoustic velocity differences between blood and vessel wall are such that this effect is unlikely to occur with angles of insonation above about 25° (13).

Even with a uniform beam and perfect processing of the signal to yield its mean frequency, this still may not correspond to the mean velocity. Spectral components whose presence is the result of transit-time broadening phenomenon described earlier distort the mean frequency, whereas the high-pass filter tends to raise the flow estimate by eliminating signals for low-flow elements (especially significant when the velocity profile is parabolic) (Fig. 28). These errors are often determined by factors that are hard to control, such as the ultrasonic path and system frequency and bandwidth. Electrical noise in the receiver also affects the mean frequency estimate; because the Doppler bandwidth changes over the cardiac cycle, the signal-

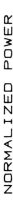
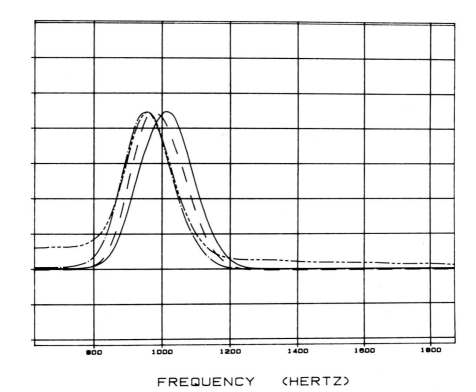

FREQUENCY (HERTZ)

FIG. 27. The effect of frequency-dependent attenuation (dispersion) on a pulsed Doppler signal. High ultrasound frequencies suffer greater attenuation in tissue than do low frequencies. A pulse consisting of a range of frequencies thus has its center frequency lowered as it travels through tissue. This results in a lower Doppler shift frequency from a moving target separated from the transducer by tissue. In this example, the center frequency of the Doppler spectrum has decreased by 10% after a 12-cm path through tissue-equivalent material. Thus, an estimate of average flow velocity based on the Doppler shift would suffer a similar error.

to-noise ratio is unlikely to be constant. Gill (12) has analyzed the effect of noise, both intrinsic to the receiver and as a result of high-amplitude, low-frequency clutter, and derives a mathematical expression that allows correction for the former (unfortunately usually less severe) source of noise. These considerations have led to the design of specialized equipment that, in spite of the obstacles, has produced measurements of flow with an overall accuracy of about 15% (11,14,23).

Finally, it should be noted that the central assumption of the uniform insonation method is itself predicated on the notion that the scatterers in moving blood are distributed uniformly throughout the fluid. It is widely believed that there is a paucity of red blood cells in the boundary layer immediately adjacent to the vessel wall, but since these do not give rise to Doppler signals, this is of little consequence for the method. In fact, uniform scattering of ultrasound by whole blood has been demonstrated over a range of hematocrits and laminar flow profiles (2). Shung (28) has shown, however, that the intensity of ultrasound scattered from a volume of blood changes in the presence of turbulence. These results suggest that the even insonation method should not be used in circumstances in which laminar flow may have given way to turbulence.

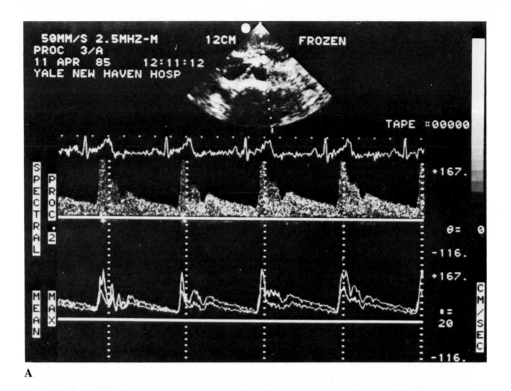

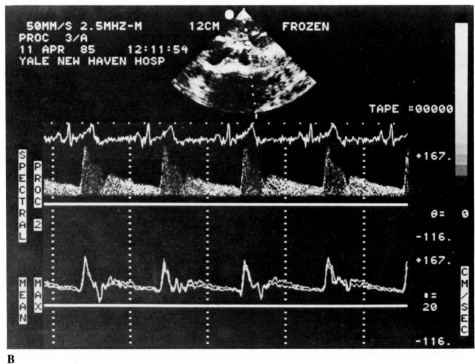

FIG. 28. A: Duplex scan of the celiac trunk. Note that in diastole the mean frequency is between the maximum and one-half the maximum (consistent with blunted velocity profile). **B:** The same examination. A high-pass filter of 400 Hz has caused the mean frequency estimator to yield a higher value.

Assumed Velocity Profile Method

In the face of difficulties in achieving insonation of an entire vessel such as the descending thoracic aorta, some workers have made measurements at one point in the vessel and assumed a given velocity profile to exist over the regions of flow not interrogated by the sample volume. Usually the assumption is that of a constant "plug" flow, that is, a perfectly flat velocity profile. In this case the spatial mean flow velocity is simply equal to the maximum velocity near the center of the vessel, an easy quantity to measure. In other circumstances the mean frequency has been estimated by simply multiplying the maximum frequency by a constant factor, determined from an experimental "calibration" (25). There is no need to employ special beam geometry or even a processor capable of calculating the mean Doppler shift frequency.

Both theory and invasive measurements in experimental animals, however, suggest that this assumption is of very limited validity. Hot-wire anemometer measurements in the aortic arch of a dog, for example (8,9), reveal velocity profiles at peak systole that are skewed, as described in Chapter 3. In other locations the velocity profile changes over the cardiac cycle and is dependent on location, so that the mean velocity bears no predictable relationship to the maximum velocity. As seen in Chapter 3, in no part of the vascular system is a perfectly flat profile seen. However, the assumptions of this method probably verge on acceptability for the case of the aortic root in the normal adult. Here good correlation has been reported with invasive cardiac output estimates based on dye dilution (20,21).

Attenuation-Compensated Method

One novel and appealing Doppler method for the measurement of volume flow rate eliminates the need to measure either the beam Doppler angle or the cross-sectional area of the vessel yet makes no severe assumptions about the velocity profile.

In the "attenuation-compensated" flowmeter two ultrasonic beams are used, the first with a uniform sample volume large enough to embrace the entire vessel and the second with a narrower beam along the same path. The power of the backscattered Doppler signal is simply proportional to the number of red blood cells in the sample volume (1). This power is difficult to measure directly because of the attenuating effect of an unknown quantity of intervening tissue. The second, smaller sample volume (situated entirely within the vessel) provides a signal with which to compare the first, subject to the same ultrasonic path and therefore the same attenuation. The difference between the two signal power levels is accounted for entirely by the volume of blood in the large sample volume, which can thus be deduced without recourse to the direct measurement of the vessel diameter. Furthermore, the dependence of this estimate on the beam–vessel angle is eliminated when it is multiplied by the mean Doppler shift frequency, which has an exactly reciprocal dependence on angle. Thus, in principle, volume flow may be measured with knowledge of neither the vessel area nor the angle of insonation. The method was proposed and results of *in vitro* trials were reported in 1979 (19), but further application has had to await practical realization of the required beam geometries. As described in

Chapter 1, these have become available, and clinical results (from flow measurements in large vessels such as the ascending aorta) are beginning to confirm the validity of the method.

REFERENCES

1. Atkinson, P., and Berry, M. V. (1974): Random noise in ultrasonic echoes diffracted by blood. *J. Phys. A.,* 11:1293–1301.

2. Atkinson, P., and Woodcock, J. P. (1982): *Doppler Ultrasound and Its Use in Clinical Measurement.* Academic Press, London.

3. Brown, P. N., Johnston, K. W., Kassan, M., and Cobbold, R. S. C. (1982): A critical study of ultrasound Doppler spectral analysis for detecting carotid artery disease. *Ultrasound Med. Biol.,* 8:515–523.

4. Burns, P. N., Halliwell, M., Webb, A. J., and Wells, P. N. T. (1982): Ultrasonic Doppler studies of the breast. *Ultrasound Med. Biol.,* 8:127–143.

5. Eik-Nes, S. H., Marsal, K., and Kristoffersen, K. (1984): Methodology and basic problems related to blood flow studies in the human fetus. *Ultrasound Med. Biol.,* 10:329–337.

6. Evans, D. H. (1982): Some aspects of the relationship between instantaneous volumetric blood flow and continuous wave Doppler ultrasound recordings. The effect of ultrasonic beam width on the output of maximum, mean and rms frequency processors. *Ultrasound Med. Biol.,* 8:605–609.

7. Evans, D. H., Barrie, W. W., Asher, M. J., Bentley, S., and Bell, P. R. F. (1980): The relationship between ultrasonic pulsatility index and proximal arterial stenosis in a canine model. *Circ. Res.,* 46:470–475.

8. Falsetti, H. L., Kiser, K. M., Francis, G. P., and Belmore, E. R. (1972): Sequential velocity development in ascending and descending aorta of the dog. *Circ. Res.,* 31:328–338.

9. Farthing, S., and Peronneau, P. (1979): Flow in the thoracic aorta. *Cardiovasc. Res.,* 13:607–620.

10. Fish, P. J. (1981): A method of transcutaneous blood flow measurement—accuracy considerations. In: *Recent Advances in Ultrasound Diagnosis, Vol. 3,* edited by A. Kurjak and A. Kratochwil, pp. 110–115. Excerpta Medica, Amsterdam.

11. Gill, R. W. (1979): Pulsed Doppler with B-mode imaging for quantitative blood flow measurement. *Ultrasound Med. Biol.,* 5:223–235.

12. Gill, R. W. (1979): Performance of the mean frequency Doppler demodulator. *Ultrasound Med. Biol.,* 5:237–247.

13. Gill, R. W. (1982): Accuracy calculations for ultrasonic pulsed Doppler blood flow measurements. *Aust. Phys. Eng. Sci. Med.,* 5:51–57.

14. Gill, R. W. (1985): Measurement of blood flow by ultrasound: Accuracy and sources of error. *Ultrasound Med. Biol.,* 4:625–641.

15. Gosling, R. G., King, D. H., Newman, D. L., and Woodcock, J. P. (1969): Transcutaneous measurement of arterial blood velocity by ultrasound. In: *Ultrasonics for Industry Conference Papers,* pp. 16–32. IPC, Guildford, England.

16. Hatle, L., and Angelsen, B. (1985): *Doppler Ultrasound in Cardiology: Physical Principles and Clinical Applications,* 2nd ed. Lea & Febiger, Philadelphia.

17. Hatle, L., Brubakk, A., Tromsdal, A., and Angelsen, B. (1978): Noninvasive assessment of pressure drop in mitral stenosis by Doppler ultrasound. *Br. Heart J.,* 60(2):131–140.

18. Holland, S. K., Orphanoudakis, S. C., and Jaffe, C. C. (1984): Frequency-dependent attenuation effects in pulsed Doppler ultrasound: experimental results. *IEEE Trans. Biomed. Eng.,* 9:626–631.

19. Hottinger, C. F., and Meindl, J. D. (1979): Blood flow measurement using the attenuation-compensated volume flowmeter. *Ultrasonic Imag.,* 1:1–15.

20. Huntsman, L. L., Stewart, D. K., Barnes, S., Franklin, S. B., Colocousis, J. S., and Hessel, E. A. (1983): Noninvasive Doppler determination of cardiac output in man: clinical validation. *Circulation,* 67:593.

21. Lewis, J. F., Kuo, L. C., Nelson, J. G., Limacher, M. C., and Quinones, M. A. (1984): Pulsed Doppler echocardiographic determination of stroke volume and cardiac output: clinical validation of two new methods using the apical window. *Circulation,* 70(3):425.

22. Lunt, M. J. (1975): Accuracy and limitations of the ultrasonic Doppler blood velocimeter and zero crossing detector. *Ultrasound Med. Biol.,* 2:1–10.

23. Magnin, P. A., Stewart, J. A., Myers, S., von Ramm, O., and Kisslo, J. A. (1981): Combined Doppler and phased-array echocardiographic estimation of cardiac output. *Circulation,* 63:388–392.

24. Namekawa, K., Kasai, C., and Omoto, R. (1983): Real-time two-dimensional bloodflow imaging using ultrasound Doppler. *J. Ultrasound Med.,* 2:10–15.

25. Ohnishi, K., Saito, M., and Sato, S. (1987): Portal hemodynamics in idiopathic portal hypertension (Banti's syndrome). Comparison with chronic persistent hepatitis and normal subjects. *Gastroenterology*, 92:751–758.

26. Rittgers, S. E., Thornhill, B. M., and Barnes, R. W. (1983): Quantitative analysis of carotid artery Doppler spectral waveforms: diagnostic value of parameters. *Ultrasound Med. Biol.*, 9:255–264.

27. Sheldon, C. D., Murie, J. A., and Quinn, R. O. (1983): Ultrasonic Doppler spectral broadening in the diagnosis of carotid artery stenosis. *Ultrasound Med. Biol.*, 9:575–580.

28. Shung, K. K. (1983): Physics of blood echogenicity. *J. Cardiovasc. Ultrasonogr.*, 2:401–406.

29. Shung, K. K., Sigelmann, R. A., and Reid, J. N. (1976): Scattering of ultrasound by blood. *IEEE Trans. Biomed. Eng.*, 6:460–467.

30. Uematsu, S. (1981): Determination of volume of arterial blood flow by an ultrasonic device. *J. Clin. Ultrasound*, 9:209–216.

5 / Clinical Applications of Carotid Doppler Ultrasound

Kenneth J. W. Taylor

Department of Diagnostic Radiology, Yale University School of Medicine, New Haven, Connecticut 06510

Stroke is the third leading cause of death in the United States despite a 40% decline in incidence reported in recent years. Stroke results from ischemic injury to the motor or sensory tracts, usually in the region of the internal capsule, as a result of cerebral hemorrhage or embolization. Stroke was described by Hippocrates, who named it "apoplexy" meaning "to strike down." Morgagni, in the 18th century, recognized a nonhemorrhagic cause of cerebral softening, and Abercrombie, in the 1830s, realized that cerebral softening could result from narrowing of the arteries near a lesion. He also suggested that the extracranial arteries could be important. However, subsequent authors stressed the importance of local vascular factors, and it was not until 1951 that Fisher suggested that internal carotid disease could be important in the production of cerebral infarction and that occlusion could occur on the basis of progressive atheroma from which emboli could arise.

Thus, it is only in the last 40 years that the importance of the extracranial arteries has been appreciated as a cause of cerebral ischemic events. Emboli may arise from the left atrium, especially in mitral valve stenosis or prolapse, from the ventricular cavity after a myocardial infarction, from the aortic valve in subacute bacterial endocarditis or atherosclerotic disease, or from the extracranial vessels. Of these, the carotid bifurcation is most prone to atherosclerotic disease, with embolization or occlusion accounting for approximately half of such events.

PATHOGENESIS

Atherosclerosis is a widespread, generalized arterial degeneration that tends to occur selectively at bifurcations because of the disturbed hemodynamics and non-laminar flow at such locations. The anatomic site of atheromatous plaques appears to be dictated by the specific flow disturbance of the carotid bifurcation since both the earliest lesions and the mature lesions have a predeliction to occur on the posterior wall of the carotid sinus where there is a reverse component associated with flow separation. The arterial wall can become damaged by any noxious influence, which might include hypertension, the effects of smoking, high serum lipoprotein level, or diabetes.

Fatty streaks may occur very early in life, but the relationship of this to the mature atheromatous plaque is not clear. The evolution of the mature plaque includes proliferation of smooth muscle cells producing a fibrous plaque. Subsequently, there may be degeneration and calcification, necrosis, and increasing lipid content with deposition of cholesterol crystals followed by varying degrees of hemorrhage and ulceration.

The pathogenesis of embolization or occlusion arising in the carotid bifurcation is summarized in Fig. 1. There is a buildup of atherosclerotic plaque, which may ulcerate and give rise to emboli to the cerebral arteries (Fig. 1A). The importance of intraplaque hemorrhage has recently been recognized as a possible precipitating factor in the initiation of embolization. The exposed, roughened surface of the atherosclerotic ulcer may cause platelet aggregation (Fig. 1B) or clot formation (Fig. 1C), which also may embolize. Finally, there may be progressive encroachment of the carotid lumen, resulting in occlusion by superimposed thrombus as the blood flow slows and stasis occurs (Fig. 1D).

It is conventional to term a stenosis significant when luminal diameter reduction exceeds 60%. This is usually assessed radiographically and is, at best, an estimation. Busuttil et al. (4) reported that the risk of stroke and death was only 2.2% in patients with nonsignificant stenosis compared with a 16.2% incidence of stroke in those with significant stenosis on whom endarterectomy was not performed. In patients with significant stenosis who underwent endarterectomy, the incidence of subsequent stroke was reduced to 1.9%.

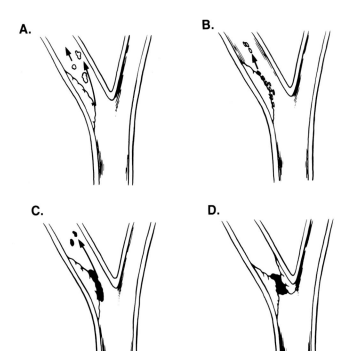

FIG. 1. Scheme to show pathogenesis of thromboembolic lesions at the carotid bifurcation. **A:** An atheromatous lesion may ulcerate, especially after intraplaque hemorrhage, giving rise to distant embolization. **B:** A platelet clot on the roughened surface may give rise to distal embolization. **C:** Thrombosis on the roughened ulcer may give rise to distal embolization. **D:** Progressive thrombosis may result in complete occlusion.

NEUROLOGIC DEFICITS

The neurologic deficit resulting from carotid vascular events varies with the size and site of the embolus. The following clinical syndromes are recognized.

Amaurosis Fugax

Amaurosis fugax refers to the temporary loss of vision in one eye. The patient usually describes this as a curtain descending over the eye. This visual disturbance may be quite transient. The anatomical basis for this phenomenon lies in the fact that the ophthalmic artery, which gives off the central artery of the retina, is the first branch of the internal carotid artery (ICA). Thus, emboli from the carotid bifurcation may pass into the retinal vessels, resulting in transient retinal ischemia.

Transient Ischemic Attack or Reversible Ischemic Neurologic Deficit

A transient ischemic attack (TIA) is a temporary stroke characterized by a motor or sensory disturbance of less than 24 hr and usually less than 15 min duration occurring on the side opposite the affected hemisphere. A right hemispheric event, therefore, results in transient left hemiparesis and vice versa. Typically, this leads to a temporary paralysis in the arm or leg, tingling and anesthesia, speech disturbance, and, perhaps, dizziness or transient loss of consciousness. Since these symptoms are very common from other causes in the elderly, a large number of patients are referred for duplex scanning as a triage procedure for any sign of carotid artery disease. Dizziness and transient loss of consciousness may also occur as a result of vertebrobasilar disease. Because of the intravertebral course of the vertebral arteries, these cannot adequately be assessed by ultrasonic duplex scanning techniques.

A TIA is significant in that it is associated with an increase in the risk of stroke during the subsequent 5 years to 17 times that of the unaffected population. The annual incidence of a first TIA is one in 6,000 for those aged 45 to 54 years and one in 1,000 for those 55 years or older. Patients with a history of TIA face a risk of stroke or death of 10% per annum.

A reversible ischemic neurologic deficit (RIND) is characterized by temporary neurologic loss similar to a TIA. Here, however, the deficit is of longer than 24 hr but less than 3 weeks duration.

Progressive Stroke

A progressive stroke or stroke in evolution is the term used to indicate a neurologic deficit that progresses over minutes or hours and is caused by an extending area of ischemia. This condition should be distinguished from the late worsening that accompanies cerebral edema complicating infarction.

Completed Stroke

A completed stroke is characterized by motor and/or sensory deficits that are stable, without progressive worsening, and fail to resolve within 24 hr, resulting in

TABLE 1. *Causes of acute stroke*

Hemorrhagic (15%)		Intracerebral
		Subarachnoid
		Atheroma
		occlusive
		embolic
	Cerebrovascular	Lacunar
	diseases (80%)	Other
Infarction	Cardiac (15%)	
	(Cardiogenic embolism)	
	Other, unusual (5%)	

From Sherman et al. (39).

permanent neurologic loss. Acute stroke has many different causes, which are summarized in Table 1.

The average age of patients with cerebral ischemia is 64 years, with males affected twice as often as females. Hypertension is found in 50%, and diabetes in 15%. A history of ischemic events is found in 75% of patients with completed strokes.

ANATOMY

The internal carotid artery (ICA) gives off no branches in the neck and at the base of the skull traverses the sinuous carotid canal in the petrous temporal bone. Passing anterior to the anterior clinoid process, it gives off the ophthalmic artery and then terminates by dividing into the middle and anterior cerebral arteries. The two anterior cerebral arteries are connected across the midline by the anterior communicating artery (Fig. 2). This provides a potential anastomosis for supply across the midline in the event of a unilateral occlusion.

The vertebral arteries arise from the subclavian arteries and pass cranially and posteriorly to enter the foramen in the transverse process of the cervical vertebrae. Each vertebral artery passes superiorly to the atlas, through the transverse foramen of each cervical vertebra, winding around the lateral mass of the atlas to enter the vertebral canal anterior to the spinal cord. The two vertebral arteries enter the cranium through the foramen magnum and join to form the basilar artery, which supplies structures in the posterior fossa. At the upper border of the pons, the basilar artery divides into the two posterior cerebral vessels, which communicate with the internal carotid system via the posterior communicating arteries. Thus, a continuous anastomotic ring around the base of the brain, the circle of Willis, can potentially shunt blood from the vertebral to the carotid territory and from one side to the other. The adequacy of these communicating channels varies, however, and flow in the vertebral arteries may be insufficient to supply the needs of the carotid circulation in the event of a sudden unilateral or bilateral carotid occlusion. The neurologic deficit occurring subsequent to a complete occlusion varies, therefore, from none to a dense, permanent stroke. These symptomatic variations reflect the existence and varying adequacy of both intracranial and extracranial collateral pathways.

Extracranial anastomoses may open in response to progressive vascular disease. Potential collateral pathways exist between two branches of the external carotid, the facial and superficial temporal arteries, with the supratrochlear and supraorbital

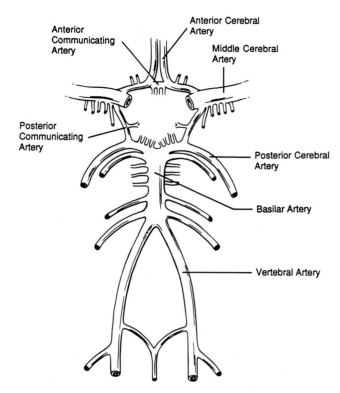

FIG. 2. Circle of Willis. This vascular anastomosis consists of the bifurcation of the basilar artery into the posterior cerebral arteries, the posterior communicating arteries, the middle and anterior cerebral branches of the internal carotid, and the anterior communicating artery.

arteries, which arise from the ophthalmic artery, the first branch of the internal carotid. This collateral circulation can be assessed by periorbital continuous-wave (CW) Doppler examination.

Anatomic Variants

Considerable technical difficulty in CW Doppler examination may be produced by anatomic variants related to tortuosity and coiling of the ICA. The occurrence of tortuosity and coiling is frequently bilateral and often symmetrical. These conditions are considered to be congenital, developmental abnormalities that become exaggerated with age but do not produce clinical symptoms. On any given tomogram, however, they can produce confusing appearances such as apparent reversal of flow. Careful tracing with real-time imaging is essential to appreciate the true course of these vessels.

In contrast, kinking of the vessels results from a sharp angulation, with stenosis of the ICA usually occurring 5 cm or more above the carotid bifurcation. It may be unilateral, is usually found in older patients, and is caused by atherosclerosis and hypertension. Unlike tortuosity and coiling, kinking may be symptomatic.

ANGIOGRAPHY VERSUS DUPLEX SONOGRAPHY

Radiologists have been slow to become involved with duplex sonographic techniques, largely leaving this field to vascular surgeons and preferring the definitive image provided by angiography. With the introduction of digital intravenous angiography (DIVA), the future of Doppler imaging appeared doubtful. Foley et al. (13), using intravenous angiography, obtained adequate studies in 73% of patients overall and in 50% of presurgical patients. They concluded that intravenous angiography was a valuable screening procedure. Further experience with DIVA, however, has disclosed severe limitations in its application, especially in the elderly (14,37). The many problems and limitations associated with DIVA include the following:

1. A swallowing reflex, initiated in response to a bolus injection of contrast, degrades the resolution of digital subtraction angiography since the technique depends on subtracting the initial film from the film taken after contrast.
2. Digital subtraction techniques result in subtraction of calcified plaque, which is, therefore, not apparent on the final image.
3. Despite early enthusiasm, more recent realistic reports have shown that injection of contrast directly into a peripheral vein provides inadequate opacification. The DIVA techniques now employ large volumes of contrast, which are injected rapidly into the central veins. However, poor cardiac output may still result in inadequate opacification of the carotid arteries.
4. The DIVA techniques require a large volume of contrast (60 ml per run), which, in elderly patients with marginal renal function, may precipitate renal failure.
5. There is a limitation on the number of runs because of the volume of contrast required for each, and hence it may not be possible to image both bifurcations in two planes. Significant disease, especially on the nonsymptomatic side, may be missed in up to 15% of patients.

In view of these limitations, most angiographers now use intra-arterial digital subtraction angiography (DSA). This technique allows the use of small intra-arterial catheters and a small amount of contrast so that the procedure may be performed on an outpatient basis and multiple views can be obtained. However, it must be realized that DSA is still invasive and less accurate than standard contrast angiography.

At this institution, we use duplex sonography as a completely noninvasive technique for screening, which is therefore welcomed by internists, neurologists and their patients, leaving definitive preoperative evaluation to angiography, of which 90% are digital intra-arterial studies. To appreciate the relative contributions of the two modalities, it should be noted that approximately 1,200 duplex scans are performed each year as compared with 60 angiograms.

It appears that DSA and duplex Doppler techniques have similar accuracy in the evaluation of the proximal common carotid arteries (CCA) and the bifurcations. Some surgeons now advocate surgery on the basis of the duplex scan alone in selected patients, as detailed in Table 2 (7). Flanigan et al. (12) found that the decision regarding surgical therapy could be made on the basis of the duplex scan alone in 90% of his patients. However, as a general rule we advocate a preoperative angiogram to search for disease more proximal or distal than that found in the bifurcation alone. In addition, the serious prognosis resulting from a classic TIA constitutes a good indication for angiography in all such patients. In practice, however, many of these patients are unacceptable operative risks and will be given antiplatelet therapy unless the stenosis is critical. A noninvasive examination is therefore still preferred in these patients.

TABLE 2. Indications for endarterectomy without angiography

1. Serial scans of known plaques
2. Critical stenosis
3. Contrast sensitivity
4. Patient refusal to undergo angiography
5. Renal failure
6. Crescendo TIA
7. Other urgent surgery (CABG) performed concurrently
8. Symptomatic intraplaque hemorrhage
9. Positive ultrasound but negative angiography in symptomatic patient

From Crew et al. (7).

INDICATIONS FOR CAROTID DUPLEX SCANNING

These are summarized in Table 3 and are now considered in detail.

Carotid Bruit

A carotid bruit must be differentiated from a neck bruit. A neck bruit may result from a wide variety of causes including a venous hum, valvular stenosis, vascular disease in the great vessels, anemia, thyrotoxicosis, and arteriovenous malformations. A carotid bruit is accurately localized over the carotid bifurcation (38) and results from audible turbulence.

Whereas a neck bruit may occur in 12.6% of the general population aged 49 and up, a true carotid bruit is limited to only 4.3% (38). The prevalence of carotid bruit increases with age, occurring in fewer than 1% of those aged 45 to 54 years and 5% of those aged 75 and older. A carotid bruit is more common in females and hypertensives. The sensitivity of a carotid bruit for the presence of carotid artery disease is only 27% overall for all grades of carotid disease and 44% for stenosis greater than 50% (27).

The prognostic significance of a carotid bruit is nonspecific. On follow-up, such individuals have a higher mortality rate and an increased incidence of stroke compared with the normal population. However, the stroke may occur in a different vascular territory, and there is increased mortality from other manifestations of vascular disease, especially myocardial infarction. Thus, a carotid bruit is an indicator of widespread vascular disease and dictates the need for a general vascular evaluation, including the carotid arteries (43). Angiography as an initial diagnostic procedure is unjustified in these patients.

TABLE 3. Indications for carotid duplex scanning

1. Carotid bruit
2. Atypical TIA
3. To monitor progression of known disease
4. Follow-up post-endarterectomy
5. Prior to major vascular surgery
6. Cholesterol emboli
7. Routine examination of the elderly

Fell et al. (10) used duplex Doppler on 81 patients with a carotid bruit. Angiography was performed in 13, and of these, 11 had significant stenoses. A total of five endarterectomies were performed.

Atypical TIA

It has been argued that a typical TIA is an absolute indication for angiography. However, even in patients with TIAs, duplex scanning may have a role in those not suited for eventual surgery or to characterize the nature of the plaque and to exclude the possibility of intraplaque hemorrhage.

Elderly patients frequently have symptoms similar to those associated with a TIA. There may be paresthesia in a limb associated with cervical spondylosis, and this may be difficult to distinguish from symptoms related to carotid artery disease. Visual disturbances are common and may simulate amaurosis fugax. Dizziness and transient confusion or dysphasia may all occur from many causes. A noninvasive imaging procedure is especially valuable in those patients in whom there is low clinical suspicion of disease but significant carotid arterial disease must be excluded. In practice, this is one of the most common indications for referral for duplex evaluation.

To Monitor Progression of Known Disease

A vascular laboratory generates its own referrals as patients are followed with longitudinal studies for known disease. Disease may be diagnosed by prior angiography or by duplex examination. In an asymptomatic patient, a unilateral 70% stenosis will be followed, as will bilateral disease that is nonsignificant (less than 60%). Even symptomatic patients may be followed without surgery if medically unfit, and treated by antiplatelet therapy.

Longitudinal studies have indicated that carotid disease is slowly progressive in most patients. Javid et al. (18) followed patients with varying degrees of internal carotid stenosis with serial angiograms over an average period of 3 years, noting that the severity of stenosis progressed in two-thirds of them. A recent study also documented progression of carotid disease followed by duplex scans and noted that patients usually became symptomatic when the stenosis exceeded 80% (35). Surgical intervention was recommended when the patient became symptomatic or when the stenosis exceeded 80%.

Follow-up Post-Endarterectomy

Restenosis may occur after endarterectomy in a significant number of individuals. Restenosis within 24 months is characterized by fibrous hyperplasia, whereas after 2 years it is usually caused by atheroma (5). Cantelmo et al. (6) reported a 12% incidence of restenosis based on routine postsurgical noninvasive testing. This rate was higher than that recently reported by other investigators who studied only clinically symptomatic restenoses. They advocated follow-up scans at 1, 3, and 12 months after surgery. Such serial examinations should employ a noninvasive and economic modality.

Nicholls et al. (30) followed 140 postendarterectomy patients for 4 years. During this period, 22% developed a recurrent, high-grade stenosis, which regressed in seven patients, giving a persistent rate of 17.1%. Most restenoses occurred within 24 months after surgery, and there was no consistent correlation between the development of symptoms and the occurrence of stenoses.

Prior to Major Vascular Surgery

Major vascular surgery, such as coronary bypass graft, may produce significant hypotension leading to stroke in individuals with predisposing severe stenosis. Kartchner and McRae (20) reported a 17% incidence of stroke in patients undergoing major cardiovascular surgery with a stenosis exceeding 60%. Such reports have encouraged combined surgical procedures in patients with severe carotid artery disease. In such patients, the coronary bypass procedure is preceded by a carotid endarterectomy. The efficacy of such procedures is controversial, and conventional wisdom holds that the combined operation is not justified. However, the author believes it is important that the patency of the carotid vessels be evaluated prior to such major surgery in order to counsel the patient adequately concerning the risks of surgery, thereby minimizing the chance of subsequent litigation in the event of a postoperative stroke. Hypotension may be avoided if the anesthesiologist is aware that severe carotid artery disease is present. Duplex techniques are entirely adequate for this purpose. Occlusion and stroke will only occur in the presence of severe stenosis, so the diagnosis of minor degrees of pathology is not a concern. Multiple studies attest to the efficacy of duplex techniques to diagnose significant disease with a sensitivity of over 90% (11,19,34).

Cholesterol Emboli

Cholesterol emboli detected on routine ophthalmic examination appear as bright plaques caused by cholesterol fragments associated with embolization from an atheromatous lesion and may be the first indicator of significant atherosclerosis. Alternatively, there may be white platelet plugs.

The anatomical basis for the occurrence of retinal emboli lies in the origin of the central artery of the retina from the ophthalmic artery, which is the first branch of the internal carotid.

A retinal embolus is a highly significant sign that ulceration and embolization are occurring from the proximal vessels. The patient is at risk for TIAs and/or stroke from larger emboli occluding the cerebral vessels, and vascular evaluation is, therefore, required.

Cholesterol emboli to the retina are very small. The entire optic disk is only 1.5 mm in diameter, and the central artery of the retina only 150 μm. Thus, cholesterol emboli lodged in one of the branches of the retinal artery will be smaller than 0.1 mm.

Routine Examination of the Elderly

There is no evidence yet that routine duplex examination of the carotid arteries would be cost effective as a screening procedure. However, it may be electively performed where so requested, for example, during an executive physical examination. There is no doubt that routine examination of the elderly would disclose significant carotid disease in many but would lead to a dilemma of therapy. Autopsy studies have shown that carotid disease is very common, even in asymptomatic patients. Martin et al. (29) studied 100 consecutive autopsies in patients over the age of 50 years. Fifteen occlusions were detected in 11 patients, six of whom had no symptoms or signs of vascular disease. A stenosis greater than 50% diameter reduction was found in 77 vessels in 29 patients. In all, 40 of these patients had significant stenoses or occlusion of the great vessels, of whom 24 were without clinical signs or symptoms of disease. It is clear that more needs to be known about the prevalence of this disease in the apparently healthy population and about other factors that account for its transition into a life-threatening condition. Recent observations on the occurrence of intraplaque hemorrhage promise to be helpful in identifying those patients who are prone to embolization. Certainly before there is any widespread application of surgical techniques for prophylaxis of stroke, further epidemiological studies of this commonplace disease will be required.

INSTRUMENTATION

The first Doppler instruments were simple CW devices used for periorbital directional Doppler examinations. Although capable of detecting severe disease, these tests were insensitive for disease of moderate severity. Continuous-wave imaging systems for the entire cervical carotid system were then introduced. In these systems, a CW Doppler probe was mounted on the end of an arm (like that of a B-scanner), and a dot was stored on an oscilloscope when a normal velocity from the carotid artery was detected. The probe was gradually moved up the artery, thereby building up a low-resolution flow image of the entire carotid system (40,41). Turnipseed et al. (42) detected 14 of 18 occlusions with this equipment.

A further development of this system was the addition of color modulation. In this equipment, high velocities were noted in different colors, simplifying detection of high-velocity jets (8). The major disadvantages of this equipment were its insensitivity to mild or moderate stenoses and its failure to diagnose atheroma and plaque that caused turbulence but normal velocities. This equipment is of historic interest, as we are now, again, considering color modulation, albeit with greatly enhanced scanning speed, sensitivity, and resolution.

Meanwhile, the conventional method for assessing the carotids is now the duplex scan, a combination of high-resolution imaging and Doppler ultrasound to reveal the hemodynamic significance of wall abnormalities and flow reduction. High-resolution scanning is used, preferably at a frequency of 7.5 to 10 MHz, with 4- to 5-MHz Doppler scanning. Some vascular surgeons use CW Doppler ultrasound alone. This requires great experience and may lead to errors regarding the origin of a vascular signal. Furthermore, a small amount of plaque or an ulcer may give rise to no hemodynamic disturbance in the Doppler signal. In these cases, a diagnosis can be made only by high-resolution scanning. High-resolution imaging is increasingly important also in the characterization of plaque and detection of intraplaque hemorrhage.

High-resolution imaging alone, however, is insufficient to characterize the hemodynamic significance of a stenosis that produces a disturbed flow pattern or to diagnose an occlusion. The carotid may appear patent on the high-resolution image. But Doppler ultrasound is required to reveal that flow is absent, indicating an occlusion. The characteristics of the Doppler signal as described below allow quantitation of flow area reduction. A two-dimensional image alone, like a single angiographic view, can be highly misleading about the area reduction.

CONTINUOUS-WAVE OR PULSED DOPPLER

Duplex evaluation of carotid artery disease is still such an art that almost every practitioner has developed his/her own criteria for quantitating pathology. Some operators are very comfortable with CW Doppler ultrasound, but it must be recalled that this technique gives no axial resolution, and therefore accurate anatomic localization of signals is not possible. Continuous-wave Doppler scanning may be useful in carotid evaluation. However, in the opinion of the author, pulsed Doppler ultrasound is a very valuable addition. The ability to locate accurately the origin of the signal in relation to its position in the lumen enhances the diagnostic accuracy of the duplex scan. Some operators use CW while tracing the course of the carotid arteries and then use pulsed Doppler ultrasound to locate the maximum peak velocity most accurately, since this peak velocity may be limited to a small pinhole in the vessel lumen.

TECHNIQUE AND ANATOMY

The carotid arterial anatomy is variable, with the bifurcation occurring anywhere from low in the neck to high under the ramus of the mandible. Most frequently it is

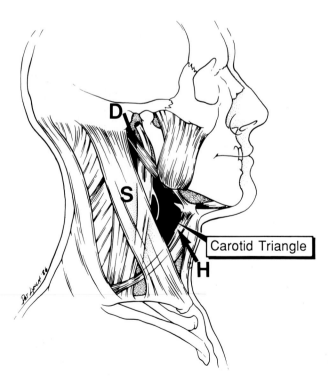

FIG. 3. The carotid triangle is a depression in the neck in which the carotid bifurcation is most frequently found. The carotid triangle is limited by the surrounding muscle bellies of the digastric (D), omohyoid (H), and sternomastoid muscles (S).

situated in the carotid triangle, a depression in the neck that can be appreciated in the majority of individuals. This depression is formed by the elevation of the surrounding muscles, the sternomastoid, omohyoid, and digastric (Fig. 3). Inspection of this carotid triangle reveals vascular pulsation. This triangle is the site of the bifurcation and origin of the first branches of the external carotid artery.

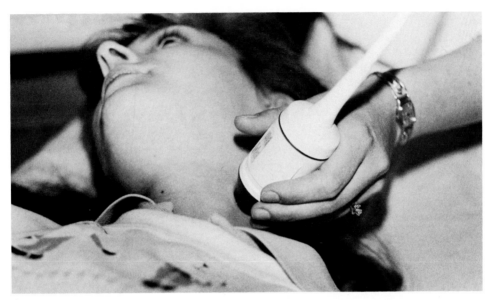

A

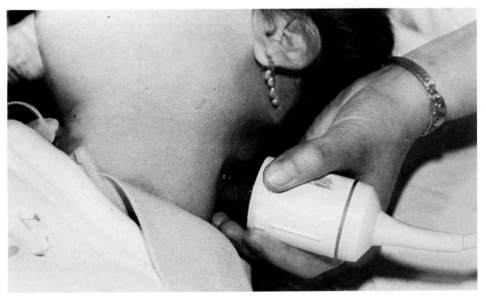

B

FIG. 4. A: The operator is seated at the patient's head, which is turned away from the side being examined, and an anterolateral approach is being used. **B:** A posterolateral approach to the carotid employs the sternomastoid muscle as an acoustic window.

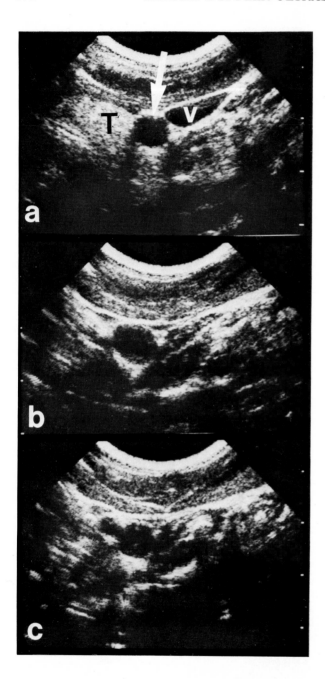

FIG. 5. Transverse scans of the neck show (**A**) the common carotid (*arrow*), (**B**) the carotid sinus at the bifurcation, and (**C**) the branches of the common carotid. The internal carotid is the larger branch. Note the lateral lobe of the thyroid (T) is anterolateral, and the jugular vein (V) is lateral.

The position of the operator and patient during the procedure is one of personal preference. If the patient is supine, it is often best for the operator to be seated on a stool at the patient's head, thereby providing access to both carotids (Fig. 4). The patient should be deprived of the pillow and requested to extend the head and turn it away from the side being examined. An alternative position, especially useful in a small room, employs a dental chair with the operator sitting behind the patient. In patients who are unable to cooperate, orthopneic, or have intractable cough or other involuntary neuromuscular movement, successful examination may be impossible. Also, the presence of thick, "bull necks" or high bifurcations may preclude successful scanning. In practice, however, all these difficulties apply to no more than 1% of the total patients referred for evaluation.

A rapid transverse scan of the carotid arterial system allows the bifurcation of the carotid arteries to be located and the general relationship between the two vessels to be appreciated (Fig. 5). The relationship between the external and internal carotid arteries can be quite variable, and the anatomy can be further complicated by marked tortuosity of the vessels.

The carotid arteries are then scanned in the longitudinal plane. In general, there are two good approaches: the anterior oblique and the posterior oblique. In the former, the probe is separated from the common carotid artery and its bifurcation only by skin, platysma, and fascia. In thin patients, this may put the probe too close to the carotid for optimal evaluation, and a posterolateral approach using the sternomastoid muscle as an acoustic window improves the resolution (Fig. 6).

On a longitudinal scan, the lateral lobe of the thyroid gland is usually easily identified, as is the neurovascular bundle lying posterolateral to the thyroid. The jugular vein is easily identified lying lateral to the CCA. The vein should never be mistaken for the artery since, on real-time examination, it displays characteristic movements that vary with both respiratory and cardiac activity. The luminal variations can be exaggerated when the patient sniffs or performs a valsalva maneuver (Fig. 7). The corresponding changes in flow velocity are also easily identified on the Doppler waveform (Fig. 8).

The line of the transducer is adjusted until the entire carotid artery is seen in its longitudinal axis. Rotating the transducer and moving it up the neck allows the common carotid to be traced to the bifurcation (Fig. 9). This is identified as a dilatation (the carotid sinus) (Fig. 6) and division of the common carotid into internal and external branches (Fig. 9). The internal carotid is usually the larger of the two

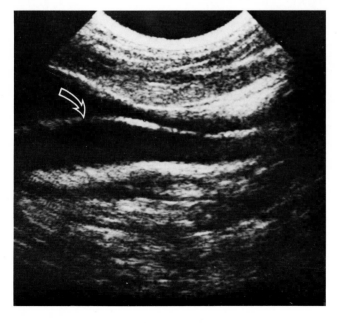

FIG. 6. Longitudinal scan of common carotid showing carotid sinus (*arrow*) as a dilatation at the bifurcation

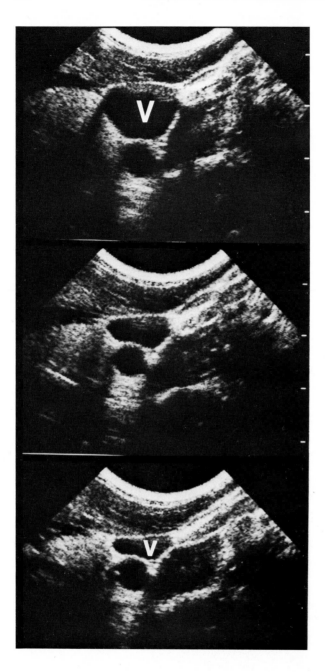

FIG. 7. A transverse section of the neck demonstrating variations in the diameter of the jugular vein (V). The jugular distends with a valsalva maneuver (**upper figure**) and collapses with a sniff (**lower figure**).

branches, and some of the branches of the external carotid may occasionally be identified, such as the superior thyroid, lingual, or facial arteries.

Where plaque is seen, its size and location are documented and recorded in at least two longitudinal and one transverse projection. This allows an appreciation of the area reduction as opposed to merely the diameter. It is important to differentiate between these two parameters of lumen reduction. As shown schematically in Fig. 10A, plaque may yield a diameter reduction of 50% but the area reduction may be 25% (Fig. 10B), 50% (Fig. 10C), or 75% (Fig. 10D). This difference must be recalled

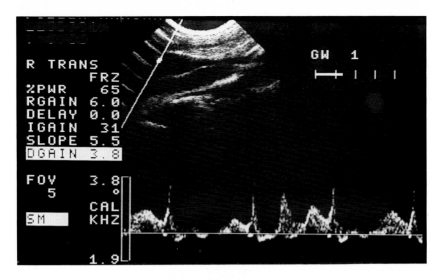

FIG. 8. Duplex scan showing longitudinal section through the jugular vein. The characteristic complex variations in venous velocity are seen on the Doppler tracing.

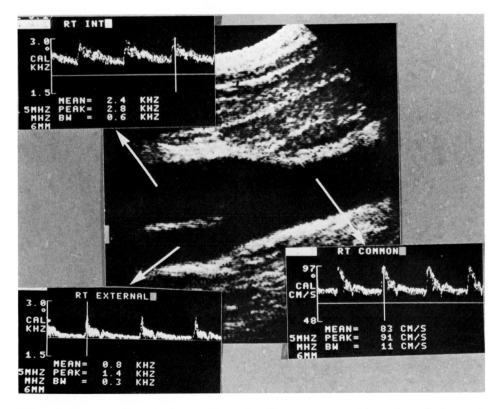

FIG. 9. Doppler waveforms in the carotid arteries. The common carotid waveform displays a clear window below the systolic envelope because all the red cells move at a similar velocity (i.e., plug flow). There is diastolic flow, and the pattern in the common carotid is half-way between the pattern in the external and internal carotid arteries. Note that there is some spectral broadening during diastole, shown as a thickening of the time–velocity envelope. The external carotid artery shows little flow in diastole, indicating a high-impedance circulation. The internal carotid artery shows a well-marked window under the systolic part of the envelope and high diastolic flow associated with the low impedance of the cerebral vasculature. The differences between the internal and external waveforms allow easy differentiation between the two vessels.

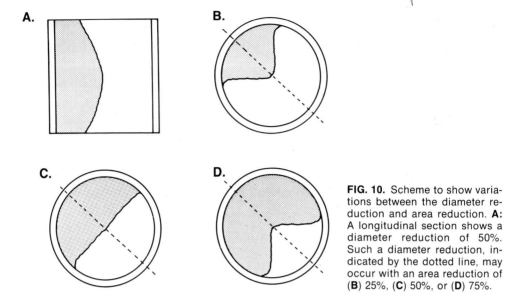

FIG. 10. Scheme to show variations between the diameter reduction and area reduction. **A:** A longitudinal section shows a diameter reduction of 50%. Such a diameter reduction, indicated by the dotted line, may occur with an area reduction of **(B)** 25%, **(C)** 50%, or **(D)** 75%.

when comparing the results of duplex scanning with angiography. In general, the Doppler waveform allows better quantitation of the hemodynamic significance of lumen reduction.

The relationship between the two vessels is variable and further complicated by tortuosity. The apparent relationship of the internal to the external carotid artery on any scan depends on whether an antero- or posterooblique scan has been used. The Doppler waveform is, however, characteristic and allows easy differentiation between the two vessels.

With the probe rotated upward, the internal carotid is traced as high as possible, searching for visual abnormalities such as a plaque or ulcer. Following this visual inspection of the B-scan, all the vessels are interrogated by Doppler scanning.

NORMAL DOPPLER WAVEFORMS

In the initial evaluation of the Doppler waveforms, some operators use a CW Doppler technique. We prefer to use pulsed Doppler ultrasound with a sufficiently long gate to encompass the entire vessel, such as a 5-mm gate.

Different machines allow the use of different methods. In some machines there is simultaneous imaging and Doppler scanning, whereas in others the use of the two modalities must be alternated. As long as the operator's hand is steadied by resting on the patient's bed or other fixed structure, it is not difficult to alternate between the two modalities. The Doppler angle is adjusted between 30 and 60°, and the common carotid artery (CCA) is first interrogated.

The CCA has a characteristic waveform that is half-way between the external and internal carotid (ICA) waveforms. There is a ''window'' under the systolic component and a moderate amount of diastolic flow (Figs. 9 and 11). Indeed, during the systolic upstroke, the velocity envelope is virtually a single line without spectral spread. This implies that during systole the red cells are moving at a single, uniform

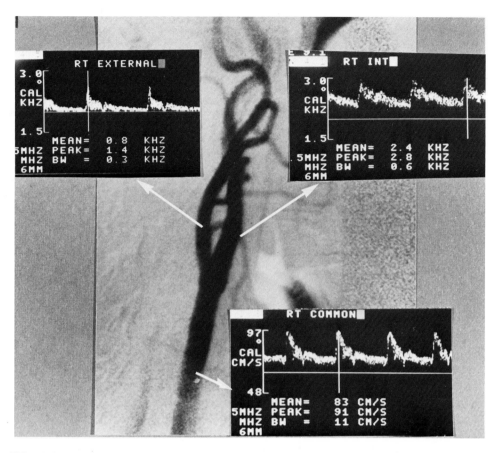

FIG. 11. Normal angiogram of carotid bifurcation with superimposed normal Doppler waveforms.

velocity. With the decrease in velocity that characterizes the downstroke, viscous drag on the cells nearest the walls produces lower frequencies, giving rise to a frequency spread manifest as a thickening of the time–velocity envelope. This "spectral broadening" persists during diastole.

The sample length is then reduced to a minimum (1.5 mm) and moved across the vessel lumen to establish the peak frequency or velocity. Since this excludes the slower cells on the periphery of the vessel, this maneuver increases the extent of the "window." The maximum Doppler shift frequency is established. With equipment that has an insonating frequency of 4.5 MHz, the returned Doppler signal should be less than 4 kHz. The absolute velocity can be computed from the Doppler shift frequency by multiplying by the cosine of the angle between the ultrasound beam and the vessel. In most equipment, a cursor is provided and can be aligned with the vessel. This corrects the measured Doppler shift frequency for this angle and computes the absolute velocities of red cells in the vessel (Fig. 12). The maximum normal velocity in the internal carotid artery is 110 cm/sec, but there is a wide range of normal velocities between 30 and 110 cm/sec.

Recent experimental work has indicated the presence of turbulence in the normal carotid bulb (32). Using a model to simulate the hemodynamics of the carotid bi-

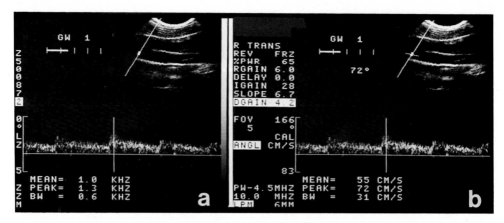

FIG. 12. Correction for the transducer angle to compute absolute velocity from the Doppler-shifted frequency. **A:** The Doppler-shifted frequency is 1.3 kHz. **B:** The cursor is aligned with the vessel lumen, parallel to its walls, and corrects for cos θ. The absolute velocity of 72 cm/sec is independent of the angle or the frequency of insonation.

furcation, Ku et al. (26) showed that there was flow separation in the carotid bulb with a central jet passing into the branches but reversed flow near the posterolateral wall of the carotid sinus caused by turbulence within the dilated carotid bulb. The site of this flow disturbance corresponds to the earliest site for atheroma (44). This reverse component can now be clearly visualized on a color-modulated scan (Plate I).

Doppler waveforms are then taken from the ICA with the sample volume progressively moved up the vessel while recording the peak velocities. The normal waveform in the ICA consists of a high diastolic flow associated with low impedance in the cerebral vessels (Figs. 9 and 11). The maximum velocity is measured and compared to that of the common carotid. The ratio should be less than unity.

The process is then repeated in the external carotid, mainly for the sake of completeness. The normal waveform shows little or no diastolic flow, indicating a high impedance of the vascular tree, and reliably differentiates the external from the internal carotid waveform (Figs. 9 and 11).

ABNORMAL DOPPLER WAVEFORMS

Findings indicative of disease vary with the extent of the process, and many different criteria have been used. Each laboratory tends to have evolved its own criteria and validated them by comparison with angiographic findings over the years. Summarized here are the criteria used by other authors in addition to those that we use.

Spectral Broadening

As stated previously, the smallest lesions that cause no hemodynamic disturbance are appreciated only by high-resolution imaging. Minimal lesions, such as atheromatous plaques, may give rise to turbulence with loss of laminar flow characterized by filling in of the systolic "window" under the time–velocity envelope (Fig. 13). This is termed "spectral broadening" (11). It is important to differentiate between

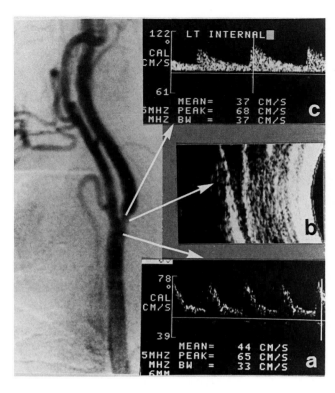

FIG. 13. Montage to show waveforms associated with minimal disease of the internal carotid artery. This 68-year-old woman presented with probable TIA. **A:** The common carotid waveform is normal. **B:** A small plaque (*arrow*) is seen on the scan at the origin of the right internal carotid. **C:** The waveform at this point displays "spectral broadening," producing complete filling in of the time–velocity spectrum.

true spectral broadening and similar appearances caused by technical factors. The novice can easily be confused by the filling in of the normal "window," which occurs in the presence of too much gain. Thus, whenever "spectral broadening" seems apparent, the gain should be lowered to see if this causes a "window" to clear (Fig. 14).

Some machines allow the operator to measure the bandwidth, that is, the spectral spread between the maximum- and minimum-velocity envelopes, and thus quantitate "spectral broadening." This is shown in the waveform for the internal carotid seen in Fig. 13. The presence of the atheromatous plaque (arrow) gives rise to marked spectral broadening measured by the bandwith (BW). We prefer to use velocity ratios to quantitate nonsignificant stenoses.

Kassam et al. (21) quantitated spectral broadening using a spectral broadening index (SBI), which is given by the term $100 (1 - f_{mean}/f_{max})$. This calculation can be implemented simply on a microcomputer and provides a quantitative estimator that is relatively insensitive to artifacts. In an *in vitro* model, Douville et al. (9) found a linear relationship between the SBI and the severity of stenoses for lesions causing greater than a 40% area reduction. The SBI was found to be maximal when recorded immediately beyond the stenosis and returned to normal within 4 to 5 cm downstream from the stenosis.

Velocity Ratios

To avoid confusion caused by spectral broadening arising from technical factors, additional parameters may be used to diagnose nonsignificant stenoses (less than

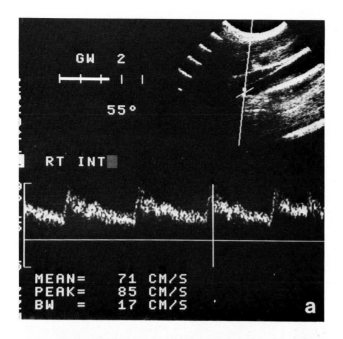

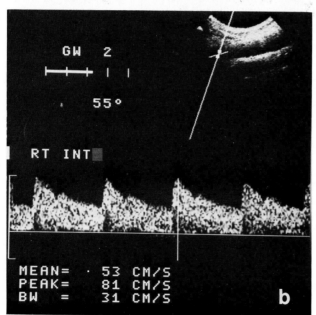

FIG. 14. A: Internal carotid artery waveform showing normal pattern at the correct gain of 4.1. **B:** Artifactual spectral broadening associated with excessive gain of 8.1. These two figures are derived from the same examination to illustrate the production of artifactual spectral broadening as a result of excessive gain.

60%). One such parameter is the ratio of the peak velocity in the internal carotid compared to that found in the common carotid. It has already been noted that in the normal arteries, the ratio V_i/V_c is unity or less. It has been further estimated by Blackshear et al. (1) that there is a linear relationship for this ratio between 1 and 2, which corresponds to zero to 50% stenosis. Thus, if the velocity of the internal carotid artery is twice that in the common carotid artery, this translates to an approximate 50% stenosis (Fig. 15). Similarly, a ratio of 1.5 corresponds to approxi-

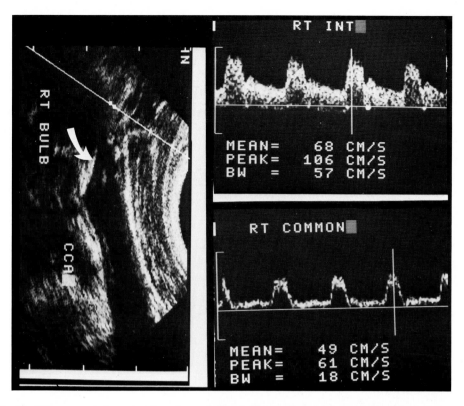

FIG. 15. Fifty-percent stenosis (diameter reduction). This patient presented with a bruit. There is apparent narrowing on the B-scan (*arrow*), but the Doppler waveforms allow better quantitation of the severity. The waveform in the internal carotid artery shows spectral broadening and a peak velocity of 106 cm/sec. The common carotid waveform is normal, but the peak velocity is only 61 cm/sec, giving a V_i/V_c ratio of approximately 2:1 consistent with a 50% stenosis.

mately 25% or a minor degree of stenosis (Fig. 16). Other signs of nonsignificant stenosis, such as spectral broadening, should be noted at the same time (Fig. 17).

In clinical practice, peak systolic ratios in the internal and common carotids are extremely helpful and correlate very well with angiographic findings. However, it is essential to find the maximum velocity, which requires a very careful search of the entire carotid artery system. Imaging is helpful in locating the sample volume in the area of maximal stenosis as apparent on the B scan. The peak velocity must then be measured with the smallest sample volume, remembering that any high-velocity jet may be only 1 or 2 mm in its maximum width.

In these respects color flow imaging is likely to be most helpful in allowing immediate appreciation of the flow dynamics in the entire carotid system and guiding the operator rapidly toward the maximum-velocity jets seen as white streaks on the image (see Plate I). The ratios, or some other quantitative parameter, will still be necessary to estimate the degree of stenosis for immediate patient management and for comparison in longitudinal studies. It is essential to remember that ratios of peak velocities (or frequencies) should only be used for nonsignificant stenoses, since the presence of turbulence produces invalid results for more severe stenotic lesions. It should also be recalled that it is not essential to convert the returned frequency to

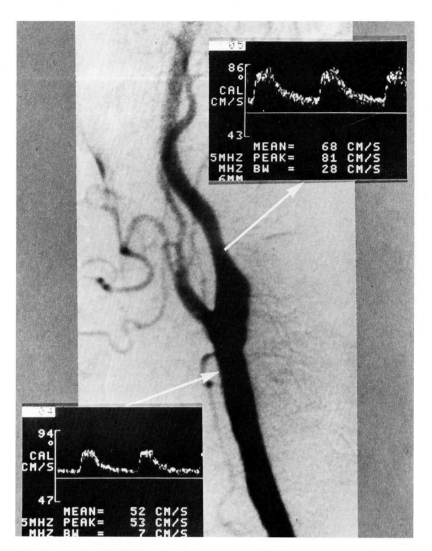

FIG. 16. Nonsignificant degree of stenosis of around 25% (diameter reduction). The peak velocity in the internal carotid is 81 cm/sec, whereas that in the common carotid is 53 cm/sec, yielding a velocity ratio of approximately 1.5. Notice that in this example there is no evidence of spectral broadening. The corresponding angiogram shows a minimal stenosis.

velocity but that one can use ratios, since a ratio is without units. However, if the ratio of the returned frequencies is used, it is essential that the angle of insonation be the same for both vessels. If the angle is different, then the ratio of the frequencies is no longer valid, and the cursor should be used to convert the frequencies to velocities. With increasing experience using this conversion, we use velocities almost exclusively, although most of the literature on the quantitation of stenosis is on the basis of shift. A further advantage of the use of velocities is that they are independent of the insonating frequency. The frequency shifts quoted in the literature are only appropriate if the same insonating frequency is used. Keagy et al. (24) compared the ratio of the peak systolic frequency in the ICA and CCA to two new criteria for the analysis of carotid arterial waveforms: (a) a parameter based on measuring the diastolic frequencies at three points since higher frequencies occur in stenosis and (b) another parameter based on the spectral area since both systolic and diastolic frequencies are increased in stenosis. In a subsequent evaluation of the two new parameters, they prospectively correctly identified 94% of vessels with less than 50% diameter reduction and 89% with greater than 50% diameter reduction, yielding an overall accuracy rate of 93% (23). These results were superior to those obtained using the ratio of the peak systolic frequencies in the ICA and CCA.

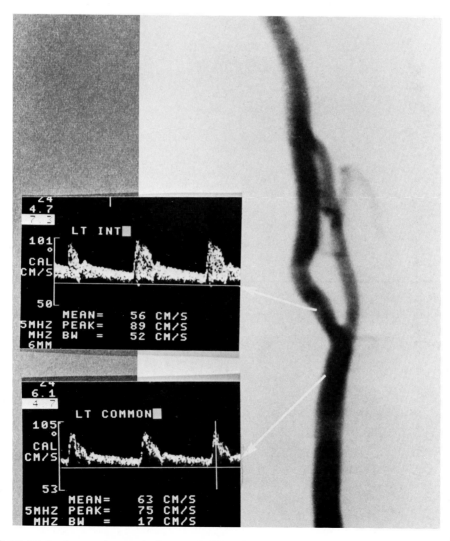

FIG. 17. Minimal narrowing producing spectral broadening in the internal carotid artery and slightly increased velocities (89 cm/sec) over the common carotid artery (75 cm/sec). This 71-year-old male was admitted for coronary artery bypass graft and was noted to have a carotid bruit. He was referred for duplex scanning to exclude a significant stenosis.

Increased Velocities (Significant Stenoses)

Significant stenoses are those lesions causing a lumen reduction exceeding 60%. Indeed, as stated previously, lesions do not generally become symptomatic until they have exceeded 80%. Spencer and Reid (40) have shown that lumen reduction exceeding 60% is associated with an increase in velocity beyond the normal range (36). For the internal carotid system, with an insonating frequency of 4.5 or 5 MHz, this corresponds to a returned frequency exceeding 4 kHz or an internal carotid velocity exceeding 112 cm/sec. The increase in the Doppler shift is approximately proportional to the degree of stenosis. Thus, a returned frequency of 5 to 6 kHz or a velocity up to 175 cm/sec corresponds to a moderate stenosis of around 80% (Fig. 18). A severe stenosis of 90% or more corresponds to returned frequencies of 7 to 8 kHz (17) (Fig. 19) and velocities of 200 to 600 cm/sec (Fig. 20). The very high Doppler shift that occurs in a significant stenosis produces "aliasing," which results in the inability to detect the true peak velocity because the sampling rate is too low. This results in the top of the time–velocity spectrum being cut off and the tip of the

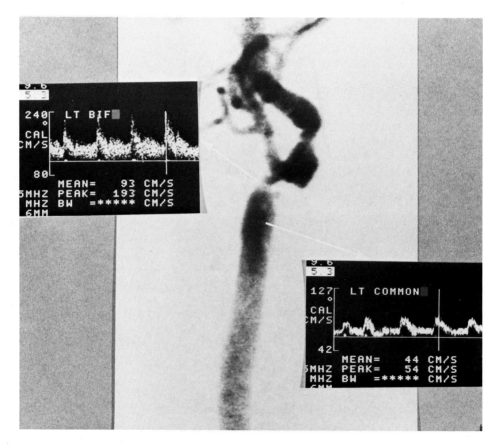

FIG. 18. Significant stenosis in the left carotid bifurcation of around 90% (diameter reduction). This 70-year-old male presented with TIA. There is spectral broadening of the waveform in the left bifurcation, and the peak velocity is approximately 193 cm/sec, whereas that in the common carotid is only 54 cm/sec.

spectrum appearing below the zero line (Fig. 20). Thus, the detected and measured velocity is less than the true velocity, and the cut-off portion of the spectrum should be added to the part measured by the spectrogram. Where possible, the sampling rate should be increased or the returned Doppler frequency diminished by increasing the angle of insonation. Alternatively, CW ultrasound can be used, in which case there is no aliasing, and the true maximum frequency shift or velocity can be measured (Fig. 21). If a CW device is used, higher frequencies, up to 14 kHz, may be found. This allows better quantitation of the severity of the stenosis. However, no method allows precise differentiation between, for example, a 70% and a 75% stenosis. It is important that estimates of severity be kept within broader limits such as 50 to 75%, 75 to 90%, 90 + %, occlusion which are adequate for purposes of patient management.

Knox et al. (25) used the ratio of the peak systolic velocity in the ICA to the end-diastolic velocity in the CCA to quantify the severity of arteriosclerosis, comparing normal and diseased vessels. With increasing stenosis, the diastolic velocity in the CCA decreased, and the peak systolic velocity in the ICA increased. The resulting ratios corresponding to varying degrees of stenosis are summarized in Table 4. The criteria formulated by the Seattle group for quantifying stenoses based on frequency change are provided in Table 5. Briefly stated, if the peak systolic frequency shift in the internal carotid artery is greater than 4 kHz (using an insonating frequency of 5 MHz and a 60° angle) or greater than a velocity of 120 cm/sec, then there is a significant stenosis exceeding 50% diameter reduction. If the systolic Doppler frequency is very high, and the end-systolic frequency exceeds 4.5 kHz (using a 5-MHz insonating beam) or 135 cm/sec Doppler angle-corrected velocity, then there is greater than 80% diameter reduction in the internal carotid artery.

Occlusion

The ultrasonic diagnosis of carotid arterial occlusion can only be made reliably by Doppler techniques. A vessel may appear patent on the B-scan yet be occluded if Doppler interrogation reveals no evidence of arterial flow (Fig. 22). It should be noted that systolic wall motion transmitted from the proximal artery may give rise to a low-amplitude, low-frequency signal that does not indicate true flow. In addition, there may be severely damped flow in the common carotid artery proximal to the occlusion (Fig. 23).

TABLE 4. *Quantitation of stenosis*

Stenosis[a]	Ratio[b]	Accuracy
Normal	1–3	100%
60%	7.5	95%
65%	11.0	97%
90%	18.0	100%

[a] "Stenosis," as used here, means diameter reduction.
[b] Peak systolic velocity in the ICA over end-diastolic velocity in the CCA.
From Knox et al. (25).

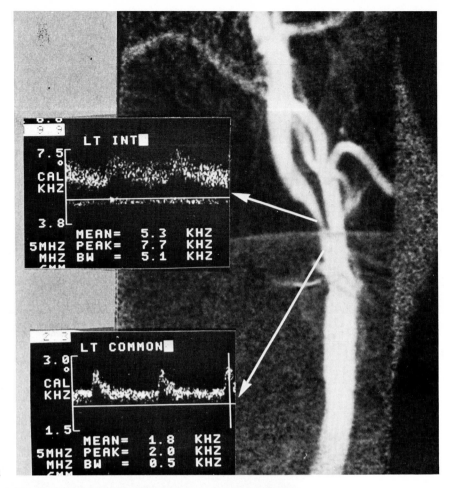

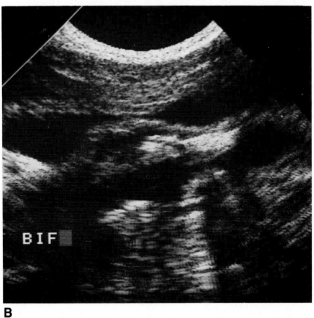

FIG. 19. Severe stenosis of around 90% (diameter reduction). This 51-year-old male presented with a right TIA and amaurosis fugax. Examination revealed bilateral carotid bruits. An outpatient DIVA was unsatisfactory. **A:** Montage to show peak frequencies of 7.7 kHz in the internal carotid artery. This corresponds to the severe narrowing as seen on the angiogram. **B:** Corresponding tomogram confirming the presence of severe stenosis (*arrow*).

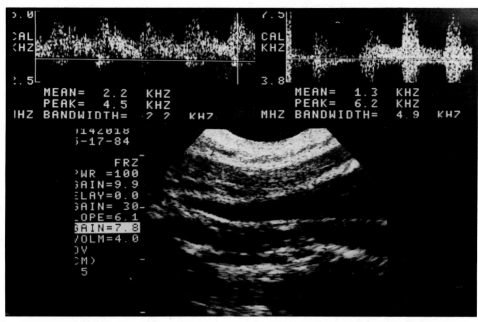

C

FIG. 19. (*continued*). **C:** Severe stenosis in another patient. Heavy calcified plaque is seen in the internal carotid, producing a high-velocity jet (6.2 kHz). Note there is gross spectral broadening with reversed flow from turbulence and eddy currents.

TABLE 5. *Classification of carotid Doppler signals*

Angiographic description	Doppler criteria	Clinical interpretation
Normal	Peak systole 125 cm/sec or 4 kHz[a] No spectral broadening	
0–15% diam reduction	Peak Systole 125 cm/sec or 4 kHz[a] Clear window under systole Minimal spectral broadening in deceleration phase of systole	Minimal disease
16–49% diam reduction	Peak systole 125 cm/sec or 4 kHz[a] No window under systole Spectral broadening throughout systole	Moderate disease
50–79% diam reduction	Peak systole 125 cm/sec or 4.5 kHz[a] Increased diastolic flow Marked spectral broadening throughout cardiac cycle	Severe disease, hemodynamically significant
80–99% diam reduction	End-diastole 135 cm/sec or 4.5 kHz[a] Spectral broadening throughout systole	Severe disease, hemodynamically significant
Occluded	ICA: no signal CCA: unilateral flow to zero or reversal	Occluded

[a] Assumes insonating frequency of 5 MHz and 60° insonating angle.
From Roederer et al. (36).

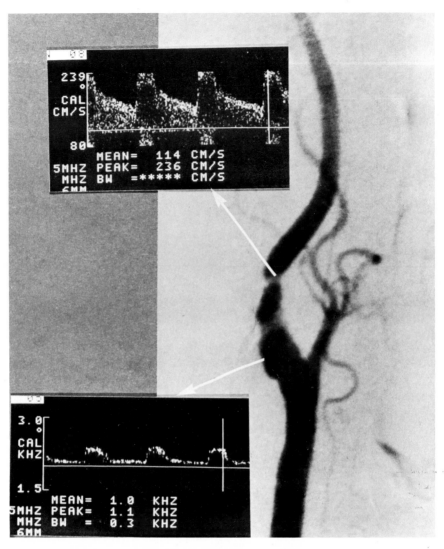

FIG. 20. Severe stenosis with measured peak frequencies up to 236 cm/sec. Note, however, that aliasing has occurred, and the top of the time–velocity spectrum has been cut off and appears below the zero line. Thus, the real velocities are higher than those measured.

Breslau et al. (3) described this further criterion for ICA occlusion or severe stenosis. The waveform of the CCA returns to zero during diastole instead of the usual continuous diastolic flow because the normal low impedance of the cerebral circulation has been replaced by the high-impedance pattern of a stenosis or occlusion (Fig. 23). They noted that this occurred in some patients bilaterally in the absence of disease but, when unilateral, was a useful indicator of high-grade stenosis or occlusion of the ICA.

The major difficulty in the diagnosis of occlusion is in differentiating between complete occlusion and minimal flow. Although stenosis causes a high-velocity jet, it is obvious that the most severe stenosis will reduce the flow volume rate to a

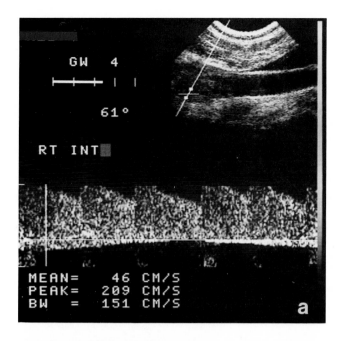

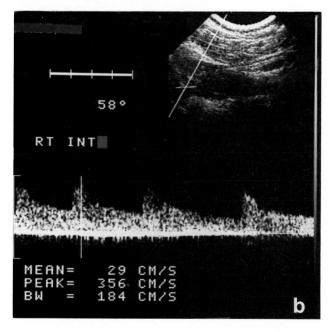

FIG. 21. The use of CW to obviate aliasing. **A:** Pulsed Doppler technique does not allow accurate measurement of the peak velocity (209 cm/sec), although the lesion appears to be severe. **B:** Use of CW scanning allows the true velocity (356 cm/sec) to be measured.

trickle and, therefore, demonstrate reduced Doppler-shifted frequencies. Since the surgical treatment of an almost occluded vessel is potentially different from that of an occluded one, this differentiation is critical and, in the author's opinion, justifies an angiogram in any patient suspected of having an occlusion or almost complete occlusion. Even with angiography, it may be difficult to differentiate between these two diagnoses (Fig. 24).

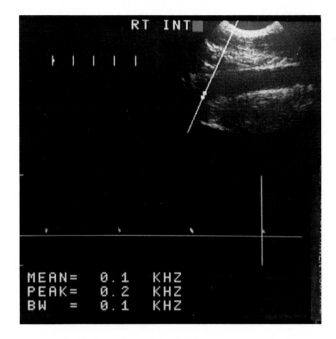

FIG. 22. Occlusion of the internal carotid artery. This 65-year-old male presented with amaurosis fugax. The lumen appears to be patent on the B-scan, but the only Doppler signal elicited is a wall thump, and no true flow is present.

Periorbital Doppler examination can be extremely helpful as a confirmatory test for severe disease or complete occlusion. It will be recalled that the normal flow in the periorbital arteries is out of the cranium from the terminal branches of the ophthalmic, the supratrochlear and supraorbital branches. As the pressure in these branches falls because of either complete occlusion or near occlusion, flow becomes

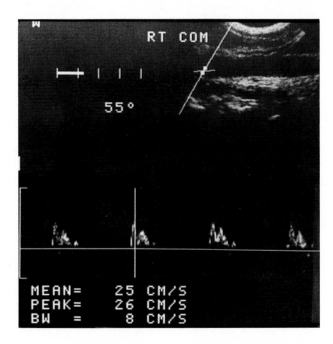

FIG. 23. Waveform in the common carotid artery proximal to severe stenosis or occlusion. Flow is of low amplitude, and the waveform returns to zero during diastole. This indicates high distal impedance associated with the stenosis or occlusion and is in contrast to the low impedance with high diastolic flow characteristic of the normal common carotid (Figs. 9 and 11).

reversed, since the pressure in the anastomosing branches from the facial and superficial temporal arteries becomes greater than that in the ophthalmic branches. Thus, the direction of flow in the supraorbital and supratrochlear vessels reverses into the cranium.

The direction detecting ability of Doppler can be most helpful here. Normal flow is out of the cranium and, therefore, towards the transducer in the supratrochlear or supraorbital arteries. In Fig. 25 it is noted that flow is reversed and thus below the zero line. By compressing the facial or superficial temporal arteries, the source of the collateral circulation can be determined. The facial artery is easily located anterior to the masseter muscle as that vessel crosses the mandible. The superficial temporal artery can be palpated at the temple anterior to the pinna. To perform the compression test, the supraorbital (or, less satisfactorily, the supratrochlear) artery is first located immediately above the eye, and the direction of flow determined to be reversed. Compression of the facial artery stops this reversed flow and produces forward flow of diminished amplitude. Padayachee et al. (31) reported a 90% sensitivity and 89% specificity for this test when performed on the supraorbital artery but only 36% sensitivity using the supratrochlear artery, though here a specificity of 96% was achieved.

As discussed previously, the adequacy of these extracranial anastomoses from the facial and temporal arteries of one side or the other is extremely variable and accounts for the presence or absence of ischemic symptoms, which also vary greatly from one individual to another. These collaterals develop slowly and become functional as progressive ischemic changes occur. However, in applying periorbital Doppler ultrasound, it should be stressed that it is an insensitive means of detecting carotid arterial disease, and flow is only reversed in cases of very severe stenosis or occlusion.

Despite the apparent simplicity of the diagnosis of complete carotid occlusion, reports in the literature indicate that it is one of the more difficult diagnoses to make by Doppler techniques (45). However, in this author's experience, this diagnosis has not presented a problem, and Flanigan et al. (12) recently reported an accuracy of 99%. Sensitivities as low as 70% have been reported by other investigators. Zwiebel and Crummy (45) reported 30 false positives or negatives versus 31 true positives. Some of these difficulties were the result of misdiagnosis of an occlusion as a very severe stenosis. Technical factors such as the sensitivity of the Doppler device and the use of CW ultrasound alone, without imaging, also contributed to this error. Other factors may contribute as well, notably, mistaking the external carotid branches for the internal, especially where the course of the internal carotid is complicated by marked tortuosity. To confound this issue further, where the external carotid branches anastomose freely with the internal carotid terminal branches to supply the cerebral circulation, the external carotid signal can simulate the internal carotid signal with decreased impedance and increased diastolic flow.

A technique has been described that helps to identify the external carotid artery when there is doubt. During insonation of the artery in the neck, the external carotid is sharply tapped over the temple. Obvious deflection can be seen in the insonated vessel if it is the external carotid artery. There is no infallible way to avoid the error of missing an occlusion or near occlusion. Several criteria are helpful, although operator experience is the single most important factor. First, the low-amplitude

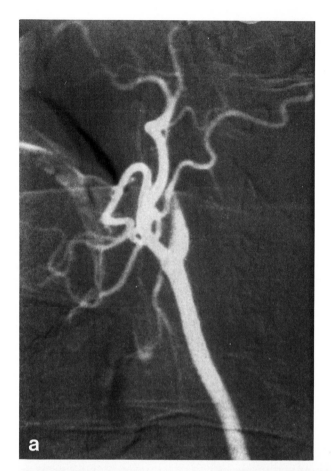

FIG. 24. A: Angiogram displaying apparent occlusion of the
internal common carotid.
B: Duplex examination demonstrating very low flow but indicating some patency of the internal carotid.

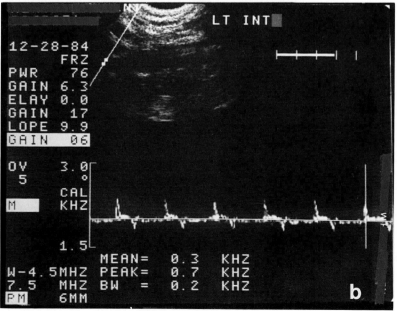

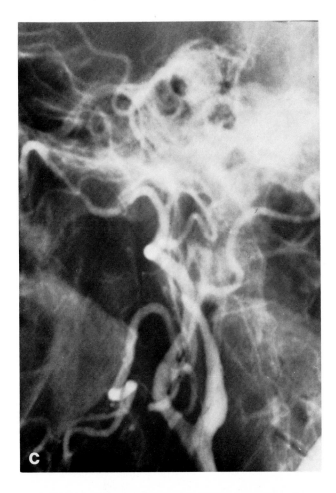

FIG. 24. (*continued*). **C:** Repeat angiogram confirms the presence of a thin column of flow that previously had been missed.

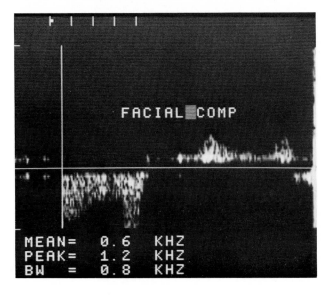

FIG. 25. Normal flow in the periorbital arteries is out of the cranium and towards the transducer. Reversed flow is seen here in the periorbital arteries in a patient with occlusion of the common carotid. Flow is below the zero axis, indicating flow away from the transducer or from the extracranial arteries into the orbit. Compression of the facial artery reverses this flow and allows a low-amplitude flow from the intracranial vessels.

signal seen in the common carotid proximal to the occlusion, especially if unilateral, should raise a strong suspicion of occlusion or near occlusion. Second, periorbital Doppler signals showing reversal of flow with the compression test of the facial and superficial temporal arteries of both sides further strengthen the suspicion of the diagnosis. Finally, very careful reevaluation of the bifurcation will demonstrate when or where a branch of the external, such as the facial artery, has been mistaken for the ICA. It should be remembered that the external carotid signal, with its usual high diastolic flow, may be modified to a lower impedance in the presence of extensive cerebral collateral flow.

Calcified Plaque

Dense calcification of carotid atheroma with distal shadowing may preclude visualization of the vessel lumen and the acquisition of any Doppler-shifted signals (Fig. 26). When this occurs, attempts should be made to visualize the vessel from a different angle in order to "image around" the plaque. If the flow characteristics still cannot be determined, they must be inferred from the signals immediately proximal and distal to the shadowing plaque. For example, the presence of a high-velocity jet obscured by calcified plaque can be inferred if severe turbulence is seen immediately distal to the plaque. A severe stenosis is suggested by the presence of very low flow proximal to the plaque with a return to zero during diastole. However, when these secondary signs of stenosis are used, it is important to look for other causes for low flow such as cardiac failure or aortic stenosis. In these conditions, there are bilateral low-amplitude signals as well as the other signs.

Atheromatous Ulcers

Three types of atherosclerotic lesions are recognized: (a) The fatty streak, which appears to be of no clinical significance, (b) the smooth, fibrous plaque, which may cause flow disturbance, and (c) the complicated plaque with endothelial ulceration and mural hemorrhage, with or without necrosis (18). The detection of an atheromatous ulcer is important because it is postulated that platelet thrombi and plaque emboli from these may be the causes of TIAs and strokes. Katz et al. (22) compared the sensitivity of high-resolution ultrasound and angiography for the detection of ulcerated plaques, using specimens obtained at endarterectomy as the "gold standard." For small ulcers (less than 2 mm), the sensitivity was 33% for ultrasound and 58% for angiography. For large ulcers (greater than 2 mm), ultrasound detected 58% and angiography 74% (Fig. 27). This study showed that both ultrasound and angiography had limited sensitivity for the detection of these important entities (22).

When considering the size at which an ulcer can successfully be imaged, it is important to appreciate and compare the small size of an embolus that can cause neurologic devastation. The central artery of the retina is only 150 μm in diameter. Thus, an embolus of 0.2 mm can cause unilateral blindness. The central perforating branches from the middle cerebral artery that supply the internal capsule are 1 to 2 mm in diameter. Thus, a 1-mm embolus can cause localized motor or sensory deficit by ischemic injury to the nerve fibers traversing the internal capsule. A 2-mm em-

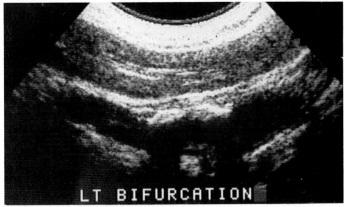

A

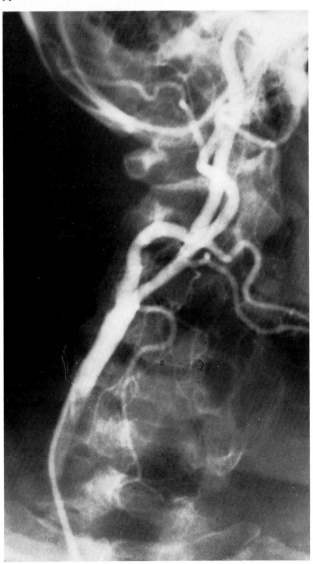

B

FIG. 26. A: Dense calcification of the bifurcation prevents Doppler examination of the flow characteristics. Other approaches, such as an anterolateral approach, should be tried. Otherwise, flow within the shadowed region must be inferred from the waveforms proximal and distal to the area of shadowing. **B:** Angiogram of same patient showing irregular scalloping of the wall of the bifurcation by the calcified plaque.

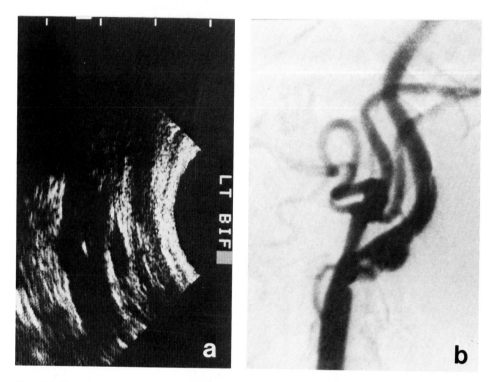

FIG. 27. Comparison of ultrasound with angiogram to show a large ulcer. The ultrasound (**A**) is a mirror image of (**B**) the angiogram. There was no flow disturbance from this ulcer.

bolus is sufficiently large to occlude an entire cerebral artery and cause a dense and permanent hemiplegia.

Intraplaque Hemorrhage

To date, most studies of carotid artery disease have concentrated on the detection and quantitation of flow reduction. For many reasons, there is a poor correlation between the degree of stenosis and the onset of symptoms. The Framingham study produced increasing evidence of the importance of thromboembolic phenomena in the production of cerebral ischemia. This focused attention on plaque morphology and, especially, the presence of intraplaque hemorrhage. Recent studies have indicated that the ultrasonic appearance of the plaque may be correlated with the presence of intraplaque hemorrhage. For the purpose of this classification, the presence of calcification is ignored, and the plaque is classified as homogeneous or heterogeneous. Reilly et al. (33) reported that ultrasound detected the presence of intraplaque hemorrhage with an overall accuracy of 82%, a sensitivity of 91%, and a specificity of 65%. This lower specificity was caused by the presence of other structures including lipid, cholesterol, and protein deposits, which can contribute to heterogeneity. Smooth fibrous plaque always appeared homogeneous. Imparato et al. (15,16) and Bluth et al. (2) have demonstrated that the finding of heterogeneous plaque with intraplaque hemorrhage is more common in symptomatic patients than in the asymptomatic, suggesting its importance as a factor in embolization. Lusby

(28) found a 92.5% incidence of intraplaque hemorrhage in symptomatic patients compared with a 27% incidence in the nonsymptomatic.

These reports indicate that factors in addition to the degree of stenosis or size of an ulcer are important in the production of cerebral ischemia. Sonographers should carefully document plaque appearances in addition to searching for ulcers and quantitating the degree of stenosis.

Volume Flow Estimation

The estimation of absolute volume flow to the brain initially appears rewarding. The size of the internal carotids, approximately 6 mm, is large enough to allow a reasonably accurate measurement. Even in the normal individual, with luminal flow, estimates of volume flow in any particular vessel could vary greatly depending on the size of the other major vessels supplying the brain and the adequacy of the anastomoses around the circle of Willis. In the abnormal individual, the value of the technique would be even less. The presence of turbulent flow and high-velocity jets makes accurate estimation of mean velocity impossible. In addition, the presence of intracranial anastomoses is augmented by the presence of extracranial collaterals in which flow could not be estimated. For these reasons, estimation of absolute brain flow by Doppler techniques cannot be simply attained.

MISCELLANEOUS INDICATIONS FOR CAROTID SCANNING

Trauma

Traumatic occlusion of the carotid artery is relatively rare but may occur in young, athletic individuals. After a trivial injury, hemiplegia and sensory loss may occur

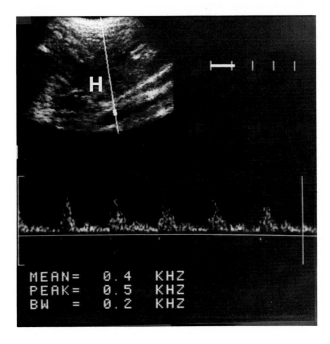

FIG. 28. Normal carotid signal in patient with a fractured mandible and large hematoma (H).

over an interval of time. This may result from hemorrhage into the wall of the common or internal carotid artery, or injury to the wall may give rise to embolization to the anterior or middle cerebral artery. This would usually be diagnosed by CT or angiography. However, we are occasionally asked to evaluate such a patient in whom clinical suspicion is low or in whom other injuries coexist, necessitating portable examination. Patients with neck trauma are difficult to examine because of neck

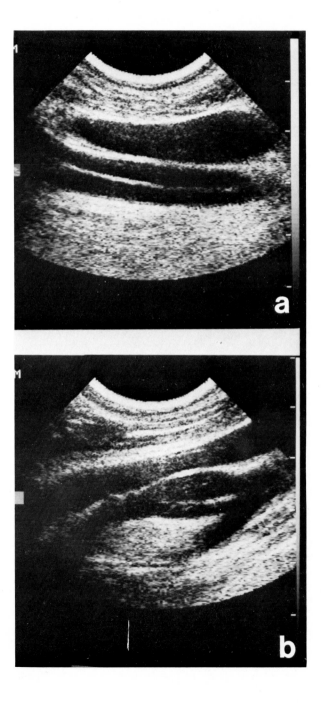

FIG. 29. Longitudinal scan of common carotid artery (**A**) and the carotid bifurcation (**B**) showing a large dissection.

bruising. A fractured mandible may be present to complicate the test further. Figure 28 demonstrates a normal carotid waveform in the examination of a patient with a fractured mandible and gross neck swelling following a motorcycle accident.

Carotid Artery Dissection

Carotid dissections may produce TIAs and stroke, either by a direct effect on the carotid wall caused by encroachment of the lumen or by embolization. There may be no predisposing factors, or dissection may be secondary to trauma or associated with abnormality of the arterial wall such as atherosclerosis, fibromuscular dysplasia, or cystic medial necrosis. This entity should be considered in a young, normotensive patient presenting with TIA or stroke with or without a history of trauma to the neck. Dissections and flaps should be searched for carefully with ultrasound. Figure 29 shows a dramatic dissection in a patient presenting with chest pain radiating to the root of the neck.

CONCLUSION

In summary, carotid artery duplex imaging is now both a mature art and a science, although too few experienced operators exist to date to make it universally available. Its diagnostic accuracy for assessing the cervical carotids is generally equal to or greater than that of angiography, and the problem of operator dependence will be lessened by the availability of color-modulated imaging. Such equipment will aid observer perception of focal stenoses, but the quantitative criteria discussed here for grading the severity of the lesion will still be required. It appears that duplex sonography, with or without color imaging, has an assured place as the initial economic and noninvasive modality for evaluating most patients with suspected carotid artery disease.

REFERENCES

1. Blackshear, W. M., Jr., Phillips, D. J., Chikos, P. M., Harley, J. D., Thiele, B. L., and Strandness, D. E., Jr. (1980): Carotid artery velocity patterns in normal and stenotic vessels. *Stroke,* 11:67–71.

2. Bluth, E. I., Kay, D., Merritt, C. R. B., Sullivan, M., and Farr, G. (1985): Sonographic characterization of carotid plaque. *Radiology,* 157(P):352.

3. Breslau, P. J., Fell, G., Phillips, D. J., Thiele, B. L., and Strandness, D. E., Jr. (1982): Evaluation of carotid bifurcation disease. *Arch. Surg.,* 117:58–60.

4. Busuttil, R. W., Baker, J. D., Davidson, R. K., and Machleder, H. I. (1981): Carotid artery stenosis—hemodynamic significance and clinical course. *J.A.M.A.,* 245:1438–1441.

5. Callow, A. D. (1982): Recurrent stenosis after carotid endarterectomy. *Arch. Surg.,* 117:1082–1085.

6. Cantelmo, N. L., Cutler, B. S., Wheeler, H. B., Herrmann, J. B., and Cardullo, P. A. (1981): Noninvasive detection of carotid stenosis following endarterectomy. *Arch. Surg.,* 116:1005–1008.

7. Crew, J. R., Dean, M., Johnson, J. M., Knighton, D., Bashour, T. T., Ellerton, D., and Hanna, E. S. (1984): Carotid surgery without angiography. *Am. J. Surg.,* 148(1):217–220.

8. Curry, G. R., and White, D. N. (1978): Color coded ultrasonic differential velocity arterial scanner (Echoflow). *Ultrasound Med. Biol.,* 4:27–35.

9. Douville, Y., Johnston, K. W., and Kassam, M. (1985): Determination of the hemodynamic factors which influence the carotid Doppler spectral broadening. *Ultrasound Med. Biol.,* 11:417–423.

10. Fell, G., Breslau, P., Knox, R. A., Phillips, D., Thiele, B. L., and Strandness, D. E., Jr. (1981): Importance of noninvasive ultrasonic-Doppler testing in the evaluation of patients with asymptomatic carotid bruits. *Am. Heart J.,* 102(2):221–226.

11. Fell, G., Phillips, D. J., Chikos, P. M., Harley, J. D., Thiele, B. L., and Strandness, D. E., Jr. (1981): Ultrasonic duplex scanning for disease of the carotid artery. *Circulation,* 64:1191–1195.

12. Flanigan, D. P., Schuler, J. J., Vogel, M., Borozan, P. G., Gray, B., and Sobinsky, K. R. (1985): The role of carotid duplex scanning in surgical decision making. *J. Vasc. Surg.,* 2:15–25.

13. Foley, W. D., Smith, D. F., Milde, M. W., Lawson, T. L., Towne, J. B., and Bandyk, D. F. (1984): Intravenous DSA examination of patients with suspected cerebral ischemia. *Radiology,* 151:651–659.

14. Hoffman, M. G., Gomes, A. S., and Pais, S. O. (1984): Limitations in the interpretation of intravenous carotid digital subtraction angiography. *Am. J. Roentgenol.,* 142:261–264.

15. Imparato, A. M., Riles, T. S., and Gorstein, F. (1979): The carotid bifurcation plaque: pathologic findings associated with cerebral ischemia. *Stroke,* 10:238–245.

16. Imparato, A. M., Riles, T. S., Mintzer, R., and Baumann, F. G. (1983): The importance of hemorrhage in the relationship between gross morphologic characteristics and cerebral symptoms in 376 carotid artery plaques. *Ann. Surg.,* 197:195–203.

17. Jacobs, N. M., Grant, E. G., Schellinger, D., Byrd, M. C., Richardson, J. D., and Cohan, S. L. (1985): Duplex carotid sonography: Criteria for stenosis, accuracy, and pitfalls. *Radiology,* 154:385–391.

18. Javid, H., Ostermiller, W. E., Jr., Hengesh, J. W., Dye, W. S., Hunter, J. A., Najafi, H., and Julian, O. C. (1970): Natural history of carotid bifurcation atheroma. *Surgery,* 67:80–86.

19. Johnston, K. W., Haynes, R. B., Douville, Y., Lally, M. E., Brown, P. M., and Cobbold, R. S. C. (1985): Accuracy of carotid Doppler frequency analysis: Results determined by receiver operating characteristic curves and likelihood ratios. *J. Vasc. Surg.,* 2:515–523.

20. Kartchner, M. M., and McRae, L. P. (1982): Carotid occlusive disease as a risk factor in major cardiovascular surgery. *Arch. Surg.,* 117:1086–1088.

21. Kassam, M., Johnston, K. W., and Cobbold, R. S. C. (1985): Quantitative estimation of spectral broadening for the diagnosis of carotid arterial disease: Method and *in vitro* results. *Ultrasound Med. Biol.,* 11:425–433.

22. Katz, M. L., Johnson, M., Pomajzl, M. J., Comerota, A. J., Ahrensfield, D., Mandel, L., Hayden, W., and Fogarty, T. (1983): The sensitivity of real-time B-mode carotid imaging in the detection of ulcerated plaques. *Bruit,* 8:13–16.

23. Keagy, B. A., and Pharr, W. F. (1982): A quantitative method for the evaluation of spectral analysis patterns in carotid artery stenosis. *Ultrasound Med. Biol.,* 8:625–630.

24. Keagy, B. A., Pharr, W. F., Thomas, D., and Bowes, D. E. (1982): Objective criteria for the interpretation of carotid artery spectral analysis patterns. *Angiology,* 33:213–220.

25. Knox, R. A., Breslau, P. J., and Strandness, D. E., Jr. (1982): A simple parameter for accurate detection of severe carotid disease. *Br. J. Surg.,* 69:230–233.

26. Ku, D. N., Giddens, D. P., Phillips, D. J., and Strandness, D. E., Jr. (1985): Hemodynamics of the normal human carotid bifurcation: *In vitro* and *in vivo* studies. *Ultrasound Med. Biol.,* 11:13–26.

27. Lewis, R. R., Padayachee, T. S., and Gosling, R. G. (1984): Ultrasound screening for internal carotid disease—II. Sensitivity and specificity of a single site periorbital artery test. *Ultrasound Med. Biol.,* 10:17–25.

28. Lusby, R. J., Ferrell, L. D., Ehrenfeld, W. K., Stoney, R. J., and Wylie, E. J. (1982): Carotid plaque hemorrhage. *Arch. Surg.,* 117:1479–1488.

29. Martin, M. J., Whisnant, J. P., and Sayre, G. P. (1960): Occlusive vascular disease in the extracranial cerebral circulation. *Arch. Neurol.,* 5:530–538.

30. Nicholls, S. C., Phillips, D. J., Bergelin, R. O., Beach, K. W., Primozich, J. F., and Strandness, D. E., Jr. (1985): Carotid endarterectomy. Relationship of outcome to early restenosis. *J. Vasc. Surg.,* 2:375–381.

31. Padayachee, T. S., Lewis, R. R., and Gosling, R. G. (1984): Ultrasound screening for internal carotid disease—I. The temporal artery occlusion test—which periorbital artery? *Ultrasound Med. Biol.,* 10:13–16.

32. Phillips, D. J., Greene, F. M., Jr., Langlois, Y., Roederer, G. O., and Strandness, D. E., Jr. (1983): Flow velocity patterns in the carotid bifurcations of young, presumed normal subjects. *Ultrasound Med. Biol.,* 9:39–49.

33. Reilly, L. M., Lusby, R. J., Hughes, L., Ferrell, L. D., Stoney, R. J., and Ehrenfeld, W. K. (1983): Carotid plaque histology using real-time ultrasonography. Clinical and therapeutic implications. *Am. J. Surg.,* 146:188–193.

34. Roederer, G. O., Langlois, Y., Chan, A. T. W., Breslau, P., Phillips, D. J., Beach, K. W., Chikos, P. M., and Strandness, D. E., Jr. (1983): Post-endarterectomy carotid ultrasonic duplex scanning concordance with contrast angiography. *Ultrasound Med. Biol.,* 9:73–78.

35. Roederer, G. O., Langlois, Y. E., Lusiani, L., Jager, K. A., Primozich, J. F., Lawrence, R. J., Phillips, D. J., and Strandness, D. E., Jr. (1984): Natural history of carotid artery disease on the side contralateral to endarterectomy. *J. Vasc. Surg.,* 1:62–72.

36. Roederer, G. O., and Strandness, D. E., Jr., (1984): A simple spectral parameter for the classification of severe carotid disease. *Bruit,* 8:174–178.

37. Russell, J. B., Watson, T. M., Modi, J. R., Lambeth, A., and Sumner, D. S. (1983): Digital subtraction angiography for evaluation of extracranial carotid occlusive disease: Comparison with conventional arteriography. *Surgery,* 94:604–611.

38. Sandok, B. A., Whisnant, J. P., Furlan, A. J., and Mickell, J. L. (1982): Carotid artery bruits: prevalence survey and differential diagnosis. *Mayo Clin. Proc.,* 57:227–230.

39. Sherman, D. G., Dyken, M. L., Fisher, M., Harrison, M. J. G., and Hart, R. G. (1986): Cerebral embolism. *Chest,* 89S(2):82S–98S.

40. Spencer, M. P., and Reid, J. M. (1979): Quantitation of carotid stenosis with continuous wave (C-W) Doppler ultrasound. *Stroke,* 10:326–330.

41. Spencer, M. P., Reid, J. M., Davis, D. L., and Paulson, P. S. (1974): Cervical carotid imaging with a continuous-wave Doppler flowmeter. *Stroke,* 5:145–154.

42. Turnipseed, W. D., Sackett, J. F., Strother, C. M., Crummy, A. B., and Mistretta, C. A. (1982): A comparison of standard cerebral arteriography with noninvasive Doppler imaging and intravenous angiography. *Arch. Surg.,* 117:419–421.

43. Wolf, P. A., Kannel, W. B., Sorlie, P., and McNamara, P. (1981): Asymptomatic carotid bruit and risk of stroke: The Framingham study. *J.A.M.A.,* 245:1442–1445.

44. Zarins, C. K., Giddens, D. P., Bharadvaj, B. K., Sotiuvai, V. S., Mabon, R. F., and Glagov, S. (1983): Carotid bifurcation atherosclerosis. Quantitative correlation of plaque localization with flow velocity profiles and wall shear stress. *Circ. Res.,* 53:502–514.

45. Zwiebel, W. J., and Crummy, A. B. (1981): Sources of error in Doppler diagnosis of carotid occlusive disease. *Am. J. Roentgenol.,* 137:1–12.

6 / *Gastrointestinal Doppler Ultrasound*

Kenneth J. W. Taylor

Department of Diagnostic Radiology, Yale University School of Medicine, New Haven, Connecticut 06510

High-resolution ultrasound imaging, combined with the ability to determine blood flow characteristics at any localized site, is extremely valuable in the noninvasive evaluation of many disease entities, particularly those involving the hepatobiliary system. In many instances, it is the most simplistic applications of Doppler imaging that have the greatest clinical value. For example, the ability to exclude a thrombosis by Doppler techniques is one of the most useful in patient management. The diagnosis or exclusion of a deep vein thrombosis or arterial occlusion is of the utmost importance in many disease entities in the abdomen. Such diagnoses may rapidly be made by this noninvasive modality.

It is important to note that a Doppler shift signal is returned from any moving structure. Normally we are interested only in the very low-level echoes returned from moving red cells. However, much larger echoes are returned from the moving boundaries of an organ or a lesion, which may be moving passively with transmitted cardiac oscillation or with respiratory activity. In addition, the walls of blood vessels give rise to a low-frequency but high-amplitude Doppler shift. These signals are usually removed by a high-pass filter. For abdominal applications, the high-pass filter is set as low as possible, usually 50 or 100 Hz. It must be recalled, however, that such filtering will prevent the slowest blood flow from being recorded. Large Doppler shift signals emanate from other abdominal structures as well. High-amplitude signals arise from peristalsis in air-containing viscera (Fig. 1). Such signals obliterate all of the low-amplitude signals coming from blood by overloading of the electrical circuits. In the region of the kidneys, ureteric contraction can frequently be heard. Because peristaltic signals are generally of short duration, the examination should be suspended for a few moments until the interference has died away (Fig. 1). In the examination of cysts and other lesions in organs such as the liver, Doppler shift signals from the wall of the lesion must not be misinterpreted as flow. Usually it can clearly be seen whether the Doppler signal is modulated by respiratory movement or transmitted cardiac movement.

The ability to indicate direction of flow using Doppler techniques can be quite

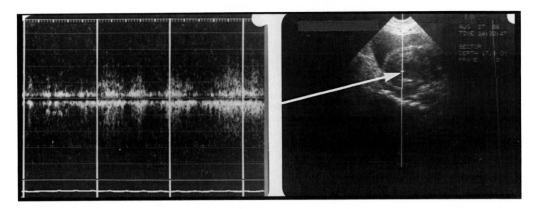

FIG. 1. Peristalsis. The B-scan demonstrates a pelvic mass, the origin of which is unclear. Definite Doppler signals are seen within this mass because of peristalsis. In this example, the peristaltic signals were helpful in identifying the nature of the pelvic mass, but peristaltic signals are usually transient ''noise'' when other waveforms are being sought.

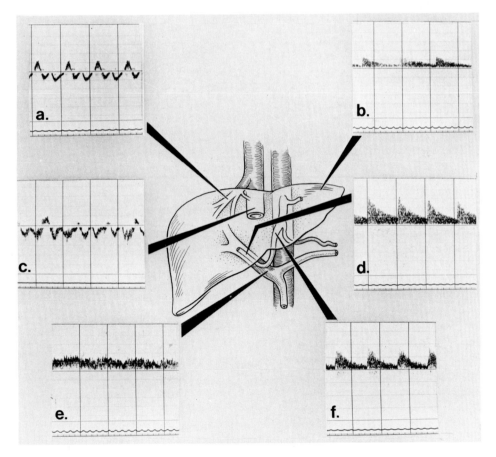

FIG. 2. Montage to show time–velocity waveforms in the vessels around the liver: (**a**) the hepatic veins, (**b**) hepatic parenchymal arterial signal, (**c**) inferior vena cava, (**d**) proper hepatic artery, (**e**) portal vein, and (**f**) common hepatic artery. (Reprinted with permission from Taylor et al., ref. 46.)

helpful in evaluating the hemodynamics of portal hypertension. Reversed flow seen in the portal vein or splenic vein strongly suggests a high portal venous pressure, usually associated with high intrahepatic venous resistance from cirrhosis. The direction of flow is indicated after spectral analysis by noting whether the flow is above or below the zero line.

NORMAL DOPPLER WAVEFORMS IN THE UPPER ABDOMEN

Normal Doppler waveforms can be obtained from all of the major vessels of the upper abdomen (Figs. 2 and 3). A frequency of 3 MHz is optimal. The technique varies with the access available in any given patient. Because of the proximity of many of the vessels to each other, a sample volume of 1.5 mm is used.

The waveform in the aorta demonstrates a clear window and a reversed flow component. The clear window under the time–velocity envelope is caused by the red cells moving at the same velocity, creating a square wavefront, so-called "plug flow." The reversed wavefront is caused by the high resistance in the lower limbs, which causes blood to bounce up the aortic vessels during diastole. This wavefront is typical of the aorta and common and external iliac arteries in the resting state.

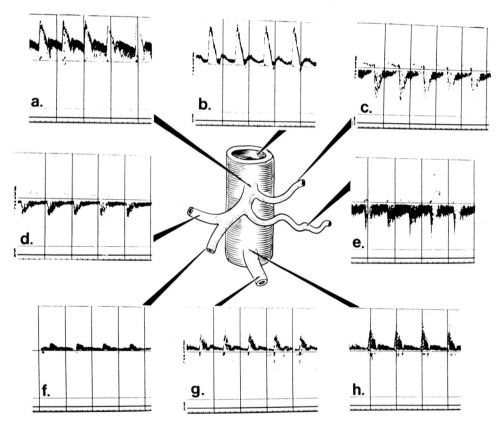

FIG. 3. Montage to show waveforms in the branches of the aorta: (**a**) celiac trunk, (**b**) upper aorta, (**c**) left gastric, (**d**) proper hepatic, (**e**) splenic (**f**) gastroduodenal, (**g**) distal superior mesenteric, and (**h**) proximal superior mesenteric. (Reprinted with permission from Taylor et al., ref. 46.)

In many patients, waveforms can be elicited from the common hepatic artery near its origin from the celiac trunk (Fig. 2). However, signals can be obtained in every patient from both the main and right hepatic arteries using an intercostal approach in the coronal plane (Fig. 4). By using the liver as an acoustic window, the portal vein is easily seen. The main hepatic artery lies anterior and to the left of the portal vein, immediately adjacent to the common duct, and the right hepatic artery can be seen between the common duct and the portal vein (Fig. 4). In this position, both the hepatic artery and portal vein can be sampled. The hepatic artery demonstrates low impedance characterized by high diastolic flow. Demonstration of this flow is vital in liver transplant recipients, since the survival of their orthograft depends on the patency of the hepatic artery.

The portal vein displays a very characteristic continuous flow pattern, which, in the normal individual, is modulated by respiratory variations. This normal variation in velocity may be reduced or lost in portal hypertension, a useful sign that is considered later.

The adjacent inferior vena cava (IVC) demonstrates a totally different waveform, and a similar complex waveform can be seen in all the large abdominal and pelvic veins. The waveform variations are complex because of the combination of regurgitation of blood from the right atrium associated with atrial systole and the variations in intra-abdominal pressure associated with the respiratory pump. Decreased intrathoracic pressure and increased intraabdominal pressure associated with inspiration produce a pressure gradient so that blood flows from the IVC into the right atrium.

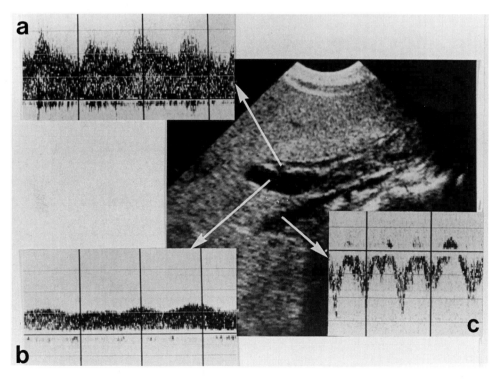

FIG. 4. Montage of vessels in the porta hepatis: (**a**) right hepatic artery, (**b**) portal vein, and (**c**) inferior vena cava. (Reprinted with permission from Taylor et al., ref. 48.)

The characteristic venous waveform, if present in the iliac and femoral veins, demonstrates continuity with the pressure variations in the IVC and, hence, patency of the communicating great veins.

The patency of the hepatic veins can be assessed by real-time imaging and by pulsed Doppler ultrasound. The Budd–Chiari syndrome, caused by occlusion of the hepatic veins or the IVC, is easily diagnosed or excluded by duplex Doppler scanning. Thrombosis of the lower IVC is seen in Fig. 5. In this patient, no flow was elicited in the middle or lower IVC, but high flow was seen above the entry of the renal vessels, demonstrating patency at that level.

An important characteristic of a sensitive pulsed Doppler device is its ability to detect signals from vessels not apparent to the unaided eye. Such signals are seen

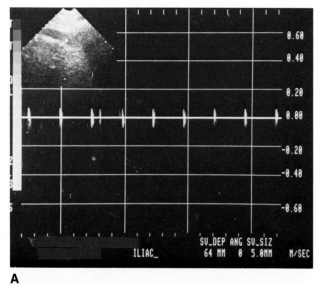

A

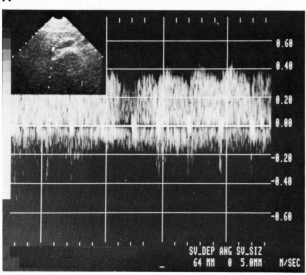

B

FIG. 5. Duplex examination of patient with indwelling Greenfield filter in the IVC. **A:** There is no flow in the lower IVC. **B:** Brisk flow is demonstrated in the upper IVC above the level of the renal veins.

within the liver parenchyma (Fig. 2b). In different positions, hepatic arterial signals as well as portal and systemic venous flow can be detected. If such parenchymal flow cannot be elicited in the normal liver, then the equipment is too insensitive for abdominal Doppler applications.

Flow can also be demonstrated in other vessels in the upper abdomen. These include the left gastric artery (Fig. 3c) and splenic artery (Fig. 3e), the remaining branches of the celiac trunk. Surprisingly high flow exists in the left gastric artery. Characteristically, the splenic arterial signal is highly turbulent with an irregular waveform and complete spectral broadening. This is assumed to arise from the tortuosity of the splenic artery. The splenic venous waveform can easily be elicited adjacent to the splenic arterial waveform and shows the same pattern as that of the portal venous system.

The superior mesenteric artery can be sampled in most individuals (Fig. 3g). When it is obscured by air in the stomach or intestine, the usual techniques, including ingestion of water and upright posture (37), should be applied to display the region of the pancreas. The signal in the superior mesenteric artery will be found to vary depending on the nutritional state of the individual. In the fasting state, a high-impedance pattern is seen with little diastolic flow. After a meal, vasodilatation and a great increase in the mesenteric circulation occur, and marked diastolic flow is seen (38,39). Indeed, attempts have been made to measure blood flow in response to a meal, and individuals with dumping syndromes have been noted to have increased blood flow after a standard test meal (2).

PORTAL VEIN

Thrombosis of Portal Vein

The normal portal venous waveform has already been considered (Fig. 2e). A most useful application of duplex imaging is the exclusion of portal or splenic vein thrombosis (45). The need for such evaluation arises frequently when a patient with cirrhosis becomes decompensated with accumulation of ascites or worsening hepatic function. Here the possibility of a hepatoma arising within a cirrhotic liver should also be considered, since this too may precipitate portal vein thrombosis. Splenic vein and portal vein thrombosis may also occur as a result of pancreatitis or pancreatic carcinoma as well as in liver transplantation. Figure 6A shows the appearance of chronic portal venous occlusion in which the lumen of the portal vein is replaced by a fibrous line and Doppler examination demonstrated no evidence of flow. An angiogram confirmed this diagnosis (Fig. 6B). Recent thrombosis of the left portal vein is shown in Fig. 7. Although thrombus may be clearly seen in the lumen of the portal vein, if the thrombus is recent, the vein may appear patent. Under these circumstances, Doppler ultrasound is essential to demonstrate occlusion.

Cavernous Transformation of the Portal Vein

Following portal vein occlusion, collateral vessels may develop with the formation of varices, most commonly in the esophageal region. However, approximately 30% of these patients develop collaterals along the course of the portal vein that appear

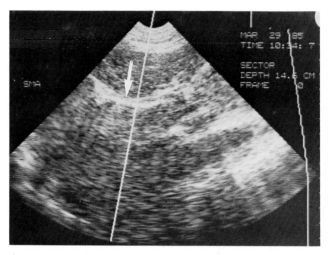

A

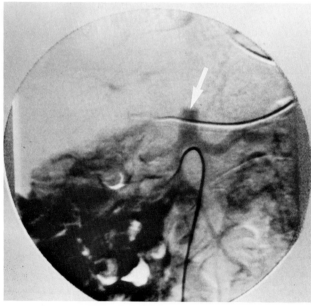

B

FIG. 6. A: Portal vein thrombosis in a patient referred for liver transplantation with cirrhosis and a hepatoma. The portal vein shows no lumen and appears as an echogenic line (*arrow*). There was no flow on the Doppler examination. **B:** Angiogram confirming the presence of portal vein thrombosis (*arrow*) in the patient shown in **A.** (Reprinted with permission from Taylor et al., ref. 48.)

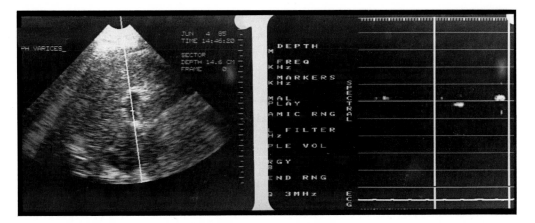

FIG. 7. Portal venous thrombosis. The Doppler cursor is located in the left branch of the portal vein, but there is no venous signal. There is a propagated arterial signal. (Reprinted with permission from Taylor et al., ref. 48.)

as periportal serpiginous channels (54). This condition is termed ''cavernous transformation of the portal vein'' (Fig. 8). Originally considered to be a primary angiomatous malformation, it is now recognized to be collateral channels. Doppler scanning aids in the diagnosis of this condition by demonstrating the typical portal venous flow in the serpiginous vessels, identifying them as collaterals of the portal venous system (54) (Fig. 8D).

Air in the Portal Vein

Air in the portal vein has been demonstrated in patients with necrotizing enterocolitis (NEC) and also in patients with mesenteric infarction and/or abscesses. Such patients are usually gravely ill and require portable evaluation and exploratory surgery (52). Bubbles passing up the portal vein can often be seen by imaging alone and give rise to a typical air pattern distributed around the periphery of the liver (Fig. 9A). This is a relatively late manifestation of NEC. It would be extremely valuable, therefore, if Doppler techniques could make this diagnosis at an earlier stage. Certainly Doppler scanning should be exquisitely sensitive to the presence of microbubbles of gas because of the high impedance mismatch at the blood/air interface. Figure 9A shows air in the portal vein and distributed throughout the liver in a child with NEC. Large-amplitude echoes emanating from the bubbles are clearly seen superimposed on the portal venous tracing (Fig. 9B). Whether Doppler ultrasound will prove to be practical and a more sensitive means of detecting air in the portal vein, permitting an earlier diagnosis of NEC, remains to be proved.

Tumor in the Portal Vein

Portal vein thrombosis may result from a tumor, especially a hepatoma, from which intravascular spread is common. Figure 10 shows a metastasis from a melanoma

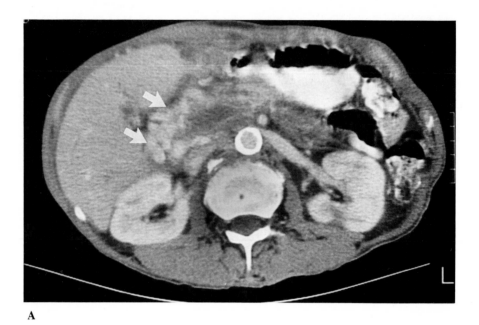

A

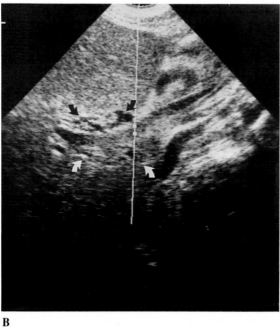

B

FIG. 8. Cavernous transformation of the portal vein. **A:** A CT scan showing a pancreatic mass consistent with pancreatitis and multiple varices (*arrow*) around the head of the pancreas. **B:** Duplex scan of the porta hepatis with the Doppler cursor in the lumen of the portal vein. No signal was elicited. Periportal serpiginous channels are seen (*arrow*).

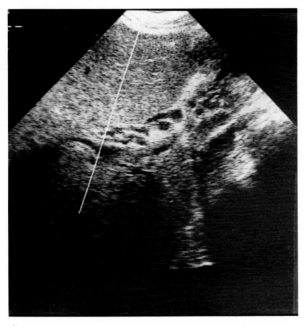

C

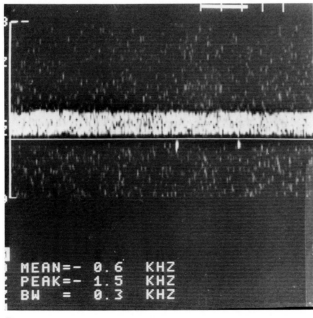

MEAN=- 0.6 KHZ
PEAK=- 1.5 KHZ
BW = 0.3 KHZ

D

FIG. 8. (*continued*). **C:** The Doppler sample volume is now in the periportal channels. **D:** A continuous portal venous signal is obtained. These appearances are diagnostic of cavernous transformation of the portal vein. (Reprinted with permission from Weltin et al., ref. 54.)

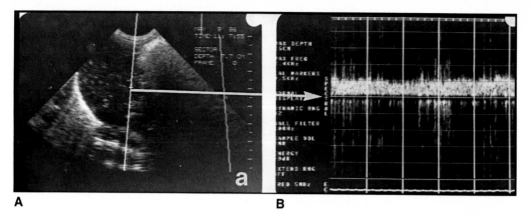

FIG. 9. Air in the portal vein. This infant had established necrotizing enterocolitis, and bubbles could be seen passing up the main portal vein. **A:** Air is seen evenly distributed throughout the liver parenchyma. **B:** The portal venous signal shows high spikes caused by air bubbles superimposed on the normal Doppler portal venous signal.

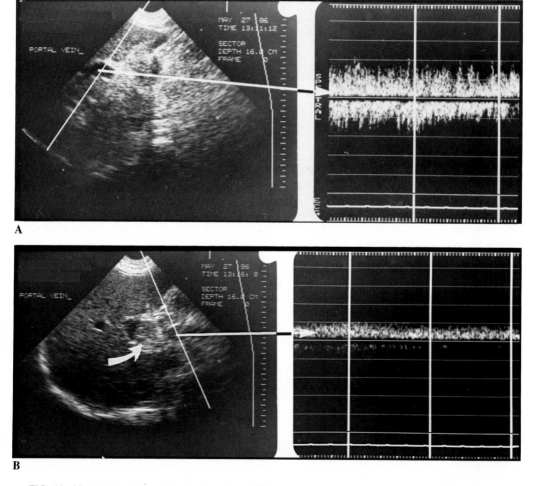

FIG. 10. Metastasis in the right portal vein. **A:** Metastasis (*arrow*) from a melanoma is seen in the portal vein. The Doppler signal before this is normal. **B:** Doppler distal to the tumor shows flow, but the waveform is irregular, and flow is in both directions, indicating turbulence associated with the prior stenosis caused by partial occlusion by the tumor.

within the right portal vein. This intravascular tumor produced turbulence around it but did not cause venous occlusion, which might have been suspected on the basis of the image alone.

DOPPLER EVALUATION OF PORTAL HYPERTENSION

Duplex examination of the portal system can be quite helpful in suggesting the diagnosis of portal hypertension and in certain instances provides definitive diagnosis (14). Multiple sonographic findings in portal hypertension have been reported in the radiologic literature, and this diagnosis can be made with increasing certainty when many of these signs are present (Table 1). Portal hypertension develops as the hepatopetal blood flow in the portal vein is impeded. The portal venous system becomes distended, the spleen engorged, and the venous pressure raised. Spontaneous portosystemic shunts develop. Rarely, there may be reversal of flow to a hepatofugal direction. Reversed flow may occur in the portal vein or splenic vein (Fig. 11) with dilatation of collateral venous pathways forming widespread portosystemic anastomoses. The most common of these and the most clinically important are the gastroesophageal collaterals present in 80 to 90% of patients with portal hypertension (9,10,35). The appearance of many other portosystemic anastomoses has been well described in the sonographic literature. The most common collateral sites are summarized schematically in Fig. 12.

Varices

Four major groups of collateral vessels are conventionally described: (a) those in the gastroesophageal region, which may result in life-threatening esophageal varices, (b) paraumbilical vein, (c) miscellaneous portosystemic anastomoses, and (d) hemorrhoidal veins, which may form extensive pelvic varices but will not be considered further here.

Gastroesophageal Collaterals

Collaterals develop in the cardiac region of the stomach from the coronary vein or right gastric veins, which drain into the esophageal veins with subsequent drainage

TABLE 1. *Sonographic findings in portal hypertension*

Dilated portal vein
Dilated splenic and superior mesenteric veins (SMV)
Patent paraumbilical vein
Varices
Splenomegaly with dilated splenic radicles
Diminished response to respiration in splenic vein and SMV
Dilated hepatic and splenic arteries
Ascites
Small liver with irregular surface or large liver with abnormal texture

From DiCandio et al. (14).

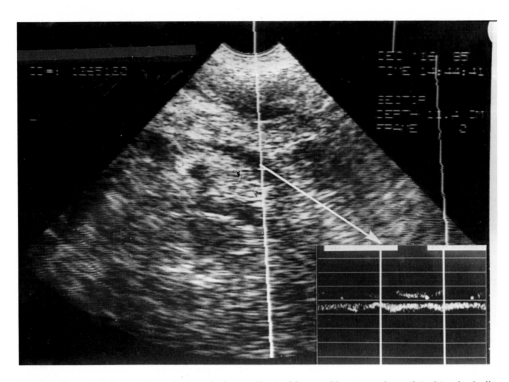

FIG. 11. Reversed flow in the splenic vein in a patient with portal hypertension related to alcoholic cirrhosis. The Doppler cursor is located in the distal splenic vein and shows very low velocity flow. The velocity spectrum is below the zero line, indicating flow away from the ultrasound beam and demonstrating reversed flow in the splenic vein.

into the azygos and hemiazygos systems (1). In a comparison with transhepatic portography, Dokmeci et al. (17) imaged the coronary vein by sonography in 85% of patients with portal hypertension but visualized the short gastric veins in only 10% (Fig. 13). Varicoceles of the coronary vein may be imaged by ultrasound as well as the gastroesophageal varices (25). In a study of 30 patients with varices, the coronary vein was 5 mm or greater in 24, yielding a sensitivity of 80% and a false negative rate of 20% (44). There was good correlation between the size of the varices and the size of the coronary vein. In this study, gastroesophageal varices were demonstrated by ultrasound in 68% of patients with large varices and in 18% of patients with small varices. Esophageal varices were small or absent on portography when the portohepatic gradient was less than 10 mm Hg (24). At higher pressures, varices tended to be larger, but their size was not proportional to the portohepatic gradient (11,30,42). Doppler technique aids in the reliable demonstration of portal venous flow in small anechoic areas seen in the submucosa of the gastroesophageal junction and thus allows their positive identification as varices. Endoscopic Doppler scanning has been used for the detection of esophageal varices (32), although direct visualization of these appears to be adequate for diagnosis.

Other vessels that are part of this collateral pathway may be seen in the lesser omentum (Fig. 14). Thickening of the lesser omentum has been described as a sign of portal hypertension in children (8). Typical portal venous flow in small anechoic areas within the lesser omentum illustrates how Doppler scanning characterizes the

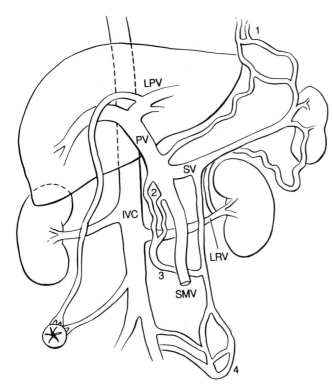

FIG. 12. Schema to show sites of portosystemic venous anastomoses. The superior mesenteric vein (SMV) and the splenic vein (SV) join to form the portal vein (PV). There may be enlargement of the coronary vein and branches of the splenic vein to form gastroesophageal varices (1), which drain via the azygos and hemiazygos veins into vena cava. Clinically, esophageal varices are the most hazardous of the portosystemic venous anastomoses for causing hemorrhage. The left portal vein may communicate with the veins draining the anterior body wall around the umbilicus by means of a patent paraumbilical vein. The portal vein and SMV may form retroperitoneal and peripancreatic anastomoses (2,3). The hemorrhoidal branches of the inferior mesenteric vein form anastomoses (4) with branches of the hemorrhoidal veins draining into the IVC. There may also be spontaneous splenorenal shunts between the left renal vein (LRV) and branches of the SV.

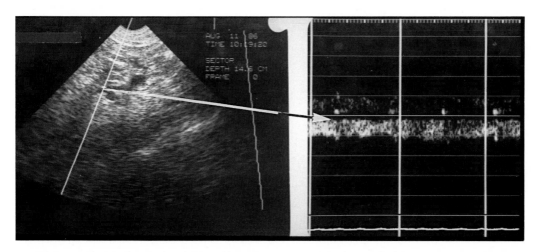

FIG. 13. The coronary vein is seen, appearing as a continuation of the portal vein in a cephalic direction. In this patient the vein is small, but typical hypertensive portal venous flow is demonstrated with no respiratory variation.

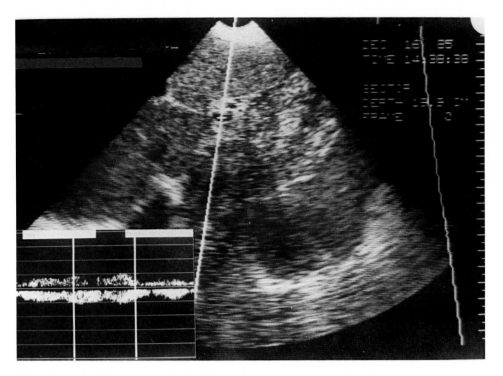

FIG. 14. Lesser omentum varices. Small anechoic areas are seen in the porta hepatis and, in particular, the lesser omentum. Interrogation of these small areas by Doppler demonstrates typical portal venous flow. The lesser omentum may be thickened because of the presence of these varices, and this allows a presumptive diagnosis of portal hypertension, especially in children.

nature of these small channels and differentiates them from other similar-appearing structures such as lymph nodes.

Paraumbilical Vein

One of the most notable portosystemic communications is the paraumbilical vein (27), originally described erroneously as a recanalized umbilical vein (18). This vessel is seen in continuity with the left portal vein and extending through the ligamentum teres down the anterior abdominal wall to the umbilicus (Fig. 15). These appearances are quite clearly seen on the B-scan and were originally described by imaging alone. To evaluate the specificity of this sign, Saddekni et al. (40) reviewed 12 patients with a patent vessel in the ligamentum teres. In ten of the 12, all of whom had liver disease, the patent vein exceeded 3 mm in diameter, and of these, six had esophageal varices. In contrast, three of ten normal controls had a patent vessel, but all were less than 3 mm in diameter. The ability of Doppler examination to establish both the presence and direction of flow in the patent vessel adds certainty to the diagnosis (Fig. 16). We therefore regard the presence of typical portal venous flow in a vessel exceeding 3 mm in diameter within the ligamentum teres to be a highly specific sign of portal hypertension and have seen it only in patients with severe disease.

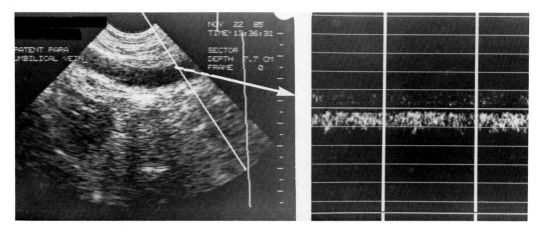

FIG. 15. Patent paraumbilical vein. A vessel is seen lying immediately deep to the anterior abdominal wall, and it could be traced from communication with the left portal vein as far as the umbilicus. Simultaneous Doppler examination demonstrates continuous portal venous flow without respiratory variation, typical of the hypertensive state.

Miscellaneous Portosystemic Anastomoses

Pancreaticoduodenal

Veins from the duodenum, pancreas, colon, spleen, and the bare area of the liver may drain into systemic veins (33,44). The pancreatico–duodenal, superior mesenteric, inferior mesenteric, and retroperitoneal veins can drain directly into the inferior vena cava, constituting a spontaneous portocaval anastomosis.

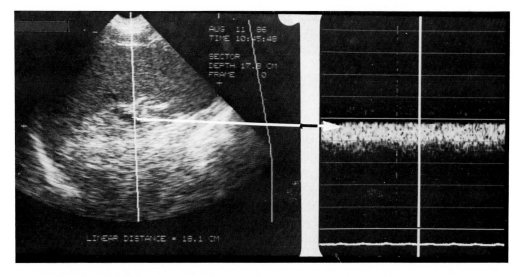

FIG. 16. Splenomegaly in portal hypertension. There is moderate splenomegaly in this patient with portal hypertension secondary to alcoholic cirrhosis. Examination of the splenic vein in the hilum spleen demonstrates continuous portal venous flow without evidence of respiratory variation, consistent with a hypertensive portal venous system.

Retroperitoneal Collaterals

Varices draining the duodenum can drain via the retroperitoneum into the paravertebral veins of the body wall (44).

Gastrorenal or Splenorenal Collaterals

There may be a direct shunt from the gastric or splenic veins into the left renal vein and thence into the inferior vena cava (12,26,44).

Cholecystic Varices

Cholecystic varices have been described and may produce the very confusing appearance of a thickened gallbladder wall (31). The true nature of these vessels can be appreciated by simultaneous Doppler examination.

Diminished Respiration Variation

Bolondi et al. (7) reported that normal respiratory variations in the branches of the portal vein were diminished or lost in the hypertensive portal vein (Fig. 16). In all normal subjects, they found a significant increase of 50 to 100% in the caliber of the splenic and superior mesenteric veins during inspiration. Bolondi reported a sensitivity of 80% and a specificity of 100% for this sign of portal hypertension (7). Although we believe this to be a highly specific sign, the sensitivity will vary with the severity of the portal hypertension. The mechanism for this effect arises from the variations in splanchnic outflow into the hepatic veins. Increased venous return in the systemic circulation occurs during inspiration, but there is increased resistance to flow in the hepatic bed as a result of mechanical collapse of the intrahepatic vessels. Therefore, decreased splanchnic flow is observed with inspiration, and increased splanchnic flow during expiration.

Size of Portal Vessels

The size of the portal venous system may be accurately measured using high-resolution imaging. However, the value of these measurements is controversial. Bolondi et al. (7) reported that the portal vein was less than 13 mm in all normal patients and 13 mm or greater in 47.8% of those with portal hypertension. They concluded that a diminished response of the splenic vein and SMV was a more sensitive indicator of portal hypertension than size of the portal vein. Weinreb et al. (53) measured the diameter of the normal portal vein in 107 subjects aged 20 to 40 years and reported a mean and standard deviation of 11 ± 2 mm. In contrast, a postmortem study of cirrhotic patients suggested that the portal vein may be normal or even decreased in size after blood flow has been diverted into collateral vessels (15,16). Lafortune et al. (28) performed an angiographic study using 64 biopsy-proven cirrhotics. They found no significant differences between the caliber of the portal vein in controls and in those of cirrhotic patients, and the caliber tended to diminish when collaterals developed. No correlation was found between the size of the SMV and the portohepatic pressure gradient. The splenic vein was nearly identical in size to the portal vein, and the caliber was unrelated to portohepatic pressure. The splenic vein was less than 15 mm in the controls and greater than 15 mm in 70% of the cirrhotics and tended to increase with increasing splenic size. The coronary vein was larger in patients with severe portal hypertension, and its size was also related to the size and number of esophageal varices.

Splenomegaly

Splenomegaly is virtually always present in portal hypertension, although sometimes of modest degree, with the spleen usually between 14 and 16 cm in its longest dimension (13). In portal hypertension, multiple distended veins are normally seen in the splenic hilum (Fig. 16), returning the characteristic portal venous Doppler signal. The splenic texture produces medium-level echoes and is completely homogeneous in texture.

Liver Appearance

The appearance of the liver itself should be evaluated carefully. Liver size may vary greatly from a small, contracted, end-stage organ to one that is enlarged as a result of extensive fatty infiltration (47). In the latter condition, increased attenuation and echogenicity are seen. It should be noted that recent ultrasonic attenuation quantitation studies have failed to document any increase in liver attenuation resulting from cirrhosis per se and that this characteristic is related to concomitant fatty infiltration (49). The surface of the liver is often noted to be irregular and is easily evaluated in the presence of ascites, which is common in end-stage liver disease. In contrast to the normal liver, there is usually prominence of the caudate lobe. Normally, the right lobe, measured on a transverse section, is wider than the caudate lobe. A caudate lobe/right lobe ratio exceeding 0.67 is suggestive of severe hepatocellular disease (23).

EVALUATION OF SURGICAL PORTOSYSTEMIC SHUNTS

Portal hypertension is a potentially lethal disease because of the risk of hemorrhage from esophageal varices. Numerous medical and surgical therapies for this condition have been employed, including sclerotherapy and the surgical creation of a decompressing portosystemic shunt. This great variety of procedures correctly suggests that none of them has been universally successful. The principal types of surgical shunt procedures are shown in Figs. 17–19. Questions about the patency of these shunts arise frequently, and the ability of duplex techniques to demonstrate patency noninvasively is valuable. For proper Doppler evaluation, however, it is essential that the sonographer be aware of the precise type of surgical procedure that has been performed. Both dynamic CT scanning and magnetic resonance imaging provide alternative, if more costly, methods for making such evaluations, but the presence of metallic clips may seriously degrade the quality of the CT image.

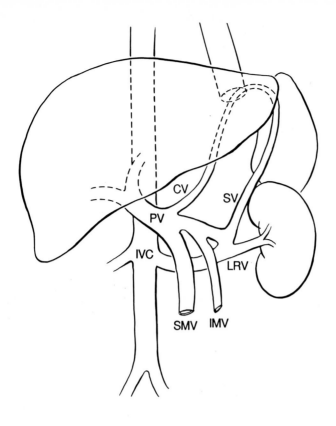

FIG. 17. Distal splenorenal shunt. Esophageal varices are present because of anastomoses between the coronary vein (CV) and the splenic vein (SV) and communications with the veins draining into the vena cavae. The splenic vein has been anastomosed with the left renal vein (LRV), producing decompression of the distended and obstructed portal venous system. IMV, inferior mesenteric vein.

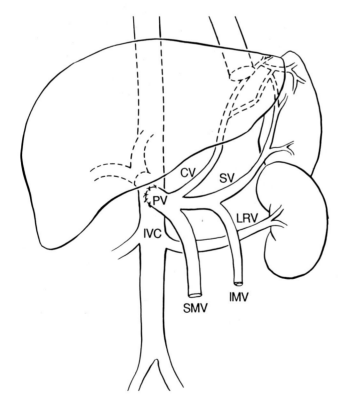

FIG. 18. End-to-side portocaval shunt. Esophageal varices are present in this hypertensive patient. The portal vein has been transected, and the distal end anastomosed to the inferior vena cava. Compare Fig. 21.

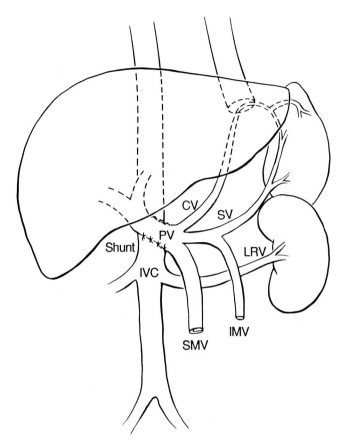

FIG. 19. Side-to-side portocaval shunt. The portal vein and inferior vena cava have been anastomosed as they lie in close proximity just before division of the portal vein into its left and right branches.

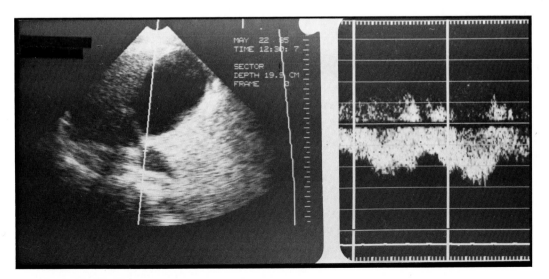

FIG. 20. Side-to-side portal venous shunt. By using the gallbladder as an acoustic window, flow can be seen through a channel into the inferior vena cava. At the site of entry of the portal venous flow, there is typically a pseudoaneurysm.

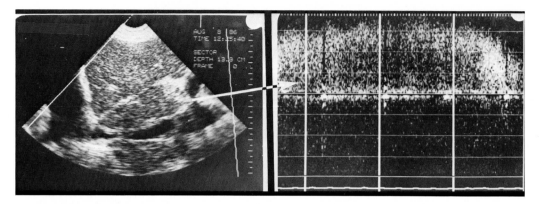

FIG. 21. End-to-side portocaval shunt. The transected end of the portal vein is clearly seen entering the inferior vena cava. Doppler examination at this point demonstrated a high-velocity flow of approximately 120 cm/sec.

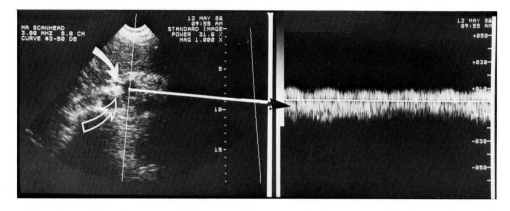

FIG. 22. Splenorenal shunt. A large patent vessel is seen between the splenic vein (*closed arrow*) and the left renal vein (*open arrow*). Typical shunt flow is seen, indicating patency of the splenorenal shunt.

The type of shunt and the body habitus of the patient suggest which patients may be optimally imaged by duplex techniques. All portocaval shunts should be amenable to duplex Doppler imaging using the gallbladder or liver as an acoustic window (Fig. 20). Portocaval shunts may be either end to side (Figs. 18 and 21) or side to side (Figs. 19 and 20). Even without Doppler scanning, patency can be suggested by the presence of a pseudoaneurysm of the IVC at the site of entry of the portal blood flow. Such an enlargement may also be seen on angiography and is caused by turbulence from the comingling blood supplies. The addition of Doppler adds certainty to the diagnosis of patency, and in this patient a stenosis was demonstrated at the anastomosis, giving a peak velocity of 120 cm/sec (Fig. 21).

Other types of surgical portosystemic shunts include proximal and distal splenorenal shunts (Figs. 17 and 22) and occasionally a mesocaval shunt. These are more difficult to display, and access is dependent on an absence of intervening gut. Techniques for imaging this area include all of those used in pancreatic sonography. Distal splenorenal shunts may be well imaged using the enlarged spleen, where present, as an acoustic window.

EVALUATION OF FLOW IN THE PORTAL VEIN

Errors in attempts to quantitate blood flow in any vessel have been addressed elsewhere (Chapter 3). In the portal vein, peculiar difficulties arise that are generally ignored in simplistic attempts to measure flow using commercially available devices. Some authors have measured the maximum blood velocity, stating quite incorrectly that the mean velocity cannot be estimated (36). In these studies, the mean velocity had been derived from the measured maximum velocity using a factor based on findings in *in vitro* experiments. Although such a method may be valid for estimation of blood flow in the normal portal vein, it is highly unlikely to be accurate in estimating flow in the hypertensive portal vein, in which flow characteristics will certainly be different. These are likely to change progressively as the portal vein increases in size, flow slows, and the vessel becomes more distended with portal hypertension. Furthermore, respiratory variations, where present, must be allowed for. Generally these variations have been ignored. Using specialized equipment, Gill (20) has made accurate estimations of portal venous flow, achieving a systematic error of only 6%. However, it is unlikely that such estimates, using commercially available equipment, will be of major clinical value. In our experience with an axial duplex scanner, the angle between the portal vein and the beam always appears to be in excess of 60°, and minor errors in this estimation will produce major errors in quantitation of flow.

SUPERIOR MESENTERIC ARTERY FLOW

The ability to demonstrate or exclude superior mesenteric artery (SMA) occlusion may be extremely valuable, for example, in elderly patients with mesenteric angina. However, flow in the inferior mesenteric artery can seldom be assessed. Figure 23 demonstrates a patient with very severe hemorrhagic pancreatitis on the basis of hyperlipidemia with serum lipid levels of 2,000 mg/dl. The abdomen was gasless and silent, and there was clinical concern that the SMA had been occluded by the severe inflammatory phlegmon. The demonstration of a normal mesenteric signal in this patient was highly reassuring.

In many of the deep abdominal vessels, variation in waveform shape with physiologic change has not been investigated. However, Qamar et al. (38,39) investigated SMA blood velocity waveforms in 82 normal subjects. The waveforms were quantitated using the pulsatility index (PI) described by Gosling and King (22). In the fasting state, the PI in the SMA was 3.57 ± 0.11, indicating a high-impedance splanchnic circulation. Following ingestion of a meal by 15 subjects, the PI decreased by 46%, and this decrease persisted for 2 hr. Qamar et al. also estimated absolute blood flow in the SMA using the duplex technique to measure the luminal area and the mean velocity. At rest, blood flow was 517 ml/min in the SMA ($n = 70$) and 703 ml/min in the celiac axis ($n = 42$) (39). Blood flow in the SMA increased by more than 100% after a solid meal and by 63% after a liquid meal (39). In contrast, the

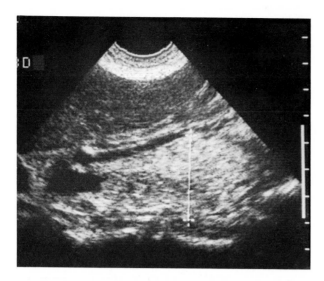

FIG. 23. Hemorrhagic pancreatitis secondary to hyperlipidemia. Longitudinal section through the head of the pancreas shows enlargement of the head of the pancreas to an AP diameter of 4 cm. This is extremely echogenic, consistent with hemorrhagic pancreatitis. Simultaneous examination demonstrated good flow in the superior mesenteric vessels.

response in the celiac axis was smaller and of shorter duration. As expected, exercise reduced both the resting and the postprandial SMA flow (39).

These estimates of SMA blood flow are consistent with other measurements using invasive methods. These include the dye-dilution method, which yielded a blood flow of 700 ml/min (34), 726 ml/min using an angiographic spillover technique (3), and 11 to 20% of the cardiac output using the videodilution technique (29).

In further experiments, quantitative estimation of blood flow in the SMA was compared in normal individuals and patients with the dumping syndrome following gastric surgery (2). At rest, patients with the dumping syndrome showed an SMA flow of 567 ± 47 ml/min compared with 493 ± 72 ml/min for the controls. Flow doubled in both groups within 5 min of a standard meal (1,232 ± 140 ml/min and 941 ± 128 ml/min, respectively). However, subsequent comparison showed increased flow in patients with the dumping syndrome (76% at 10 min, 66% at 15 min, 55% at 30 min, and 42% at 45 min) (2). These authors concluded that an abnormal redistribution of the splanchnic blood flow occurred in the dumping syndrome and may contribute to its etiology.

Doppler ultrasound has been used for assessing viability of the gut at surgery (57). When there is gangrene of the bowel it is difficult to be certain whether gut is viable, and a continuous-wave Doppler device can be quite helpful in demonstrating perfusion and hence viability.

DOPPLER EVALUATION OF PSEUDOANEURYSMS

Pseudoaneurysms of the peripancreatic arteries occur most frequently as a result of arterial wall involvement by the autolytic process occurring in pancreatitis. Such aneurysms may leak or rupture into the gut, producing melena, or into the biliary system, producing hemobilia. The possibility of a leaking pseudoaneurysm must be considered in any patient recovering from pancreatitis (Figs. 24 and 25). Since these patients are usually alcoholic, many other causes for gastrointestinal (GI) bleeding

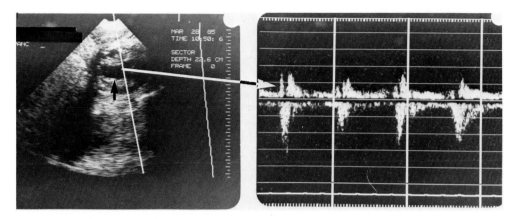

FIG. 24. Peripancreatic pseudoaneurysm. A pancreatic mass with a fluid center (*arrow*) was seen in a patient with chronic pancreatitis and a history of multiple episodes of intestinal bleeding. This was initially considered to be a pseudocyst on the basis of the B-scan appearance, but Doppler examination demonstrated a turbulent arterial signal indicating the presence of a pseudoaneurysm. (Reprinted with permission from Falkoff et al., ref. 18a.)

are possible, including esophageal varices, alcoholic gastritis, or peptic ulceration. Such patients may have numerous episodes of GI bleeding, all investigated at great cost in both time and money, before the true diagnosis is appreciated. Indeed, in one series, six of 11 patients had "blind resections" for some abnormality noted on endoscopy without improvement of their GI bleeding (6).

Patients with pancreatitis are routinely referred for ultrasound examination during their recovery to search for developing pseudocysts and to document liquefaction of the contents. Based on B-scan images alone, it is unlikely that a pseudocyst can reliably be differentiated from a pseudoaneurysm. Gooding (21) advocated the use of real-time, now almost universally applied, for the diagnosis of pseudoaneurysms, arguing that such entities showed pulsation and continuity with the surrounding vessels. However, in patients with acute or chronic pancreatitis in whom the pancreatic phlegmon is of wood-like consistency surrounded by dense, fibrous tissue and calcification, it is highly unlikely that extrinsic pulsation will be demonstrated. In fact, of the 14 cases reported in the literature, only two pseudoaneurysms exhibited pulsation (4).

An illustrative case is shown in Fig. 24. This patient was a young alcoholic with pancreatitis who had received 33 units of blood during 13 previous hospital admissions for investigation of GI bleeding. All other investigations, including endoscopy, upper and lower GI barium examinations, and two bleeding studies with ^{99m}Tc-labeled red cells, had been nondiagnostic.

An ultrasonic B-scan demonstrated an apparent thick-walled pseudocyst; meanwhile Doppler examination of the contents demonstrated turbulent flow, and the diagnosis of a pseudoaneurysm of a peripancreatic artery was made. A CT examination with a well-timed bolus injection further confirmed this diagnosis. Angiography definitively confirmed the presence of a pseudoaneurysm arising from a replaced hepatic artery (Fig. 25A), and this aneurysm was successfully embolized (Fig. 25B).

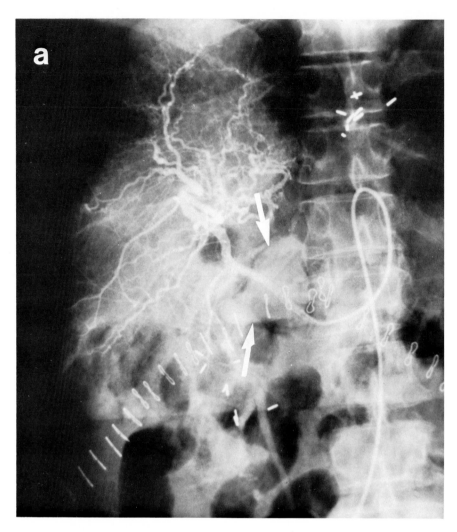

FIG. 25. A: Angiogram showing pseudoaneurysm (*arrow*) of a replaced right hepatic artery. **B:** Angiogram after successful treatment by embolization, showing obliteration of the aneurysm by coils (*arrow*). (Courtesy of D. Denny, M.D.)

Dynamic CT with a well-timed bolus may be effective as illustrated in this case. However, other reports in the literature indicate that when timing of the bolus is suboptimal, the arterial nature of the mass may be missed (41). The MRI would also be a definitive means for diagnosis of this entity because of the presence of a flow void. Nevertheless, MRI cannot compete with the economy and simplicity of a duplex Doppler examination in making this difficult diagnosis.

The clinical impact of the duplex diagnosis in this patient was extraordinarily important, permitting a noninvasive assessment of the vascular anatomy and leading to timely therapy. This case also illustrates the developing collaboration between ultrasonographers and angiographers. Duplex Doppler can be used to triage many

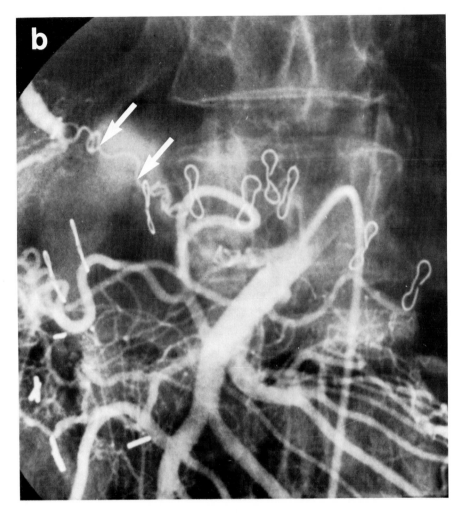

FIG. 25. (continued).

patients for vascular abnormalities, leaving angiography to confirm the diagnosis and, in many cases, also provide the definitive treatment.

LIVER TRANSPLANT EVALUATION

In our experience, duplex evaluation of liver transplants is valuable at all stages from preoperative assessment to the investigation of every potential complication with the exception of rejection (48). Because duplex Doppler equipment is portable, it is extremely valuable in the early postoperative patient who is too ill to be transported or to undergo sophisticated imaging procedures. In our first 16 patients evaluated for transplant, 84 duplex Doppler examinations were performed as compared with seven angiograms. Many of these angiograms were performed to confirm an abnormality suggested by ultrasound.

Preoperative Evaluation

In our series, we noted a number of important preoperative findings. The most common indication for liver transplantation is biliary atresia, in which the end-stage liver is small, contracted, and usually surrounded by a moat of ascites (Fig. 26). We have often seen apparent minor dilatation of the central biliary ducts, and echogenic strands extending out from the porta hepatis were seen in one patient with cholangitis. In these patients, fever, presumably caused by the cholangitis, is common but often raises the possibility of a hepatic abscess. Such an entity can reliably be excluded by ultrasound examination.

The vascular anatomy of the liver should be assessed carefully. Up to 25% of patients with biliary atresia have other major vascular anomalies including absence of the inferior vena cava or portal vein (51). To date, we have identified each of these anomalies once with angiographic confirmation in both instances. Some patients receive a liver transplant because of tumor, either a hepatoblastoma (Fig. 27) or a hepatoma. Hepatomas usually have arteriovenous shunting around the periphery, and corresponding abnormal malignant signals may be elicited on duplex examination. Particularly in patients with hepatomas, but also in any patient referred for liver transplant evaluation, it is essential to search for patency of the portal vein.

In one of our patients with a hepatoma, preoperative portal venous occlusion was noted (Fig. 6). Transplantation was finally not performed because of extrahepatic spread of hepatoma found at exploratory laparotomy and missed preoperatively by both ultrasound and CT examination. Chronic portal vein obstruction with cavernous transformation should be sought specifically. In the presence of portal vein thrombosis, subsequent transplantation may be difficult or impossible, although embolectomy of the portal vein prior to transplantation has been reported (55).

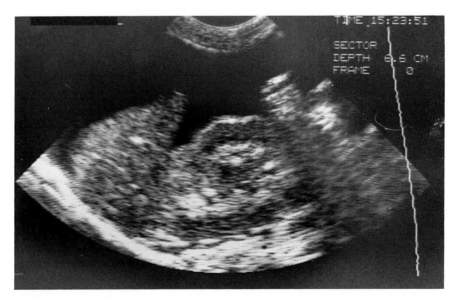

FIG. 26. End-stage liver disease in an infant with biliary atresia. A small echogenic liver is seen surrounded by a moat of ascites.

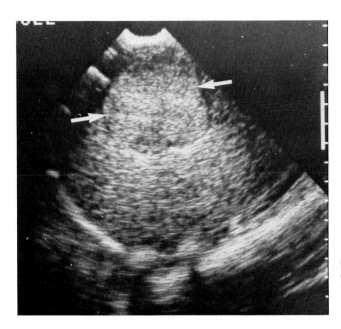

FIG. 27. Preoperative liver scan of candidate for liver transplantation showing focal echogenic mass. Biopsy revealed hepatoblastoma.

Postoperative Evaluation

One of the most critical evaluations of the postoperative liver transplant patient is that of the integrity of hepatic arterial perfusion. The anatomy of the anastomosis may vary. In our series, to facilitate anastomosis of the small hepatic artery in children, the donor aorta was also taken, permitting an aortoaortic anastomosis (Fig. 28). The anastomosed aorta demonstrating a highly unusual waveform is seen in Fig. 29. The very short duration of systole is probably related to the acoustic mismatching of the transplanted artery. Although the contribution of the hepatic artery is not essential to the viability of the normotopic liver, the orthograft, at least in adults deprived of any collateral circulation, is heavily dependent for its viability on oxygenated blood from the hepatic artery. Therefore, posttransplant hepatic arterial occlusion will lead to liver necrosis and death.

In our series of 12 completed liver transplants, hepatic arterial occlusion was diagnosed emergently in one child (Figs. 28 and 30A). A repeat scan following successful surgery showed good arterial flow (Fig. 30B). On many other occasions, however, a duplex scan, prompted by a patient's deteriorating condition, permitted prompt reassurance concerning the integrity of the hepatic arterial anastomosis. Concern about the adequacy of this anastomosis is by no means an esoteric one. The overall incidence of hepatic arterial occlusion in liver transplants is 11%. However, in children and patients with complex arterial reconstructions, the incidence may be as high as 23%.

In a series of 104 angiograms in recipients of liver orthografts, 70% were abnormal (56). The most common abnormality was hepatic arterial thrombosis, which occurred in 42% of 50 pediatric grafts. Twenty-four percent of these children survived without retransplantation because of the development of collaterals. Twelve percent of adult grafts showed hepatic arterial occlusion, and all required retransplantation. Patients

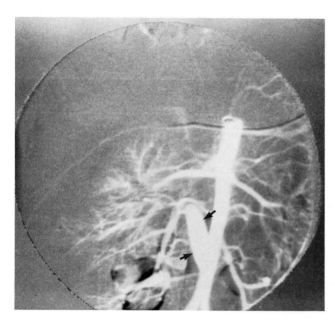

FIG. 28. Angiogram of liver orthograft recipient showing anatomy of the aortoaortic anastomosis. To avoid the need for anastomosing the small hepatic artery in children, the donor aorta has been used in the aortoaortic anastomosis, and the other branches of the celiac trunk have been ligated. In this patient, the hepatic artery is occluded. (Reprinted with permission from Taylor et al., ref. 48.)

with suspected acute hepatic arterial occlusion are invariably extremely ill and in the intensive care unit. A portable evaluation is valuable, since these patients are not fit to be taken to the CT, MRI, or angiography suite.

Portal Venous Occlusion

Wozney et al. (56) diagnosed portal vein thrombosis or stenosis in 13% of 87 patients with liver orthografts using angiography. In our series of 12 patients, portal venous occlusion occurred twice. An acute occlusion was diagnosed emergently, and a chronic obstruction was diagnosed as cavernous transformation of the portal vein. Thrombus may be seen within the portal vein (Fig. 31). However, in a recent occlusion, the portal vein may appear patent although no flow is evident on Doppler examination (e.g., Fig. 7).

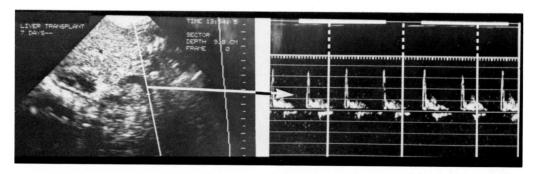

FIG. 29. B-Scan to show anastomosed aorta arching over the hilum of the right kidney. The anastamosed vessel could easily be seen on real time. Unusual waveform is seen in the anastomosed aortic graft. The pulse wave is extremely brief, probably because of mismatching. (Reprinted with permission from Taylor et al., ref. 48.)

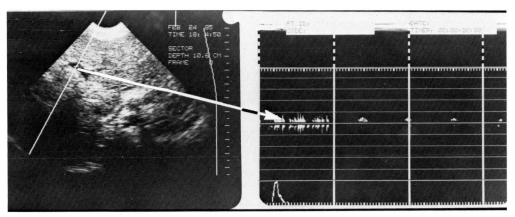

A

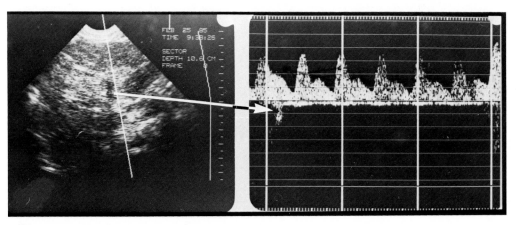

B

FIG. 30. A: Hepatic arterial occlusion in hepatic orthograft. There is absence of arterial pulsation in the hepatic artery or within the liver parenchyma. There is slight transmitted pulsation from cardiac motion. **B:** Postoperative scan after embolectomy of hepatic artery. The B-scan demonstrates air throughout the liver parenchyma, but there is normal hepatic arterial flow. (Reprinted with permission from Taylor et al., ref. 48.)

Portal Vein Stenosis

Portal vein stenosis occurred in two patients, one of whom died soon thereafter from acute rejection. The other patient is alive and well 18 months after diagnosis. Prior to our report in the literature (48), portal vein stenosis in recipients of liver orthografts had been diagnosed only by portography (43). The stenotic area was clearly seen on the B-scan (Fig. 32). As in the diagnosis of carotid artery stenosis, concomitant Doppler examination allowed quantitation of the severity of the stenosis. Before the stenosis, normal low flow was seen in the portal vein. A high-velocity jet, approximately three times the normal velocity, occurred at the site of the stenosis with distal turbulence, producing an irregular waveform with flow in both directions (Fig. 32). We considered this to be indicative of a significant stenosis, and subsequent

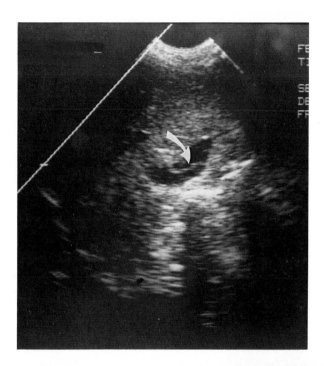

FIG. 31. Portal venous thrombosis in hepatic orthograft. Thrombus (*arrow*) is seen in the right portal vein. Doppler examination demonstrated no evidence of flow. (Reprinted with permission from Taylor et al., ref. 48.)

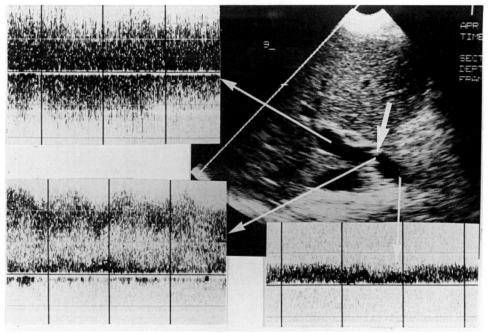

FIG. 32. Portal venous stenosis in liver orthograft recipient. The B-scan demonstrates an apparent stenosis (*arrow*) in the middle of the portal vein. Doppler examination demonstrates the hemodynamic results of this. Before the stenotic area, the waveform in the portal vein is normal. At the stenosis, there is a high-velocity jet, but more distally the waveform is irregular, and there is flow in both forward and reverse directions associated with eddy currents. (Reprinted with permission from Taylor et al., ref. 48.)

portography demonstrated a stenosis of approximately 60% diameter reduction. Since diagnosis, this patient has been followed noninvasively by duplex techniques, and the degree of stenosis has been stable during this interval. However, had there been evidence of a progressive lesion, it would have indicated the need for angioplasty to prevent subsequent thrombosis of the portal vein.

Biliary Obstruction

A number of different types of anastomoses may be used to drain the biliary system, and any of these may result in bilary occlusion caused by stricture or hemobilia. The latter may occur secondary to biopsy. Figure 33 shows the liver of a child with worsening jaundice. The differential diagnosis lay between a severe rejection episode and mechanical obstruction of the bile ducts. On B-scan imaging alone, the dilated ducts in the region of the porta hepatis could be mistaken for dilated varices, and the absence of flow in these vessels suggested biliary dilatation. At surgery, gross dilatation of the biliary system was found, and the anastomosis was refashioned.

Rejection Episodes

In some rejection episodes, it was noted that the normal diastolic component of the hepatic arterial signal was lost, giving a high-impedance signal. It was considered possible that a similar phenomenon might be seen in liver transplant rejection as we had observed in renal allografts. However, further observation demonstrated no consistent trend, and the cause of the high-impedance signal is not apparent. Isotope scanning with diisopropylacetanilide iminodiacetic acid (DISIDA) was found to be the most effective way of monitoring liver function in rejection episodes.

Effects of Biopsy

In several patients, small holes full of flocculent material were seen post-biopsy, and these were assumed to be intrahepatic hematomas associated with biopsy. Since

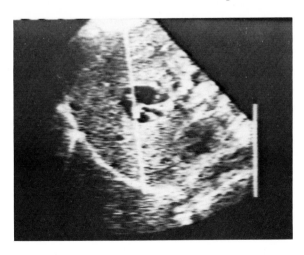

FIG. 33. Biliary obstruction in a liver orthograft recipient. This child demonstrated worsening jaundice, and the differential diagnosis lay between graft rejection and obstruction at the biliary anastamosis. The B-scan demonstrates gross dilatation of vessels in the porta hepatis. (Reprinted with permission from Taylor et al., ref. 48.) It was unclear whether this was caused by dilated biliary vessels or varices. Doppler examination demonstrated absence of portal venous flow, correctly indicating that the appearances were caused by dilated biliary vessels. The biliary anastamosis was refashioned with resolution of the jaundice.

biopsies are performed frequently in these patients, such findings are common. As noted above, biopsy may also result in hemobilia, giving rise to echogenic debris within a dilated biliary system.

Perihepatic Fluid Collection

Perihepatic fluid collections were common in our patients, occurring in 25% of those examined. By imaging alone it was impossible to differentiate among hematomas, seromas, bilomas, and abcsesses. Where infections were suspected, the patient was usually extremely toxic and in the intensive care unit. In these patients it was usual to aspirate the fluid collection under ultrasound guidance and, if it proved purulent, to proceed to catheter drainage at the bedside. In severely immunosuppressed patients, overwhelming sepsis can occur easily and quickly. Duplex scanning is valuable in these patients for localization of fluid collections and their guided aspiration.

TUMORS

Doppler examination of tumors appears to be particularly valuable in some tumors related to the gastrointestinal tract.

Liver

Echogenic lesions of the liver frequently present a diagnostic dilemma, especially in patients with diffuse hepatocellular disease. The differential diagnosis includes focal fat, hemangiomas, hepatomas, metastases, and, very rarely, "regenerating nodules." Birnholz (5) described the sonographic appearance of regenerating nodules, but our clinical experience has been that these are very seldom visualized. Indeed, in 22 patients with biopsy-proven cirrhosis, focal lesions were seen in five patients, and biopsy revealed tumor in all (47). Thus, we do not feel that focal liver lesions should ever be dismissed as regenerating nodules but should be biopsied to exclude a hepatoma or metastases. This was further investigated by Freeman et al. (19). It was shown that regenerating nodules were clearly seen when scanned *in vitro* at a frequency of 7.5 MHz but could not be delineated when scanned either *in vitro* or *in vivo* at a frequency of 3 MHz.

Duplex Doppler examination, using a frequency of 3 MHz, provides another way to evaluate these lesions since to date we have found high-velocity signals in all hepatomas (Fig. 34). Of 14 hepatomas to date, two have had signals of 3 kHz, whereas the remaining 12 have given rise to signals of 5 kHz or higher (Fig. 35). In contrast, hemangiomas have yielded little or no signal. The reason for this is readily apparent. In hepatomas, there is arterioportal shunting around the periphery of these tumors. Thus, the resulting Doppler shift is of high velocity because of the relatively large pressure gradient between the arteries and veins. In contrast, hemangiomas display cavernous spaces in which blood flows very slowly, hence the need for a delayed CT examination after contrast administration. This low-flow signal is removed in Doppler signal processing by the high-pass filter.

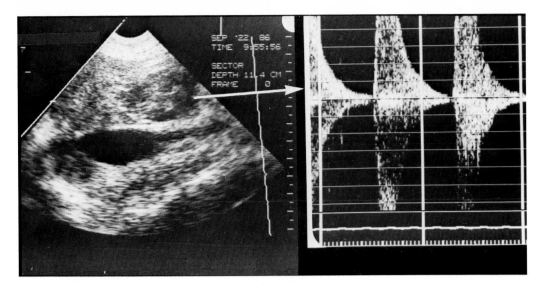

FIG. 34. Tumor signals in a hepatoma. A 4-cm hypoechoic mass is seen in the liver. Tumor signals exceeding 5 kHz and producing aliasing are demonstrated at the periphery of a focal liver mass. Our experience to date indicates that this evidence of arterioportal shunting is highly suggestive of a hepatoma. (Reprinted with permission from Taylor et al., ref. 50.)

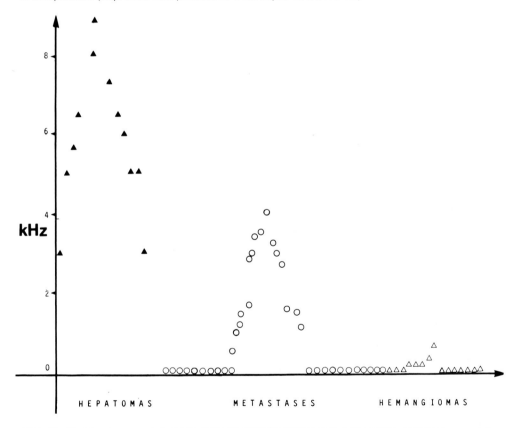

FIG. 35. Plot to show peak systolic Doppler shift frequencies in hepatomas, metastases, and hemangiomas. The mean systolic velocity is 5.8 ± 1.8 kHz for hepatomas, 0.9 ± 1.3 kHz for metastases, and 0.1 ± 0.2 for hemangiomas. Hepatoma signals are significantly different from both metastases and hemangioma signals ($p < 0.001$).

In contrast to hepatomas, two-thirds of metastases give rise to no detectable Doppler signals. The remaining one-third give Doppler signals up to 4 kHz, overlapping with the lowest signals seen in hepatomas. However, in our work to date, signals of 5 kHz or above have always proved to be associated with hepatomas (50).

Pancreas

In ten of 12 pancreatic malignant tumors examined to date, Doppler shift signals of 3 to 10 kHz have been elicited. One such example is given in Fig. 36. This is more surprising than the presence of similar signals in hepatomas, since pancreatic cancers are typically hypovascular on angiography.

Colon

Most colonic primary tumors are obviously not amenable to ultrasonic examination. However, we have found typical neovascular Doppler signals in several patients with recurrent colonic tumors in areas with ultrasonic access.

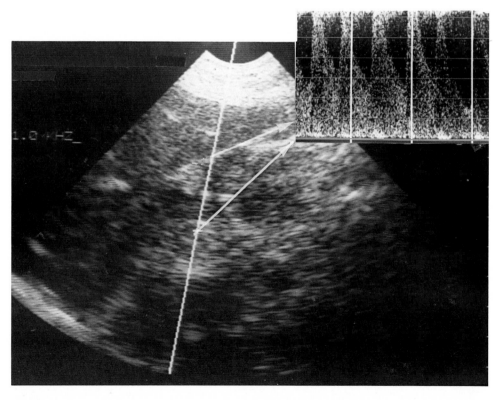

FIG. 36. Tumor signals in a pancreatic tumor. A pancreatic mass is apparent and was considered to result from chronic pancreatitis on a CT scan. Doppler examination demonstrated 9-kHz tumor signals. To date, we have not seen such arteriovenous shunting in pancreatitis, indicating the high probability of tumor. Subsequently, this patient developed liver metastases and died soon after.

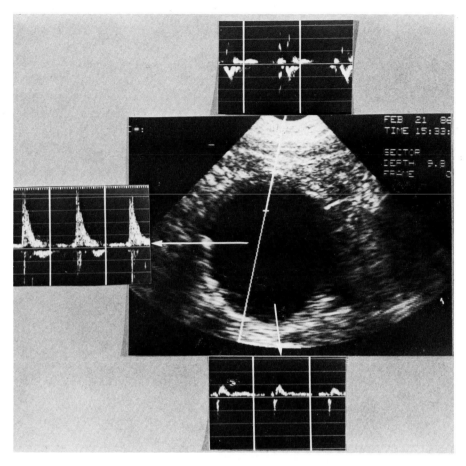

FIG. 37. Transverse scan of abdominal aortic aneurysm. Waveforms within the aneurysm show a central high-velocity jet, which slows within the dilated segment, producing reversed flow and eddy currents nearer the wall. Areas of virtual stasis may be noted.

ABDOMINAL AORTIC ANEURYSM

Doppler examination allows differentiation of the flow characteristics within aortic aneurysms and may be helpful in the diagnosis of a dissection. The flow within an aneurysm may be extremely complex (Fig. 37). A central high-velocity jet into the central axis of the aneurysm slows within it and gives rise to eddy currents with a reversed component or even absence of flow near the aneurysm wall.

COLOR FLOW MAPPING

The eventual importance of color flow mapping in gastrointestinal applications of Doppler ultrasound is difficult to predict. Most of these machines have been designed for cardiac applications and are relatively insensitive for use in the abdomen. These machines do, however, image flow in the larger vessels. It is important, however, that insensitivity of a machine not be mistaken for a thrombosis. Much more sensitive machines are becoming available.

It is also important to understand that color allocation is on the basis of direction of flow with respect to the transducer. Thus, hepatic arterial flow, portal venous flow, caval flow, and hepatic venous flow during atrial systole will all be displayed in the same color.

Certainly, color Doppler displays would be most helpful in locating the high-velocity jets in tumors. Tumor signals are of very low amplitude, so sensitivity is paramount. The value of a new generation of sensitive color imaging devices for the demonstration of neovascularity awaits evaluation.

CONCLUSION

Duplex Doppler ultrasound is an important new modality for use in the abdomen. It extends the use of ultrasound from the mere display of morphology to the simultaneous evaluation of function and perfusion. Simplistic applications, such as the diagnosis of deep venous thrombosis or arterial occlusion, are extraordinarily valuable, especially since they can be performed portably. Doppler examination aids identification of the nature of a structure because of its specific perfusion characteristics. Finally, much more work needs to be done on tumor signals, since this promises to be one of the most rewarding areas for future tissue characterization.

REFERENCES

1. Aagaard, J., Jensen, L. I., Sorensen, T. I. A., Christensen, U., and Burcharth, F. (1982): Recanalized umbilical vein in portal hypertension. *Am. J. Roentgenol.,* 139:1107–1109.

2. Aldoori, M. I., Qamar, M. I., Read, A. E., and Williamson, R. C. N. (1985): Increased flow in the superior mesenteric artery in dumping syndrome. *Br. J. Surg.,* 72:389–390.

3. Anderson, J., and Gianturco, C. (1981): Angiographic spillover technique for estimating blood flow. In: *Measurement of Blood Flow, Applications to the Splanchnic Circulation,* edited by D. N. Granger, G. B. Buckley, pp. 401–424. Williams & Wilkins, Baltimore.

4. Athey, P. A., Sax, S. L., Lamki, N., and Cadavid, G. (1986): Sonography in the diagnosis of hepatic artery aneurysms. *Am. J. Roentgenol.,* 147:725–727.

5. Birnholz, J. C. (1979): Ultrasound evaluation of diffuse liver disease. In: *Clinics in Diagnostic Ultrasound, Vol. 1,* edited by K. J. W. Taylor, pp. 23–33. Churchill-Livingstone, New York.

6. Bivens, B. A., Sachatello, C. R., Chuang, V. P., and Brady, P. (1978): Hemosuccus pancreatitis (hemoductal pancreatitis): Gastrointestinal hemorrhage due to rupture of splenic artery aneurysm into the pancreatic duct. *Arch. Surg.,* 113:751–753.

7. Bolondi, L., Gandolfi, L., Arienti, V., Caletti, G. C., Corcioni, E., Gasbarrini, G., and Labo, G. (1982): Ultrasonography in the diagnosis of portal hypertension: Diminished response of portal vessels to respiration. *Radiology,* 142:167–172.

8. Brunelle, F., Alagille, D., Pariente, D., and Chaumont, P. (1981): An ultrasound study of portal hypertension in children. *Ann. Radiol. (Paris),* 24:121–130.

9. Burcharth, F. (1979): Percutaneous transhepatic portography. I. Technique and application. *Am. J. Roentgenol.,* 132:177–182.

10. Burcharth, F., Nielbo, N., and Andersen, B. (1979): Percutaneous transhepatic portography. II. Comparison with splenoportography in portal hypertension. *Am. J. Roentgenol.,* 132:183–185.

11. Burcharth, F., Sorensen, T. I. A., and Andersen, B. (1979): Percutaneous transhepatic portography. III. Relationships between portosystemic collaterals and portal pressure in cirrhosis. *Am. J. Roentgenol.,* 133:1119–1122.

12. Dach, J. L., Hill, M. C., Pelaez, J. C., LePage, J. R., and Russell, E. (1981): Sonography of hypertensive portal venous system: Correlation with arterial portography. *Am. J. Roentgenol.,* 137:511–517.

13. De Graaff, C. S., Taylor, K. J. W., and Jacobson, P. (1979): Grey scale echography of the spleen: follow-up in 67 patients. *Ultrasound Med. Biol.*, 5:13–21.

14. Di Candio, G., Campatelli, A., Mosca, F., Santi, V., Casanova, P., and Bolondi, L. (1985): Ultrasound detection of unusual spontaneous portosystemic shunts associated with uncomplicated portal hypertension. *J. Ultrasound Med.*, 4:297–305.

15. Doehner, G. A., Ruzicka, F. F., Hoffman, G., and Rousselot, L. M. (1955): The portal venous system: Its roentgen anatomy. *Radiology*, 64:675–689.

16. Doehner, G. A., Ruzicka, F. F., Rousselot, L. M., and Hoffman, G. (1956): The portal venous system: On its pathological roentgen anatomy. *Radiology*, 66:206–217.

17. Dokmeci, A. K., Kimura, K., Matsutani, S., Ohto, M., Ono, T., Tsuchiya, Y., Saisho, H., and Okuda, K. (1981): Collateral veins in portal hypertension: Demonstration by sonography. *Am. J. Roentgenol.*, 137:1173–1177.

18. Fakhry, J., Gosink, B. B., and Leopold, G. R. (1981): Recanalized umbilical vein due to portal vein occlusion: Documentation by sonography. *Am. J. Roentgenol.*, 137:410–412.

18a. Falkoff, G. E., Taylor, K. J. W., and Morse, S. (1986): Hepatic artery pseudoaneurysm: Diagnosis with real-time and pulsed Doppler US. *Radiology*, 158:55–56.

19. Freeman, M. P., Vick, C. W., Taylor, K. J. W., Carithers, R. L., and Brewer, W. H. (1986): Regenerating nodules in cirrhosis: Sonographic appearance with anatomic correlation. *Am. J. Roentgenol.*, 146:533–536.

20. Gill, R. W. (1979): Pulsed Doppler with B-mode imaging for quantitative blood flow measurement. *Ultrasound Med. Biol.*, 5:223–235.

21. Gooding, G. A. W. (1981): Ultrasound of a superior mesenteric artery aneurysm secondary to pancreatitis: A plea for real-time ultrasound of sonolucent masses in pancreatitis. *J. Clin. Ultrasound*, 9:255–256.

22. Gosling, R. G., and King, D. H. (1974): Arterial assessment by Doppler-shift ultrasound. *Proc. R. Soc. Med.*, 67(b):447–449.

23. Harbin, W. P., Robert, N. J., and Ferrucci, J. T., Jr. (1980): Diagnosis of cirrhosis based on regional changes in hepatic morphology: Radiological and pathological analysis. *Radiology*, 135:273–283.

24. Joly, J. G., Marleau, D., Legare, A., Lavoie, P., Bernier, J., and Viallet, A. (1971): Bleeding from esophageal varices in cirrhosis of the liver: Hemodynamic and radiological criteria for the selection of potential bleeders through hepatic and umbilicoportal catheterization studies. *Can. Med. Assoc. J.*, 104:576–580.

25. Juttner, H.-U., Jenney, J. M., Ralls, P. W., Goldstein, L. I., and Reynolds, T. B. (1982): Ultrasound demonstration of portosystemic collaterals in cirrhosis and portal hypertension. *Radiology*, 142:459–463.

26. Kane, R. A., and Katz, S. G. (1982): The spectrum of sonographic findings in portal hypertension: A subject review and new observations. *Radiology*, 142:453–458.

27. Lafortune, M., Constantin, A., Breton, G., Legare, A. G., and Lavoie, P. (1985): The recanalized umbilical vein in portal hypertension: A myth. *Am. J. Roentgenol.*, 144:549–553.

28. Lafortune, M., Marleau, D., Breton, G., Viallet, A., Lavoie, P., and Huet, P.-M. (1984): Portal venous system measurements in portal hypertension. *Radiology*, 151:27–30.

29. Lantz, B. M., Link, D. P., Holcroft, J. W., and Foerster, J. M. (1981): Video-dilution technique: Angiographic determination of splanchnic blood flow. In: *Measurement of Blood Flow, Applications to the Splanchnic Circulation*, edited by D. N. Granger and G. B. Buckley, pp. 425–437. Williams & Wilkins, Baltimore.

30. Lebrec, D., DeFleury, P., Rueff, B., Nahum, H., and Benhamou, J.-P. (1980): Portal hypertension, size of esophageal varices and risk of gastrointestinal bleeding in alcoholic cirrhosis. *Gastroenterology*, 79:1139–1144.

31. Marchal, G. J. R., Van Holsbeeck, M., Tshibwabwa-Ntumba, E., Goddeeris, P. G., Fevery, J., Oyen, R. H., Adisoejoso, B., Baert, A. L., and Van Steenbergen, W. (1985): Dilatation of the cystic veins in portal hypertension: Sonographic demonstration. *Radiology*, 154:187–189.

32. McCormack, T., Smallwood, R. H., Walton, R. H., Martin, T., Robinson, P., and Johnson, A. G. (1983): Doppler ultrasound probe for assessment of blood-flow in oesophageal varices. *Lancet*, 1:677.

33. McIndoe, A. H. (1928): Vascular lesions of portal cirrhosis. *Arch. Pathol.*, 5:23–40.

34. Norryd, C., Denker, H., Lunderquist, A., and Olin, T. (1974): Superior mesenteric flow in man studied with dye-dilution technique. *Acta Chir. Scand.*, 141:109–118.

35. Nunez, D., Russell, E., Yrizarry, J., Peiras, R., and Viamonte, M. (1978): Portosystemic communications studied by transhepatic portography. *Radiology*, 127:75–79.

36. Ohnishi, K., Saito, M., Koen, H., Nakayama, T., Nomura, F., and Okuda, K. (1985): Pulsed Doppler flow as a criterion of portal venous velocity: Comparison with cineangiographic measurements. *Radiology*, 154:495–498.

37. Pollack, D., and Taylor, K. J. W. (1981): Ultrasound scanning in patients with clinical suspicion of pancreatic cancer: A retrospective study. *Cancer*, 47:1662–1665.

38. Qamar, M. I., Read, A. E., Skidmore, R., Evans, J. M., and Wells, P. N. T. (1984): Non-invasive assessment of the superior mesenteric artery blood flow in man. *Gut*, 25:A546–547.

39. Qamar, M. I., Read, A. E., Skidmore, R., Evans, J. M., and Wells, P. N. T. (1986): Transcutaneous Doppler ultrasound measurement of superior mesenteric artery blood flow in man. *Gut*, 27:100–105.

40. Saddekni, S., Hutchinson, D. E., and Cooperberg, P. L. (1982): The sonographically patent umbilical vein in portal hypertension. *Radiology*, 145:441–443.

41. Shultz, S., Druy, E. M., and Friedman, A. C. (1985): Common hepatic artery aneurysm: Pseudocysts of the pancreas. *Am. J. Roentgenol.*, 144:1287–1288.

42. Smith-Laing, G., Camilo, M. E., Dick, R., and Sherlock, S. (1980): Percutaneous transhepatic portography in the assessment of portal hypertension. Clinical correlations and comparison of radiographic techniques. *Gastroenterology*, 78:197–205.

43. Starzl, T. E., Porter, K. A., and Francavilla, J. A. (1978): A hundred years of the hepatotrophic controversy. *Ciba Found. Symp.*, 55:111–129.

44. Subramanyam, B. R., Balthazar, E. J., Madamba, M. R., Raghavendra, B. N., Horii, S. C., and Lefleur, R. S. (1983): Sonography of portosystemic venous collaterals in portal hypertension. *Radiology*, 146:161–166.

45. Taylor, K. J. W., and Burns, P. N. (1985): Duplex Doppler scanning in the pelvis and abdomen. *Ultrasound Med. Biol.*, 11:643–658.

46. Taylor, K. J. W., Burns, P. N., Woodcock, J. P., and Wells, P. N. T. (1985): Blood flow in deep abdominal and pelvic vessels: Ultrasonic pulsed-Doppler analysis. *Radiology*, 154:487–493.

47. Taylor, K. J. W., Gorelick, F. S., Rosenfield, A. T., and Riely, C. A. (1981): Ultrasonography of alcoholic liver disease with histological correlation. *Radiology*, 141:157–161.

48. Taylor, K. J. W., Morse, S. S., Weltin, G. G., Riely, C. A., and Flye, M. W. (1986): Liver transplant recipients: Portable duplex US with correlative angiography. *Radiology*, 159:357–363.

49. Taylor, K. J. W., Riely, C. A., Hammers, L., Flax, S., Weltin G., Garcia-Tsao, G., Conn, H. O., Kuc, R., and Barwick, K. W. (1986): Quantitative attenuation in normal liver and in patients with diffuse liver disease: Importance of fat. *Radiology*, 158:65–71.

50. Taylor, K. J. W., Ramos, I., Morse, S. S., Fortune, K. L., Hammers, L., and Taylor, C. R. (1987): Focal liver masses: Differential diagnosis with pulsed Doppler ultrasound. *Radiology*, 164:643–647.

51. Teichburg, S., Markowitz, J., Silverberg, M., (1982): Abnormal cilia in a child with polysplenia syndrome and extrahepatic biliary atresia. *J. Pediatr.*, 100:399–401.

52. Traverso, L. W. (1981): Is hepatic portal venous gas an indication for exploratory laparotomy? *Arch. Surg.*, 16:936–938.

53. Weinreb, J., Kumari, S., Phillips, G., and Pochaczevsky, R. (1982): Portal vein measurements by real-time sonography. *Am. J. Roentgenol.*, 139:497–499.

54. Weltin, G., Taylor, K. J. W., and Carter, A. R. (1984): Duplex Doppler: An aid in the diagnosis of cavernous transformation of the portal vein. *Am. J. Roentgenol.*, 44:999–1001.

55. Williams, J. W., Britt, L. G., Peters, T. G., Vera, S. R., and Haggitt, R. C. (1984): Portal vein obstruction in patients requiring hepatic resection or transplantation. *Am. J. Surg.*, 50:465–468.

56. Wozney, P., Zajko, A. B., Bron, K. M., Point, S., and Starzl, T. E. (1986): Vascular complications after liver transplantation: A 5 year experience. *Am. J. Roentgenol.*, 147:657–663.

57. Wright, C. B., and Hobson, R. W. (1975): Prediction of intestinal viability using Doppler ultrasound techniques. *Am. J. Surg.*, 129:642–645.

7 / Renal Duplex Sonography

Christopher M. Rigsby, Peter N. Burns, and Kenneth J. W. Taylor

*Department of Diagnostic Radiology, Yale University School of Medicine,
New Haven, Connecticut 06510*

The application of Doppler ultrasound in evaluating native and allografted kidneys is an area of increasing interest and investigation. Duplex Doppler equipment, which combines on-line spectrum analysis of the Doppler shift frequency with B-scan imaging, permits simultaneous evaluation of physiologic renal blood flow velocity changes with morphologic assessment of the organ. Doppler can be used for documenting renal arterial and venous flow for the exclusion of vascular obstruction (5,14,19,21,27,31), and some success has been reported for detecting main renal artery stenosis (5,12,14,19,21,27). Doppler techniques can often show blood flow velocity changes in episodes of acute allograft rejection (2,3,7,20,25,26,28,31) and may be helpful in distinguishing this from other causes of graft dysfunction. Vascular complications in the transplanted kidney can also be identified (3,7,16,24,26,31,33).

In this chapter, we discuss the use and limitations of Doppler in evaluating native and transplanted kidneys.

NATIVE KIDNEYS

Doppler evaluation of the main renal artery and vein is best performed with the patient supine, using a 3-MHz transducer. The transducer is placed in the upper abdomen along the midline, oriented transversely. These vessels can be identified on the B-scan image in relation to the aorta and inferior vena cava (Figs. 1 and 2). Overlying bowel gas and excessive retroperitoneal fat frequently obscure portions of the retroperitoneum, particularly on the left. Therefore, insonation of the major renal vessels may be limited. Overnight fasting, however, may minimize interference resulting from bowel gas.

Doppler signals obtained from the normal main renal artery show a peak in frequency shift in systole, followed by a gradual diminution throughout diastole (Fig. 1). These changes in Doppler shift frequency reflect changes in blood flow velocity. A spectral "window" is present in systole, resulting from near uniform blood flow velocity with a blunted parabolic profile. The gradual decrease in flow velocity ob-

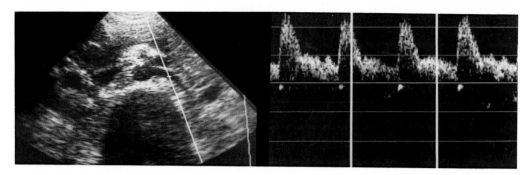

FIG. 1. Normal main renal artery. Transverse sonogram of retroperitoneum at level of renal hila. Doppler sample volume cursor (*small white bar*) is positioned in the left renal artery. Corresponding Doppler signals show a systolic peak in blood flow velocity followed by a gradual decrease in diastole. A spectral window is present in systole.

served in diastole results from the normal low peripheral vascular impedance within the kidney. Doppler signals obtained from the main renal vein show flow in a direction opposite to that of arterial flow (Fig. 2). Venous flow is continuous, and mild respiratory and cardiac variation may be identified, similar to that in the inferior vena cava.

To evaluate the intrarenal arterial system, the patient should be placed in the contralateral decubitus position, imaging the kidney in a coronal plane. Doppler signals can be obtained from the proximal arterial and segmental branches as well as the interlobar and arcuate arteries. Although these vessels may be too small to be resolved on the real-time image, the Doppler-gated cursor can be positioned in the appropriate anatomic location until spectra from the desired vessel are obtained. Doppler arterial signals obtained with the cursor positioned in the renal sinus would correspond to proximal arterial and segmental branches (Fig. 3). Arterial signals obtained along the lateral aspect of a medullary pyramid would represent interlobar arterial signals, and arcuate arterial signals would be obtained more peripherally, at the corticomedullary junction. Doppler signals obtained from these intrarenal arteries resemble those obtained from the main renal artery, although they become

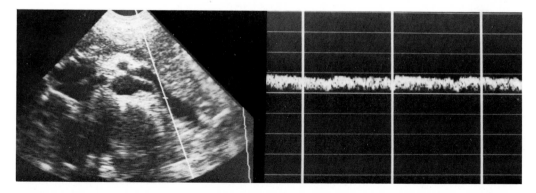

FIG. 2. Normal renal vein. Transverse sonogram of retroperitoneum at level of renal hila. Doppler sample volume cursor (*small white bar*) is located in the left renal vein. Doppler signals show continuous blood flow with minimal respiratory variation.

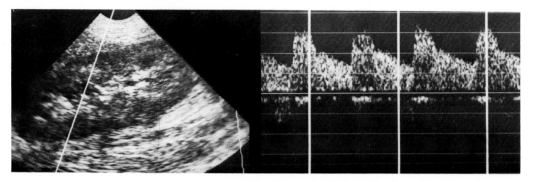

FIG. 3. Normal intrarenal arterial Doppler signals. Coronal sonogram of right kidney. Doppler sample volume cursor is positioned within the renal sinus. Doppler signals from a segmental artery were obtained. The waveform resembles that obtained from the main renal artery (Fig. 1), although no spectral window is present during systole.

more damped as they are traced distally. There is normally a systolic peak in shift frequency followed by a gradual decrease during diastole with persistent antegrade flow. A spectral window in systole, however, is generally not appreciated in signals obtained from these intrarenal arterial branches. Venous flow can be identified in the kidney that is continuous and in a direction opposite to that of arterial flow.

Renal Artery Stenosis

The reported prevalence of renovascular disease varies from less than 1% (35) up to 10% (18) of hypertensive patients. Definitive diagnosis and quantitation by measurement of pressure gradient can only be established by arteriography. However, this procedure is expensive, invasive, and, therefore, generally used for confirming suspected disease rather than for screening purposes. Screening should be selective because of the prohibitive cost of screening all hypertensive patients, the small number of patients with renovascular disease, and the even smaller number of patients who will benefit from surgical correction of such disease.

Rapid sequence excretory urography and renal scintigraphy have been used for screening patients for renovascular disease. A true positive rate for prediction of surgical cure or improvement of 60.2% has been reported by Thornbury using excretory urography (34). The probability for a favorable surgical outcome in hypertensive patients having positive studies was 24%, and reanalysis of the Cooperative Study data showed a false-negative rate for screening of at least 21.8% (34). As a result, excretory urography is no longer recommended for screening hypertensive patients. The reported sensitivity of radionuclide renal scanning in screening for renovascular disease is as high as 88% (17). However, it is less specific than the urogram as a result of difficulty in distinguishing between unilateral renovascular lesions and unilateral parenchymal disease (17). Therefore, the need for a simple and noninvasive diagnostic procedure with acceptable sensitivity and specificity for the detection of renovascular disease clearly remains.

Various studies using duplex sonography have been reported, attempting to meet the demands for a screening technique. However, it remains unclear whether Doppler examination will prove efficacious in this regard. In this clinical setting, Doppler ultrasound is used to detect flow disturbances resulting from partial vascular obstruction, specifically to identify increased blood flow velocity in a stenotic segment (jet effect) and nonlaminar disturbed flow, including turbulence, in poststenotic segments.

Duplex interrogation of the renal arteries is occasionally unsuccessful, with technically inadequate examinations occurring in 6% (21) to 21% (12) of patients studied. Factors that prevent insonation of one or both renal arteries include recent oral intake, intestinal gas, scarring from previous abdominal surgery, obesity, abdominal aortic aneurysms, ascites, and significant vessel calcification.

Greene et al. (12) reported the noninvasive characterization of renal artery blood flow variables to calculate volume flow rate in renal arteries. The data obtained were used to detect renal artery occlusive disease. A reduction in lumen cross section, measured convective increases in spatial average velocity, or increased Doppler audio spectra broadening were used as criteria for partial obstruction. Only a small number of patients were evaluated, however, and the method is cumbersome and time consuming, occasionally requiring over 1 hr to obtain technically adequate results. Subsequently, other investigators elaborated on waveform changes observed in patients with significant renal artery stenosis (greater than 60% diameter reduction) documented by arteriography (19,21,27). They observed an irregular waveform with spectral broadening, a rounded or nondistinct peak, and a localized increase in peak systolic frequency associated with a sudden decrease in frequency distally (19,21,27). In one study, the localized increased peak frequency was greater than 4 kHz with a 3-MHz transducer (21). These criteria for stenosis yielded a sensitivity of 83% and specificity of 97% in studies of 120 (21), 124 (19), and 95 patients (27).

Avasthi et al. (5) studied 68 patients for renal artery disease with duplex sonography. Eleven patients (16%) had technically inadequate studies, and 17 patients (30%) required two separate studies to obtain a technically adequate examination. Twenty-six patients were subjected to arteriography. The presence of one or more of the following hemodynamic abnormalities observed by Doppler examination was used to diagnose stenosis: peak blood velocity of 100 cm/sec, absence of blood velocity during diastole, absence of any detectable blood velocity indicating occlusion, or broad-band Doppler frequency spectra caused by focal blood velocity disturbances. In this study, calculation of absolute blood flow velocity was made after measurement of the angle between the ultrasound beam and the vessel examined. Interoperator variability for measurement of this angle was $\pm 3°$, which, at an angle of 60°, produced an error of less than 10% in the velocity calculation. The sensitivity for renal artery stenosis was 89% with a specificity of 73% using this method.

Most recently, Kohler et al. (14) reported using the ratio of peak renal artery velocity to aortic velocity (RAR) to distinguish stenotic (greater than 60% diameter reduction) from nonstenotic renal arteries in a retrospective study. Ninety percent of the duplex examinations were technically adequate, and arteriographic correlation was available for 43 renal arteries. With an RAR of greater than 3.5 taken to indicate a stenotic lesion, this method yielded a sensitivity of 91% and specificity of 95%.

In conclusion, it remains unclear whether duplex sonography will be useful for screening patients suspected of having renal artery stenosis. It is noninvasive and therefore well suited for following patients after revascularization or angioplasty. However, it is highly operator dependent, and a significant number of patients fail to have technically adequate examinations. Some of the criteria used for diagnosis are subjective and therefore difficult to apply. Sample volume size must be large to avoid signal loss from respiratory motion. This results in spectral broadening of the waveform even with normal vessels, since signals are obtained from the entire cross section of the artery and not just the center stream. Calculation of absolute blood flow velocity is limited by the need to measure the probe–vessel angle accurately, and this is often difficult to define. Use of a threshold peak frequency shift (e.g., 4 kHz) or the RAR is also probe–vessel angle dependent. However, one can manually vary the angle to achieve maximum frequency shift without necessarily measuring the incident angle. Thus far, the results of duplex sonography for identifying significant renal artery stenosis appear encouraging, but additional clinical investigation in prospective studies is required.

Vascular Occlusion

Duplex sonography can be used for providing or excluding the diagnosis of renal artery or vein occlusion (Fig. 4). Occlusion of the main renal artery can be suspected when one fails to obtain signals from the vessel (5,14,19,21,27,31). False-negative studies result when flow in a collateral vessel near the renal hilum is misinterpreted as main renal arterial flow (14). Careful examination and identification of the renal artery from its origin to the hilum are required, therefore, to avoid this pitfall. Furthermore, one should attempt to identify intrarenal arterial flow in these cases (31). The absence of intrarenal flow clearly would be a supportive finding for main vessel occlusion. However, in long-standing renal artery occlusion, collateral channels may develop to reconstitute retrograde intrarenal and even distal main renal arterial flow (1), thus posing another potential pitfall.

Avasthi and coworkers (4) have reported on the application of Doppler ultrasound in evaluating patients for renal vein thrombosis. After measuring the Doppler incident angle and renal venous luminal diameter, they calculated the mean left and right renal venous blood flow velocities in 12 normal subjects (left renal vein 40.2 ± 10.9 cm/sec; right renal vein 43.5 ± 13.9 cm/sec). The investigators then assumed a 95% confidence level value of the mean velocity of less than two standard deviations of the average value obtained from the normal subjects. As a result, a mean velocity of less than 17.0 cm/sec was used as the criterion for reduction of blood flow velocity caused by obstruction in 11 patients with nephrotic syndrome who were studied with Doppler ultrasound. These patients had a clinical suspicion for renal vein thrombosis, and each was subjected to renal venography. The sensitivity and specificity of the Doppler flowmetric technique were 85% and 56%, respectively.

The use of Doppler technique in this clinical setting is of interest, but there exist major limitations, as discussed by these investigators. The technique requires operator skill and patience, and not infrequently one fails to obtain technically adequately results. The interobserver variability in measuring the Doppler incident angle affected the calculated velocity measurements by up to 19% from the mean. In addition, renal veins are not always circular on cross section and change in diameter

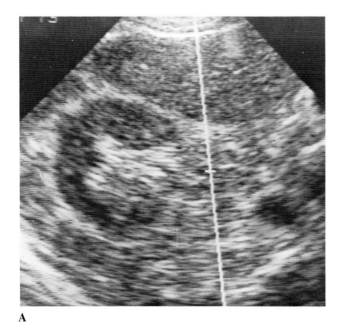

A

FIG. 4. Exclusion of main renal artery and vein occlusion. A cardiac transplant patient was admitted to the hospital with acute renal failure. Portable duplex sonography excluded obstruction of the collecting system as well as main vessel occlusion. Transverse sonograms of the right kidney (**A,C**) show the Doppler sample volume cursor positioned within the right main renal artery and vein, respectively. Normal arterial and venous signals (**B,D**) were obtained from these vessels as well as from within the kidney. The patient's renal insufficiency was subsequently shown to result from cyclosporin nephrotoxicity.

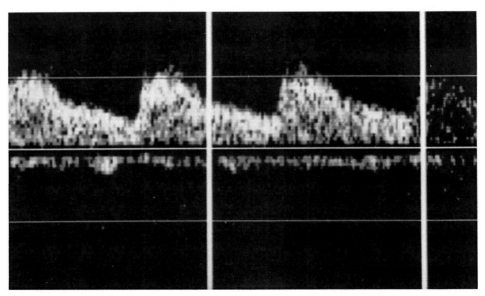

B

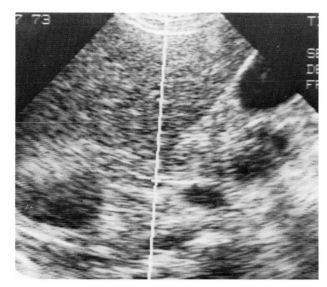

FIG. 4. (continued)

C

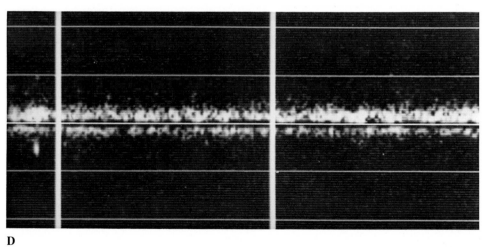

D

with respiration. Therefore, renal vein diameter measurements are only approximations. Furthermore, various conditions affecting renal arterial blood flow or renal vascular impedance may exist, reducing renal venous blood flow velocity, and hence result in false-positive studies. Because of these limitations, it would appear inappropriate to advocate this technique for screening patients for renal vein thrombosis. Conceivably, however, it could have application in following the course of known renal vein thrombosis.

Renal Tumors

Tumor signals have been demonstrated by the Doppler technique in several different tumors. New vessels may be induced in the host by substances secreted by the tumor at an early stage of its development (11). Small cancers may remain dormant until an adequate blood supply has developed (30). Once tumor vessels have appeared, the tumor can grow and has access for hematogenous dissemination (30). The tumor vessels are found on the periphery of the growing mass and tend to be abnormal in morphology, allowing presumptive diagnosis of malignancy when studied by angiography. Abnormalities include the presence of arteriovenous anastomoses. These give rise to high-velocity Doppler shift frequencies caused by the pressure gradient and are not seen in inflammatory masses or pseudotumors. These, therefore, help to identify the malignant nature of these masses. Only preliminary data are available, but we have detected abnormal tumor signals in nine of 12 hypernephromas using the pulsed Doppler technique (Fig. 5). Further work is required on this promising application.

Intraoperative Doppler Applications

Doppler studies have been reported for intraoperative use in renal surgery (8,9). Doppler examination can identify relatively avascular planes in the kidney for ne-

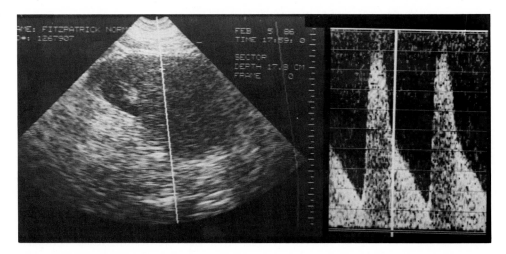

FIG. 5. Malignant renal tumor Doppler signals. Longitudinal sonogram of a kidney shows Doppler sample volume cursor positioned at the periphery of a lower pole solid mass. Doppler signals show a high blood flow velocity, which has been seen in malignant lesions of the kidney and other organs. This mass proved to be a renal cell carcinoma.

phrotomy to remove large or dendritic calculi (9). This reduces blood loss as well as operative and warm ischemia time. Doppler scanning can be helpful in localizing the main renal artery and vein when previous surgery, inflammation, or tumor invasion of the hilum or pedicle obscures normal anatomy (8). Doppler study also can identify intrarenal arteriovenous fistulas prior to excision, evaluate intrarenal blood flow to determine segmental parenchymal viability in cases of segmental obstructive disease, and document blood flow prior to wound closure at the completion of procedures requiring prolonged ischemia (8).

Doppler Estimation of Volume Flow Rate in Renal Vessels

Native Kidneys

Several investigators have succeeded in obtaining estimates of renal arterial flow in the native kidneys of normal volunteers. These experiments are hampered by the limited ultrasound access to the vessels, the difficulty in obtaining reliable cross-sectional area measurements, the lack of a correlative noninvasive method for obtaining flow rates in humans, and the difficulty of relating invasive animal studies to the human situation.

Reid et al. (23) were the first to report volume flow estimates in the renal arteries. Using a 2-MHz CW device that was able to discriminate between forward and reversed flow and a bank of filters capable of estimating the peak Doppler shift frequency to within 300 Hz, they obtained an analog trace corresponding to peak flow velocity. In two volunteers, a B-scan was used to estimate the lumen diameter and as an aid to the orientation of the CW probe. Using the assumed velocity profile method (see Chapter 3) and being unable to ascertain the beam–vessel angle, these investigators made the additional assumption that this angle was zero. The velocity profile was assumed to be that of plug flow. Because of intervening bowel gas, only right renal arteries were studied. In spite of these difficulties, plausible flow values of 340 and 380 ml/min were obtained. However, no estimate of errors was made. Instead, a comparison was made with readings obtained at surgery in a single dog using an electromagnetic flow meter. Good correlation was obtained, but here the lumen diameter was measured angiographically, and the probe–vessel angle could be controlled by placing the transducer on the artery itself.

Some of these technical limitations were addressed by Greene et al. (12), who were the first to apply a duplex scanner with pulsed Doppler ultrasound to the noninvasive estimation of renal artery flow. The instrument employed a zero-crossing detector to produce an estimate of the mean Doppler frequency and a time interval histogram to give an indication of spectral width. Because the zero crosser can give unreliable readings where there is a broad Doppler spectrum (15), and the time interval histogram is, itself, a rather crude indicator of the Doppler paraspectrum, an external fast Fourier transform spectrum analyzer was used to calibrate the analog trace needed for the calculation. Of the 16 examinations of normal subjects, 24% had to be abandoned because of technical inadequacy of the scan. In those studies that were successful, scanning times were up to 1 hr, emphasizing the difficulty of Doppler access to the renal vessels, especially on the left side. Both the vessel diameter and the beam–vessel angle were measured from the frozen real-time image.

The acquisition of this image was triggered by the EKG to ensure that it coincided with peak systole. The authors somewhat optimistically quote the precision of their diameter measurement to be ±0.2 mm (less than the wavelength of sound at 5 MHz) and that of the angle to be ±1°. The range of angles used was 50 to 80°. The actual accuracy of these physical measurements is, of course, critical to the reliability of the resulting flow values. These values were, on average, 403 ml/min with a standard deviation of 127 ml/min.

Renal Transplants

Several investigators have noted that overall renal flow, and especially flow to the cortex, decreases with allograft rejection (13,29). Samson (28) first used ultrasound to try to detect this change. He simply looked at the output of the zero-crossing meter from a 5-MHz continuous-wave flowmeter and plotted relative change of this voltage (which in fact corresponds to the approximate velocity of blood) by means of serial measurements. He documented changes that seemed to link lower flow rates with episodes of clinical rejection. He later confirmed a correlation between his Doppler frequency measurement and the flow rate using an implanted electromagnetic flowmeter in an experimental dog model (29). This remains, however, a most qualitative approach to the assessment of renal allograft flow. Reid et al. (23) used his CW technique for 16 measurements on ten transplanted kidneys, integrating the peak velocity while assuming a zero angle of insonation and a flat velocity profile. The renal artery lumen diameter was deduced from the external vessel diameter measured at surgery. His results gave values ranging from 140 to 560 ml/min. In four of these studies on two patients, a comparison was made with another estimate of renal flow based on ^{131}I-hippuran excretion analysis. The two methods showed an average discrepancy of about 190% (range 8% to 430%). This should not, however, necessarily be taken as an indication of the unreliability of their Doppler method, as the excretion analysis reflects tubular function more than actual renal blood flow.

As the imaging resolution and capacity for quantitative analysis of duplex instruments improve, more consistent and reliable methods for the measurement of renal flow may be forthcoming. However, the exceptional technical difficulty of the ultrasound examination itself is likely to remain a daunting influence on the next development.

RENAL ALLOGRAFTS

There are multiple causes of posttransplant renal failure, which include acute and chronic rejection, acute tubular necrosis (ATN), obstruction of the collecting system, renal artery stenosis, vascular occlusion, cyclosporin toxicity, and infection. The utility of B-scanning for morphologic evaluation of renal allografts is well established, particularly for determining the presence or absence of a dilated collecting system (Fig. 6) and periallograft fluid collections (Fig. 7). The application of Doppler techniques permits detection of blood flow velocity changes in the kidney, which often occur in acute allograft rejection (2,3,7,20,25,26,28,31), and evaluation of the renal arterial and venous systems to exclude vascular occlusion (3,7,16,26,31,33) and stenosis (24,31,33).

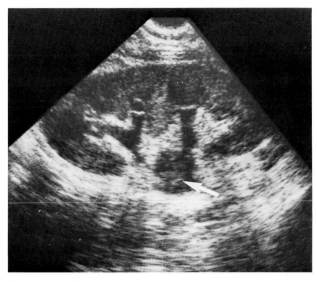

A

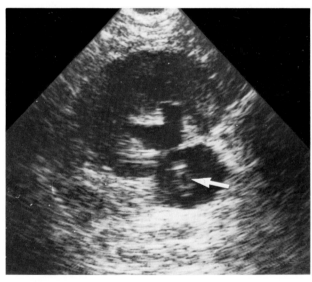

FIG. 6. Obstructed renal allograft collecting system. Longitudinal (**A**) and transverse (**B**) sonograms of a renal allograft show a dilated collecting system resulting from an obstructing blood clot (*arrow*), which developed with bleeding following percutaneous needle biopsy of the transplant.

B

Doppler evaluation of renal allografts can easily be performed because of the superficial location of the organ and absence of loops of bowel interposed between the graft and overlying skin (Fig. 8). With a 3-MHz transducer, the renal transplant can be evaluated in transverse and longitudinal planes. Doppler evaluation of the anastomosed main renal artery may be performed in a longitudinal (Fig. 9) or transverse plane depending on the orientation of the vessel. Attempts should be made to obtain signals along the entire length of the vessel, from the anastomosis to the renal hilum, particularly when there is a question of renal artery stenosis. The intrarenal vessels are generally best evaluated with longitudinal imaging of the grafted kidney (Fig. 10).

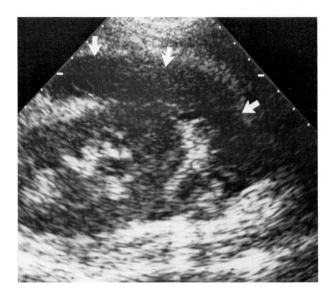

FIG. 7. Periallograft lymphocele. Longitudinal sonogram of renal allograft showing a complex fluid collection (*arrows*) adjacent to the lower pole of the graft. This was aspirated under sonographic guidance and shown to be a lymphocele.

Doppler signals obtained from the normal anastomosed main renal artery show a rapid rise in frequency shift in systole followed by a gradual decrease during diastole, reflecting persistent antegrade flow in a low-impedance microcirculation (Fig. 11). Generally, there is no identifiable spectral window below the systolic time–velocity pulse, unlike that seen in normal native main renal arteries. This probably results from the difference in arterial input. Mild turbulence is often detected in the grafted

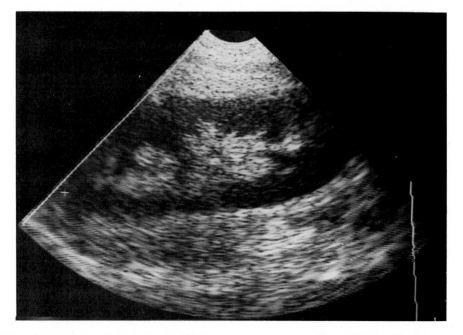

FIG. 8. Normal renal allograft. Longitudinal sonogram of a renal allograft in the iliac fossa shows its superficial location, which permits easy access for duplex evaluation.

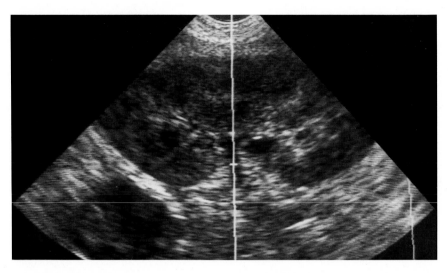

FIG. 9. Main renal artery. Longitudinal sonogram of a renal allograft showing the Doppler sample volume cursor positioned in the main renal artery as it enters the hilum.

main renal artery at the site of surgical anastomosis. Differentiation of normal anastomotic turbulence from renal artery stenosis is crucial and is discussed below. Occasionally, signals obtained from the external and internal iliac arteries may be confused with main renal arterial signals because of the relative proximity of these vessels. Doppler signals from the external iliac artery are quite different and characteristic, showing a systolic spectral window resulting from plug flow and early diastolic reversed flow velocity because of high peripheral impedance (32) (Fig. 12). Internal iliac arterial flow has a blunted parabolic profile. Doppler signals from this vessel show no spectral window or reversed component (32) (Fig. 13) and therefore may resemble main renal arterial signals. However, the inability to trace the vessel to the transplant would allow proper recognition and avoidance of a potential pitfall.

Time–velocity spectra of the intrarenal arterial system (segmental, interlobar, and arcuate arteries) resemble those obtained from normal native kidneys (Fig. 11).

Doppler signals from the renal veins show flow in a direction opposite to that of arterial flow. Venous flow is continuous in the small vessels, and mild respiratory variation may be seen in the main renal vein.

Allograft Rejection

Two histologic forms of acute renal transplant rejection are recognized—interstitial and vascular. In the former, there is inflammatory infiltration of the interstitium associated with edema (36) (Fig. 14). The inflammatory cells are found within the intertubular capillaries, venules, and lymphatics, but the glomeruli, arterioles, and arteries are usually normal (22).

In acute vascular rejection there is an alterative, proliferative endovasculitis (Fig. 15), which may be associated with or followed by a chronic sclerosing vasculopathy (36). The endothelial space is filled with a mononuclear cell infiltrate associated with

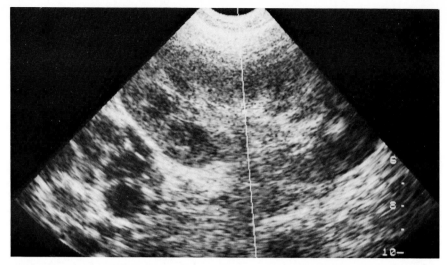

A

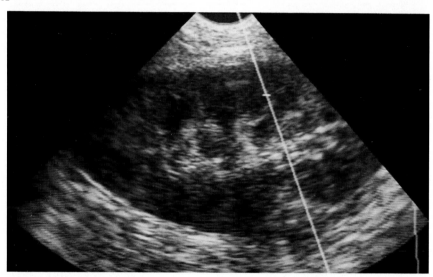

B

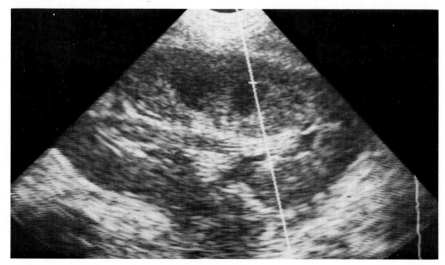

C

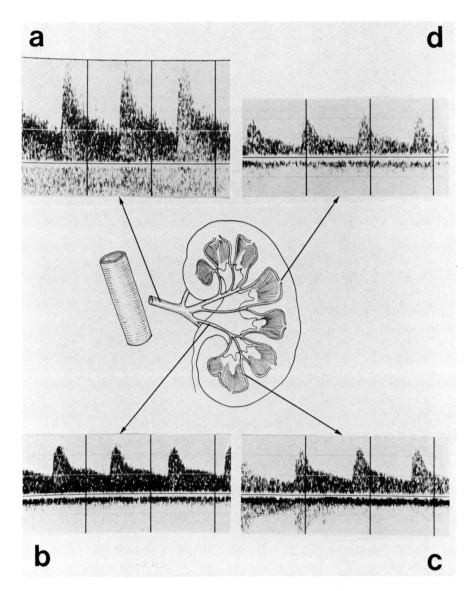

FIG. 11. Normal renal allograft arterial Doppler signals. Montage shows arterial Doppler signals obtained from (**A**) the main renal artery as well as (**B**) a segmental, (**C**) an interlobar, and (**D**) an arcuate artery. Each waveform is similar, with a peak in blood flow velocity in systole followed by a gradual decrease during diastole, remaining continuous and never approaching zero velocity. The continuous signal below the base line (**B,C,D**) represents venous flow.

FIG. 10. Intrarenal arteries. Longitudinal sonograms of a renal allograft show the Doppler sample volume cursor positioned to obtain signals from (**A**) a segmental, (**B**) an interlobar, and (**C**) an arcuate artery.

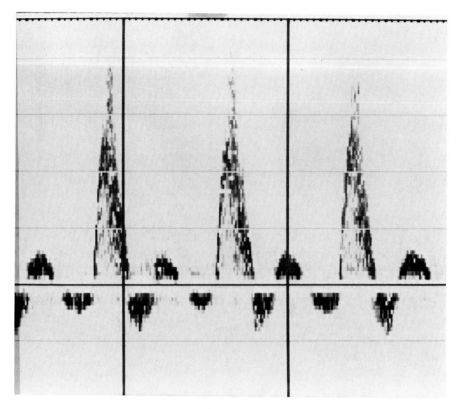

FIG. 12. External iliac arterial Doppler signals. Doppler signals from the external iliac artery show rapid acceleration and deceleration in systole, associated with a systolic spectral window. Reversed flow in early diastole is present.

swelling of the endothelium. Myofibroblast proliferation occurs in the subendothelial space, which results in intimal thickening. Platelets and fibrin may adhere to sites of vessel wall damage with subsequent thrombosis. This can progress to obliteration of the vascular lumen.

Sampson (28) was the first investigator to study renal transplant arterial flow using a Doppler flowmeter. A decrease in blood flow to the graft, expressed by a decrease in the ratio of peak renal artery to femoral artery frequency shift, correlated with episodes of acute rejection. An increase in this ratio was observed when patients responded to antirejection therapy. The absence of change, despite therapy, was seen with repeated episodes of rejection. A decrease in signal was observed in some patients recovering from ATN, although in each case the transplants subsequently rejected. No change in signal was seen in episodes of pyelonephritis or cortical necrosis. However, no recordings were made during the first 14 days following transplantation, during which time distinction of acute rejection from ATN and other causes of graft dysfunction is most vital. Furthermore, the study was limited by the inability to maintain a constant angle between the transducer and vessel for all recordings. In a second study, using canine renal allografts, Sampson et al. (29) employed a device that maintained a constant angle between the Doppler transducer and transplanted renal artery. The allografts all underwent rejection, and these investigators observed a progressive fall in renal artery blood flow. Renal artery blood flow changes were determined by a Doppler flowmeter and showed close correlation with changes recorded by an indwelling electromagnetic flowmeter. However, regulation of a constant probe–vessel angle is not possible for clinical use.

Because of the obvious limitations in attempting to maintain a constant probe–vessel angle for successive studies, subsequent investigation concentrated on the analysis of the waveform of the Doppler signal. Time–velocity spectra can be evaluated, examining the relative change of diastolic to peak systolic blood flow velocity, which is unaffected by a relatively wide variation in the probe–vessel angle. Using a directional Doppler velocimeter also prevents interference of arterial signals with venous flow.

In episodes of acute allograft rejection, there is a relative decrease in arterial diastolic-to-peak-systolic frequency shift, producing a more pulsatile Doppler waveform (Fig. 16). This represents a decrease in diastolic blood flow velocity resulting from increased peripheral vascular impedance in the graft. In severe rejection the Doppler signal becomes pulsatile, with rapid acceleration and deceleration in blood flow velocity in systole. Diastolic flow may be obliterated (Fig. 17) or reversed (Fig. 18). The increased resistance in the microcirculation results from an endovasculitis in cases of acute vascular rejection. The histologic changes produce encroachment

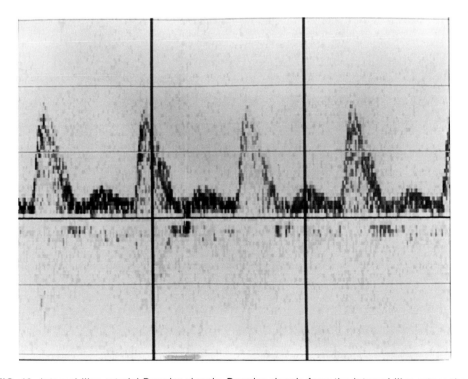

FIG. 13. Internal iliac arterial Doppler signals. Doppler signals from the internal iliac artery show a systolic peak in blood flow velocity and continuous diastolic flow. The diastolic flow velocity relative to peak systolic flow velocity is less than that observed in the normal allograft main renal artery.

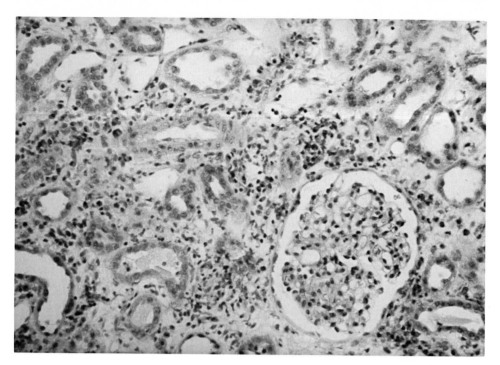

FIG. 14. Predominantly acute interstitial allograft rejection. There is a diffuse interstitial infiltrate of lymphocytes and other mononuclear cells associated with interstitial edema and focal tubular necrosis. The vessels are not significantly involved. Magnification × 450. (Courtesy of M. Kashgarian, M.D., Yale University School of Medicine.)

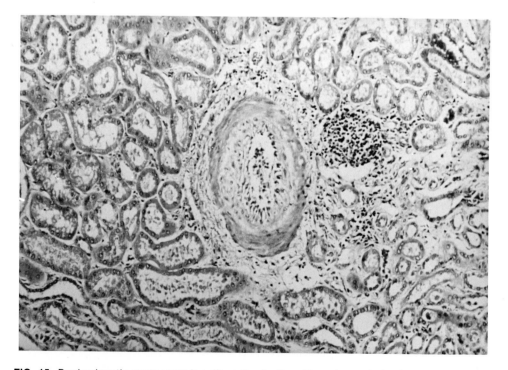

FIG. 15. Predominantly acute vascular allograft rejection. There is myointimal proliferation with narrowing of the lumen of the artery. Occasional lymphocytes are present in the arterial wall and margination along the endothelium. A minor component of interstitial infiltrate is also present. Magnification × 450. (Courtesy of M. Kashgarian, M.D., Yale University School of Medicine.)

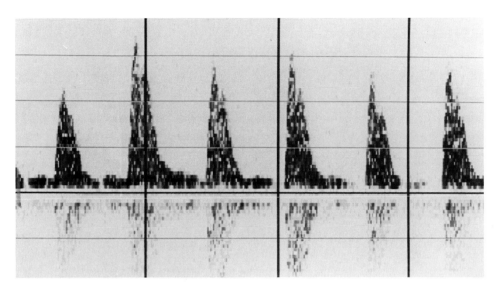

FIG. 16. Acute allograft rejection. Doppler signals obtained from a segmental artery show a relative decrease in diastolic flow in a patient with biopsy-proven rejection.

on the vascular lumen and impede the flow of blood. In interstitial rejection, there are no intrinsic vascular changes. Interstitial edema (20) or vasomotor constriction (3) may be responsible for the increased vascular resistance in these cases. Improved diastolic flow can be identified in patients who respond to rejection therapy.

Berland et al. (7) were the first to quantify Doppler signals in renal allografts using

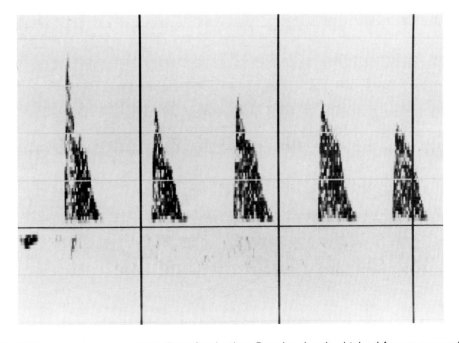

FIG. 17. Moderately severe acute allograft rejection. Doppler signals obtained from a segmental artery during an episode of acute rejection show obliterated diastolic flow.

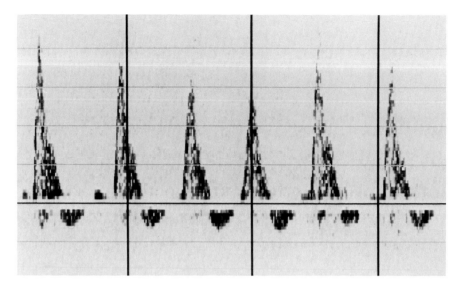

FIG. 18. Severe acute allograft rejection. Doppler signals obtained from a segmental artery during an episode of severe rejection show a pulsatile signal with reversed diastolic flow.

the pulsed Doppler index (PDI). The PDI was calculated from unspecified arterial signals obtained in the renal medulla and cortex. This index represents the area within the wave cycle divided by the height of the wave peak and multiplied by the cardiac cycle time and is inversely proportional to the peripheral vascular resistance. The PDI correlated well with radionuclide renogram studies, but no histologic confirmation of rejection was performed. Certain cases of mild rejection yielded normal PDI values. Some cases of ATN had normal PDI values, whereas others were within the abnormal range.

Most recently, Rigsby et al. (25) quantified renal allograft Doppler signals using the pulsatility index (PI) (Fig. 19). The PI represents the peak-to-peak excursion in

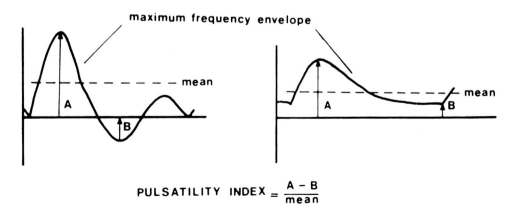

FIG. 19. Pulsatility index. The pulsatility index (PI) is the ratio of the peak systolic frequency shift (A) minus the minimum diastolic frequency shift (B) divided by the mean frequency shift (mean). (Reprinted with permission from Rigsby et al., ref. 25.)

TABLE 1. Pulsatility index in normal allografts

Vessel	Mean PI	n	SD
Mean renal artery	1.26	23	0.33
Segmental artery	1.18	21	0.33
Interlobar artery	1.19	20	0.44
Arcuate artery	1.12	22	0.30

Reprinted from Rigsby et al. (25) with permission.

frequency shift divided by the mean frequency shift and varies directly with peripheral vascular impedance. Fifty-five renal transplant patients were evaluated with Doppler ultrasound during 54 episodes of acute rejection, three episodes of chronic rejection, three episodes of ATN, and on 23 occasions with normal graft function. Each patient with graft dysfunction had percutaneous biopsy or graft nephrectomy within 24 hr of the duplex study. Normal graft function was established by clinical criteria.

In each duplex study Doppler signals were obtained from the main anastomosed renal artery and at least one segmental, interlobar, and arcuate artery. The envelope of the Doppler waveform was hand traced over four cardiac cycles using a digitizing tablet (Apple Computer Inc.). A microcomputer (Apple IIe) then calculated the mean PI for each vessel.

In normal allografts, there was little variation in the PI among the four arterial sites examined (range 1.12–1.26) (Table 1). The mean PI for each site as well as the

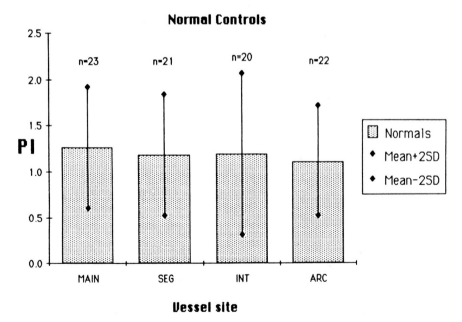

FIG. 20. Pulsatility index in normal transplants. Histograms obtained from patients with normal renal allografts, showing mean PI at each vascular site. Normal range defined by two standard deviations is indicated for each vessel. Main, main renal artery; Seg, segmental artery; Int, interlobar artery; Arc, arcuate artery. (Reprinted with permission from Rigsby et al., ref. 25.)

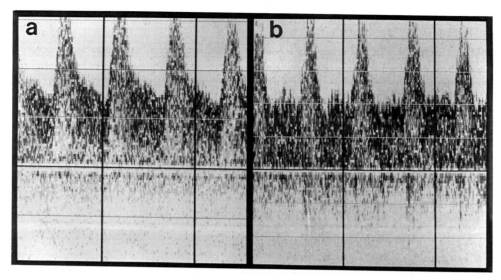

FIG. 25. Acute tubular necrosis. **A:** Normal arterial Doppler signals obtained from base-line study. **B:** Normal arterial Doppler signals (PI = 1.3) obtained during an episode of acute tubular necrosis. Changes consistent with acute tubular necrosis were demonstrated on biopsy within 48 hr of this study.

high pulsatility (e.g., PI ≥ 1.8) may prove to obviate the need for biopsy and allow a patient to be treated for acute rejection. However, a greater number of other causes of graft dysfunction must first be evaluated to confirm this specificity before this approach is advocated clinically.

Finally, Doppler ultrasound has been shown to be useful for follow-up in patients with documented acute rejection. Reappearance of diastolic flow and normalization of Doppler signals can be identified in patients who respond to immunosuppressive therapy. Persistent loss of diastolic flow has been correlated with a poor prognosis for the graft (3).

Allograft Vascular Occlusion

Vascular occlusion represents a major complication of renal transplantation and requires immediate surgical intervention.

Main renal artery thrombosis usually results from technical difficulty encountered at surgery (6). This is a correctable complication if the period of warm ischemia is less than 90 min in duration (Fig. 29). Vascular occlusive changes can also be identified within an allograft as a result of severe vascular rejection, resulting invariably in graft nephrectomy.

Arterial occlusion may be diagnosed by Doppler scanning when arterial signals from the renal artery or from within the graft cannot be obtained. If arterial occlusion is suspected, a large Doppler sample volume (approximately 5 mm axial length) should be used to facilitate identification of arterial flow, if present. When arterial signals in the graft are indeed absent, it is prudent to sample signals in adjacent major vessels (e.g., external iliac artery) to ensure adequate sensitivity of the Doppler system.

Taylor et al. (33) reported ten of 88 (11.4%) renal transplant patients who developed small vessel occlusive changes resulting from severe acute vascular rejection. A preoperative diagnosis was made in each case with Doppler examination by failure to identify intrarenal signals. At nephrectomy, small vessel occlusion was demonstrated in each patient, with retrograde extension of thrombus into the main renal artery in one case.

Illustrative Case History

A 26-year-old female received a cadaveric renal allograft for end-stage renal disease. The patient had an unremarkable early postoperative course. The serum creatinine decreased from

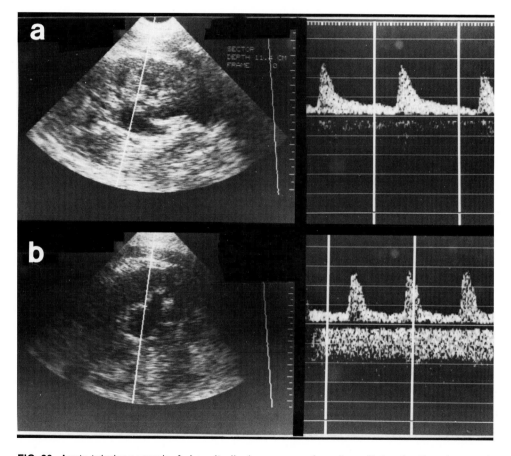

FIG. 26. Acute tubular necrosis. **A:** Longitudinal sonogram of an allograft showing Doppler sample volume cursor positioned in renal sinus where segmental arterial signals were obtained for a base-line study. These signals show slightly decreased diastolic flow. **B:** Longitudinal sonogram of allograft again shows cursor positioned to obtain segmental arterial signals. This was obtained during an episode of biopsy-proven acute tubular necrosis. There is also mild dilatation of the collecting system. The Doppler signals show persistent decreased diastolic flow with no significant change in comparison to the base-line study.

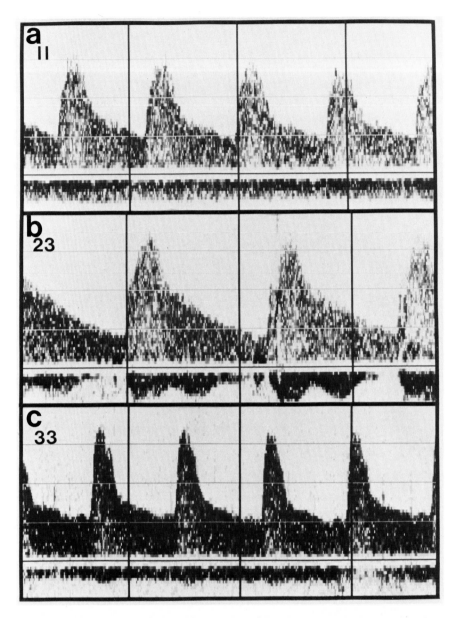

FIG. 27. Successive episodes of acute tubular necrosis and acute interstitial rejection. **A:** Normal arterial Doppler signals (PI = 1.25) obtained at a time of normal allograft function on day 11. **B:** Slightly abnormal arterial signals (PI = 1.56) obtained during an episode of biopsy-proven acute tubular necrosis on day 23. This PI value would yield a false positive result. **C:** Normal arterial signals (PI = 1.37) obtained during an episode of biopsy-proven acute interstitial rejection on day 33.

8.3 to 2.2 mg/dl in the first 9 days following surgery. Doppler signals obtained on postoperative days 0 and 9 were normal (Fig. 30). The patient's clinical condition began to deteriorate. On day 10 a biopsy was performed, which showed severe acute vascular rejection. The serum creatinine rose to 5.5 and 8.2 mg/dl on days 11 and 12, respectively, despite addition of antithymocyte globulin to the treatment regimen. Doppler signals on both days showed very

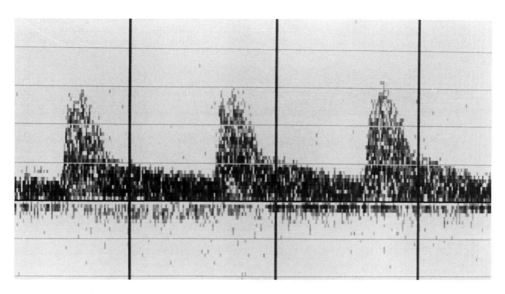

FIG. 28. Chronic rejection. Arterial signals from an allograft with biopsy-proven chronic rejection. There is only a minimal decrease in relative diastolic blood flow velocity.

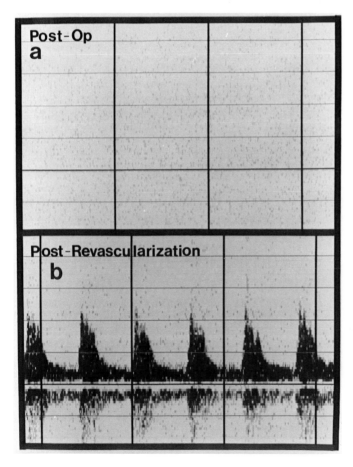

Post-Op
a

Post-Revascularization
b

FIG. 29. Main renal artery thrombosis. **A:** Portable duplex study performed in the recovery room in an anuric patient immediately following transplantation showing absence of arterial perfusion of the graft. **B:** Arterial signals were obtained from the main renal artery and from within the graft following removal of a thrombus from the main renal artery.

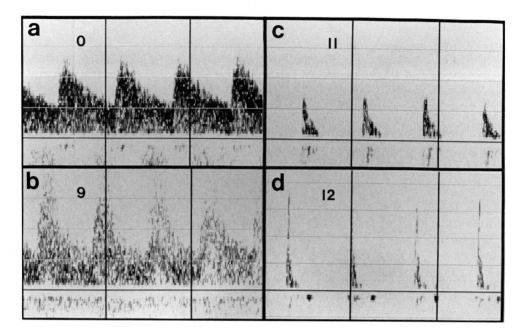

FIG. 30. Severe acute vascular rejection preceeding arterial occlusion. **A:** Normal arterial Doppler signals (PI = 0.86) were obtained on day 0 immediately following transplantation. **B:** Normal signals (PI = 1.14) were again obtained on day 9. **C:** Abnormal pulsatile signals (PI = 3.99) on day 11. **D:** Extremely pulsatile signals (PI = 10) with reversed diastolic flow were obtained on day 12.

abnormal signals, indicating severe acute rejection (Fig. 30). Aggressive therapy was continued, with no response. On day 22, a Doppler study showed no signals from the main renal artery or within the graft, indicating vascular occlusion (Fig. 31). An arteriogram was then performed and showed occlusion at the external iliac–main renal artery anastomosis (Fig. 32). Nephrectomy was performed, showing a necrotic kidney with occlusive vascular changes resulting from acute vascular rejection.

Transplant Renal Artery Stenosis

Stenosis of the grafted renal artery occurs in 1.6 to 16% of transplant patients (10). This complication should be suspected when hypertension develops in association with graft dysfunction. The presence of a bruit is a suggestive but variable finding.

In one study, Doppler findings in transplant renal artery stenosis included increased peak frequency at the site of stenosis with spectral broadening, disorganization of flow, and distal decreased peak frequency (24). Using these Doppler criteria, these investigators had five true positive and two true negative diagnoses for stenosis. Arteriographic findings were used for correlation.

Taylor and Burns (31) reported the combination of high-velocity blood flow with distal turbulence as characteristic Doppler findings in stenosis. In a subsequent report, Taylor et al. (33) observed these changes in seven patients suspected of having renal artery stenosis, all of whom later had arteriography. Among these seven patients, four were found to have significant stenosis (Figs. 33–37), one with arterial kinking (Figs. 38 and 39), one with minimal stenosis of a small accessory renal artery, and one who had a normal renal artery. However, in each of the four cases of significant stenosis and in the case of arterial kinking, the Doppler peak frequency shift exceeded 7.5 kHz and was associated with gross turbulence distally. The remaining two patients had only mild turbulence and peak frequency shifts of 4 kHz and 7.5 kHz, respectively. These authors concluded, therefore, that significant stenosis should not be considered without a peak frequency shift of greater than 7.5 kHz and must be associated with gross turbulence distally. The use of such a threshold is dependent on the frequency of the transducer and the angle between the ultrasound beam and the vessel. Taylor et al. used a 3-MHz transducer in this study. Use of any other frequency transducer would require adjustment of the cutoff peak frequency used for diagnosis. Furthermore, the angle between the vessel and the transducer is generally not known because the long axis of the vessel is never well defined. Therefore, the transducer should be angled manually to achieve the maximum Doppler peak frequency shift.

In examining the grafted main renal artery, a mild degree of turbulence at the site of surgical anastomosis is frequently observed (Fig. 40). This is a normal finding and

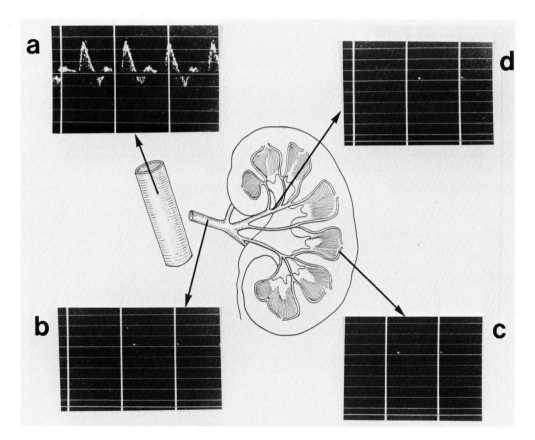

FIG. 31. Renal artery occlusion (same patient as in Fig. 30). Normal external iliac artery signals were obtained (**A**), but no signals could be obtained from (**B**) the main renal artery or (**C,D**) the intrarenal arteries. (Reprinted with permission from Taylor et al., ref. 33.)

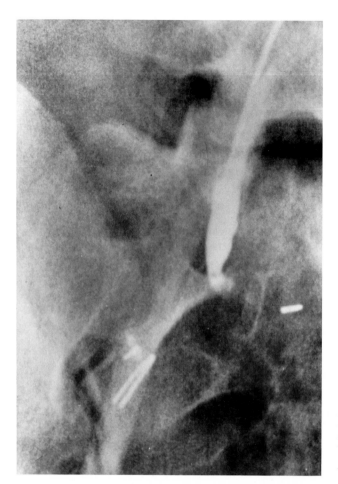

FIG. 32. Renal artery occlusion (same patient as in Figs. 30 and 31). Right external iliac arteriogram showing complete occlusion at the anastomosis with the transplanted renal artery. (Reprinted with permission from Taylor et al., ref. 33.)

should not be misinterpreted as stenosis. Comparison with a base-line study is of aid in interpreting such a finding. Furthermore, there should be no associated increased peak frequency shift more proximally.

It should also be emphasized that the entire length of the anastomosed main renal artery must be examined when stenosis is suspected. The flow aberrations described above may exist in only a relatively short segment of the vessel. Normal laminar flow with normal velocities is usually reestablished where the vessel enters the renal hilum.

Doppler evaluation of transplant renal arteries is useful in screening for stenosis when the diagnosis is suspected clinically. It is a sensitive technique but may be incapable of distinguishing arterial kinking or stenosis in an accessory vessel from significant main renal artery stenosis. The use of a threshold frequency shift (>7.5 kHz) may reduce the number of false positive findings. Doppler examination may also be helpful for follow-up in patients who have had percutaneous transluminal angioplasty of stenotic lesions when recurrent stenosis is suspected.

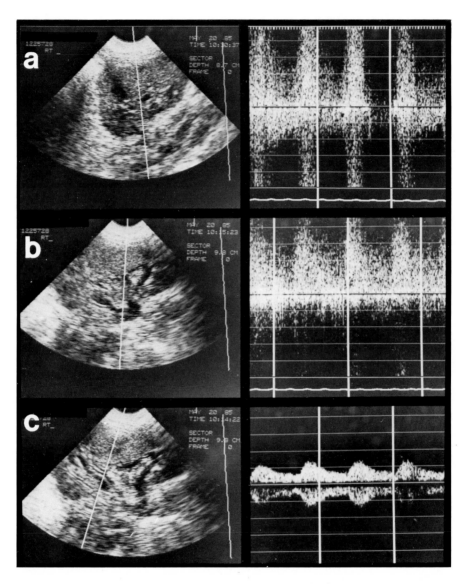

FIG. 33. Transplant renal artery stenosis. **A:** Longitudinal sonogram of renal allograft with Doppler sample volume cursor positioned in renal artery proximal to the renal hilum. An aliased Doppler signal shows a peak frequency shift of at least 9 kHz. **B:** The cursor is positioned in the renal artery as it enters the renal hilum. Doppler signals show significant turbulence. **C:** The cursor is now positioned within the graft. Segmental arterial Doppler signals show reconstitution of normal laminar flow.

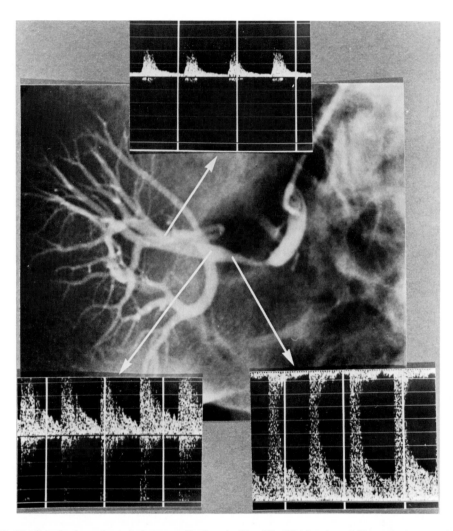

FIG. 34. Renal artery stenosis (same patient as in Fig. 33). Right external iliac arteriogram demonstrating a tight stenosis at the anastomosis and involving the transplant renal artery. Arterial Doppler signals show a peak frequency shift of 10 kHz at the stenosis with turbulence in the poststenotic segment. No turbulence was seen in the intrarenal arterial signals. (Adapted with permission from Taylor et al., ref. 33.)

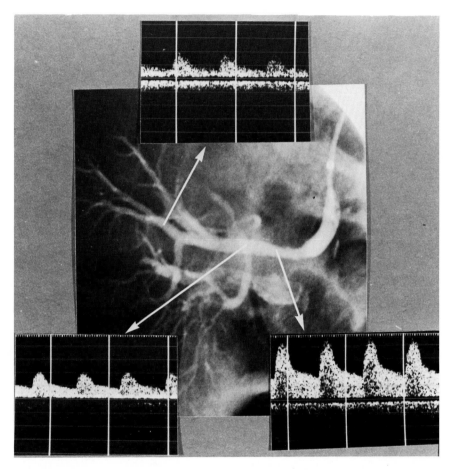

FIG. 35. Treated renal artery stenosis (same patient as in Figs. 33 and 34). Right external iliac arteriogram following angioplasty shows correction of the stenotic lesion. Doppler signals were normal with no evidence of a high-velocity jet or turbulence in the main renal artery. (Reprinted with permission from Taylor et al., ref. 33.)

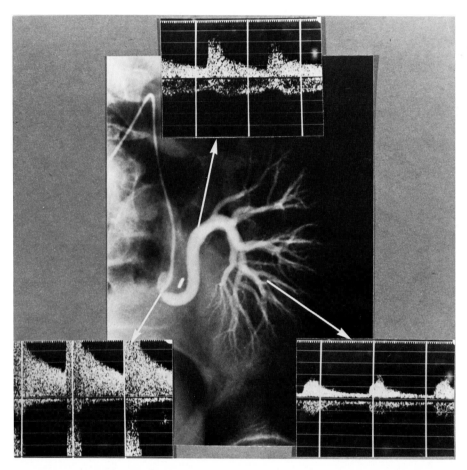

FIG. 36. Renal artery stenosis. Left external iliac arteriogram showing a tight anastomotic stenosis. The aliased Doppler signal obtained from this site shows a large frequency shift (>9 kHz). Significant turbulence in the renal artery more distally was also observed (not shown). The intrarenal arterial signals show evidence of undisturbed flow. (Reprinted with permission from Taylor et al., ref. 33.)

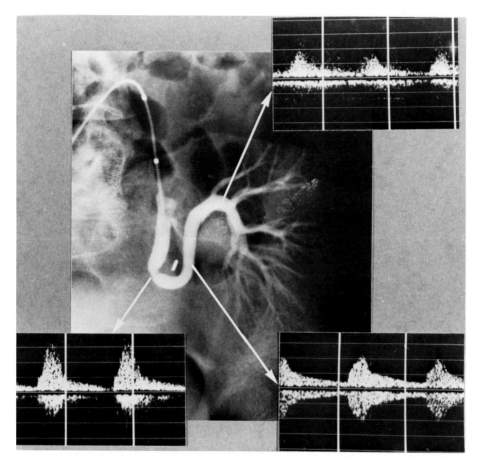

FIG. 37. Treated renal artery stenosis (same patient as in Fig. 36). A follow-up arteriogram after angioplasty showing increased luminal diameter at the stenotic segment. The Doppler signals show no high-velocity jet in the corresponding segment. The intrarenal arterial signals show undisturbed flow. (Reprinted with permission from Taylor et al., ref. 33.)

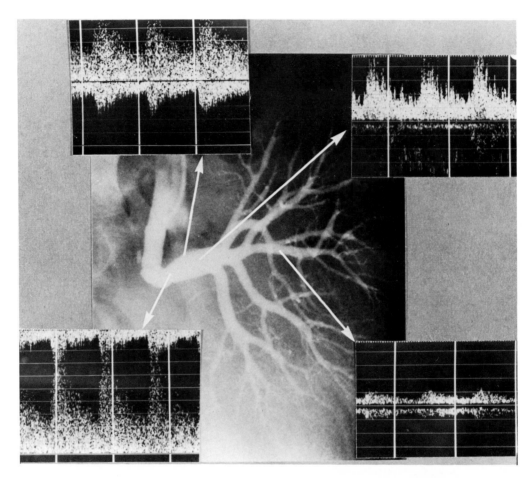

FIG. 38. False-positive Doppler study resulting from arterial kinking. Left external iliac arteriogram showing kinking of the main renal artery. The Doppler study showed a large frequency shift (10 kHz) in the corresponding segment of the vessel associated with distal turbulence, falsely suggesting a significant stenosis of the renal artery. No appreciable pressure gradient across the kinking was demonstrated at arteriography. (Reprinted with permission from Taylor et al., ref. 33.)

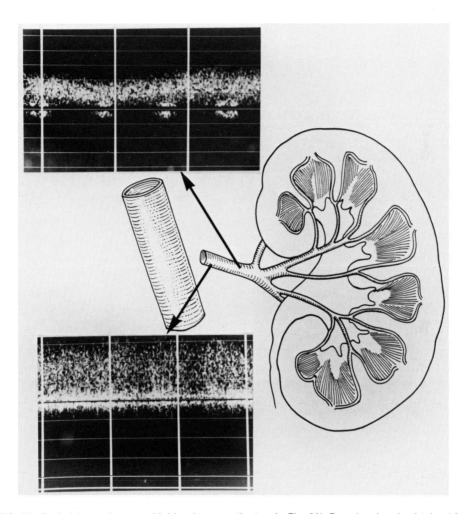

FIG. 39. Probable renal venous kinking (same patient as in Fig. 38). Doppler signals obtained from the distal transplant renal vein show increased velocities in comparison with signals obtained in the same vessel more proximally. This suggests simultaneous kinking of the renal vein. (Reprinted with permission from Taylor et al., ref. 33.)

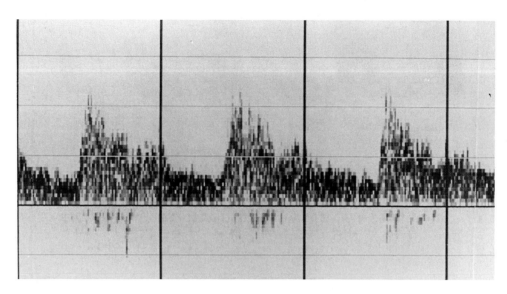

FIG. 40. Normal anastomotic turbulence. Mild turbulence may normally be observed in the Doppler signals obtained from the arterial anastomosis. As an isolated finding, this should not be misinterpreted as stenosis.

Arteriovenous Fistulas

Percutaneous needle biopsy of renal transplants is the standard by which the presence or absence of graft rejection is generally established. However, there is a low but definite risk of developing arteriovenous fistulas following such a procedure.

Taylor et al. (33) reported one case of a graft arteriovenous fistula resulting as a biopsy complication and detected by Doppler examination. Within the transplant, Doppler ultrasound demonstrated a high-velocity jet with a peak frequency shift of 10 kHz, believed to have resulted from a large pressure gradient and indicating a direct arteriovenous communication (Fig. 41).

CONCLUSION

The addition of Doppler techniques to ultrasound imaging has offered a new diagnostic tool for evaluating the kidneys. Physiologic and pathologic blood flow changes can be correlated with anatomic findings provided by B-scanning. It should be emphasized, however, that much of the material presented in this chapter is preliminary and that the use of Doppler scanning is rapidly evolving. The spectrum of applications as well as the strengths and limitations of this technique are yet to be clearly defined.

In native kidneys, Doppler scanning can be used to detect vascular occlusion, although potential pitfalls exist. Various studies report success in diagnosing renal artery stenosis. However, the personal experience of the authors in this effort has been disappointing. Excessive fat or muscle and intestinal gas represent major obstacles to obtaining technically satisfactory results. Doppler evaluation of renal

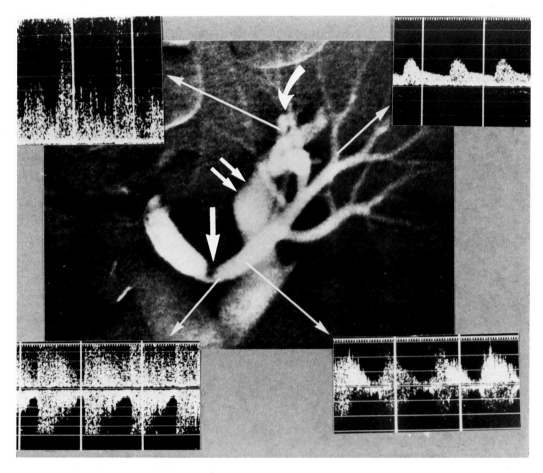

FIG. 41. Renal artery stenosis and renal arteriovenous fistula. Intrarenal digital subtraction angiogram of the right external iliac artery reveals a tight anastomotic stenosis (*straight arrow*). Doppler signals show a high-velocity jet exceeding 7.5 kHz with some reversed flow resulting from eddy currents at the same site. Turbulence is seen at the stenosis and more distally. A pseudoaneurysm is identified on the angiogram (*curved arrow*) associated with early venous filling (*double arrow*). Doppler signals from this area of the kidney demonstrate a large frequency shift of 10 kHz and turbulence resulting from the large pressure gradient. (Adapted with permission from Taylor et al., ref. 33.)

masses is an exciting new area of investigation and may prove useful in differentiating malignant tumors from benign lesions.

Grafted kidneys are well disposed to Doppler evaluation because of their superficial location. As a result, vascular complications such as occlusion and stenosis can be identified without difficulty. Doppler waveform changes can be demonstrated in most cases of acute rejection, although they are frequently absent in interstitial rejection. Further investigation is required to determine whether Doppler evaluation can help to distinguish acute rejection from other causes of graft failure. Examination of change in PI in longitudinal studies may be helpful in this effort as well as in attempting to identify interstitial rejection.

REFERENCES

1. Abrams, H. L. (1983): Renal arteriography in hypertension. In: *Abrams' Angiography—Vascular and Interventional Radiology,* edited by H. L. Abrams, pp. 1247–1297. Little, Brown, Boston.

2. Arima, M., Ishibashi, M., Usami, M., Sagawa, S., Mizutani, S., Sonoda, T., Ichikawa, S., Ihara, H., and Nagano, S. (1978): Analysis of the arterial blood flow patterns of normal and allografted kidneys by the directional ultrasonic Doppler technique. *J. Urol.,* 122:587–591.

3. Arima, M., Takahara, S., Ihara, H., Ichikawa, Y., and Ishibashi, M., Sagawa, S., Nagono, S., Takaha, M., and Sonoda, T. (1982): Predictability of renal allograft prognosis during rejection crisis by ultrasonic Doppler flow technique. *Urology,* 19:389–394.

4. Avasthi, P. S., Greene, E. R., Scholler, C., and Fowler, C. R. (1983): Noninvasive diagnosis of renal vein thrombosis by ultrasonic echo–Doppler flowmetry. *Kidney Int.,* 23:882–887.

5. Avasthi, P. S., Voyles, W. F., and Greene, E. R. (1984): Noninvasive diagnosis of renal artery stenosis by echo–Doppler velocimetry. *Kidney Int.,* 25:824–829.

6. Belzer, F. O., Glass, N., and Sollinger, H. (1984): Technical complications after renal transplantation. In: *Kidney Transplantation: Principles and Practice,* edited by P. J. Morris, pp. 407–426. Grune & Stratton, London.

7. Berland, L. L., Lawson, T. L., Adams, M. B., Melrose, B. L., and Foley, W. D. (1982): Evaluation of renal transplants with pulsed Doppler duplex sonography. *J. Ultrasound Med.,* 1:215–222.

8. Boyce, W. H. (1981): Ultrasonic velocimetry in resection of renal arteriovenous fistulas and other intrarenal surgical procedures. *J. Urol.,* 125:610–613.

9. Bryniak, S. R., and Chesley, A. E. (1981): The use of the Doppler stethoscope in anatrophic nephrotomy. *J. Urol.,* 126:295–296.

10. Faenza, A., Spolaore, R., Poggioli, G., Selleri, S., Roversi, R., and Gozzetti, G. (1983): Renal artery stenosis after renal transplantation. *Kidney Int.,* 23(Suppl. 14):S-54–S-59.

11. Folkman, J. (1986): How is blood vessel growth regulated in normal and neoplastic tissue? G. H. A. Clowes Memorial Award Lecture. *Cancer Res.,* 46:467–473.

12. Greene, E. R., Venters, M. D., Avasthi, P. S., Conn, R. L., and Jahnke, R. W. (1981): Noninvasive characterization of renal artery blood flow. *Kidney Int.,* 20:523–529.

13. Henry, W. L., Kountz, S. L., Cohn, R., Robison, S. L., and Harrison, D. C. (1969): Changes in pulsatile blood flow in autograft and homograft kidneys during rejection. *Transplantation,* 7:545–553.

14. Kohler, T. R., Zierler, R. E., Martin, R. L., Nicholls, S. C., Bergelin, R. O., Kazmers, A., Beach, K. W., and Strandness, D. E., Jr. (1986): Noninvasive diagnosis of renal artery stenosis by ultrasonic duplex scanning. *J. Vasc. Surg.,* 4:450–456.

15. Lunt, M. J. (1975): Accuracy and limitations of the ultrasonic Doppler blood velocimeter and zero crossing detector. *Ultrasound Med. Biol.,* 2:1–10.

16. Marchioro, T. L., Strandness, D. E., Jr., and Krugmire, R. B., Jr. (1969): The ultrasonic velocity detector for determining vascular patency in renal homografts. *Transplantation,* 8:296–298.

17. McAfee, J. G., Thomas, F. D., Grossman, Z., Streeten, D. H. P., Dailey, E., and Gagne, G. (1977): Diagnosis of angiotensinogenic hypertension: The complementary roles of renal scintigraphy and the saralasin infusion test. *J. Nucl. Med.,* 18:669–675.

18. McNeil, B. J., Varady, P. D., Burrows, B. A., and Adelstein, S. J. (1975): Measures of clinical efficacy: Cost–effectiveness calculations in the diagnosis and treatment of hypertensive renovascular disease. *N. Engl. J. Med.,* 293:216–221.

19. Nichols, B. T., Rittgers, S. E., Norris, C. S., and Barnes, R. W. (1984): Non-invasive detection of renal artery stenosis. *Bruit,* 8:26–29.

20. Norris, C. S., and Barnes, R. W. (1984): Renal artery flow velocity analysis: A sensitive measure of experimental and clinical renovascular resistance. *J. Surg. Res.,* 36:230–236.

21. Norris, C. S., Rittgers, S. E., and Barnes, R. W. (1984): A new screening technique for renal artery occlusive disease. *Curr. Surg.,* 41:83–86.

22. Porter, K. A. (1983): Renal transplantation. In: *Pathology of the Kidney,* edited by R. H. Heptinstall, pp. 1455–1547. Little, Brown, Boston.

23. Reid, M. H., Mackay, R. S., and Lantz, M. T. (1980): Noninvasive blood flow measurements by Doppler ultrasound with applications to renal artery flow determination. *Invest. Radiol.,* 15:323–331.

24. Reinitz, E. R., Goldman, M. H., Sais, J., Rittgers, S. E., Lee, H. M., Mendez-Picon, G., Muakkassa, W. F., and Barnes, R. W. (1983): Evaluation of transplant renal artery blood flow by Doppler sound-spectrum analysis. *Arch. Surg.,* 118:415–419.

25. Rigsby, C. M., Burns, P. N., Weltin, G. G., Chen, B., Bia, M., and Taylor, K. J. W. (1987): Doppler signal quantitation in renal allografts: Comparison in normal and rejecting transplants, with pathologic correlation. *Radiology,* 162:39–42.

26. Rigsby, C. M., Taylor, K. J. W., Weltin, G. G., Burns, P. N., Bia, M., Princenthal, R. A., Kashgarian, M., and Flye, M. W. (1986): Renal allografts in acute rejection: Evaluation using duplex sonography. *Radiology,* 158:375–378.

27. Rittgers, S. E., Norris, C. S., and Barnes, R. W. (1985): Detection of renal artery stenosis: Experimental and clinical analysis of velocity waveforms. *Ultrasound Med. Biol.*, 11:523–531.

28. Sampson, D. (1969): Ultrasonic method for detecting rejection of human renal allotransplants. *Lancet*, 2:976–978.

29. Sampson, D., Abramczyk, J., and Murphy, G. P. (1972): Ultrasonic measurement of blood flow changes in canine renal allografts. *J. Surg. Res.*, 12:388–393.

30. Schor, A. M., and Schor, S. L. (1983): *Tumour angiogenesis. Pathology*, 141:385–413.

31. Taylor, K. J. W., and Burns, P. N. (1985): Duplex Doppler scanning in the pelvis and abdomen. *Ultrasound Med. Biol.*, 11:643–658.

32. Taylor, K. J. W., Burns, P. N., Woodcock, J. P., and Wells, P. N. T. (1985): Blood flow in deep abdominal and pelvic vessels: Ultrasonic pulsed Doppler analysis. *Radiology*, 154:487–493.

33. Taylor, K. J. W., Morse, S. S., Rigsby, C. M., Bia, M., and Schiff, M. (1987): Vascular complications in renal allografts: Detection with duplex Doppler US. *Radiology*, 162:31–38.

34. Thornbury, J. R., Stanley, J. C., and Fryback, D. G. (1982): Hypertensive urogram: A nondiscriminatory test for renovascular hypertension. *Am. J. Roentgenol.*, 138:43–49.

35. Tucker, R. M., and Labarthe, D. R. (1977): Frequency of surgical treatment for hypertension in adults at the Mayo Clinic from 1973 through 1975. *Mayo Clin. Proc.*, 52:549–555.

36. Zollinger, H. U., and Mihatsch, M. J. (1978): Kidney transplantation. In: *Renal Pathology in Biopsy*, edited by H. U. Zollinger and M. J. Mihatsch, pp. 564–614. Springer, New York.

8 / Pulsed Doppler Ultrasound of the Pelvis and the First Trimester of Pregnancy

Kenneth J. W. Taylor

Department of Diagnostic Radiology, Yale University School of Medicine, New Haven, Connecticut 06510

Any application of Doppler ultrasound in the female pelvis is dominated by the issue of potential bioeffects and the safety of duplex Doppler devices. This is not an academic issue since these applications of Doppler ultrasound are experimental and as yet do not have Food and Drug Administration (FDA) approval for clinical use. This fact alone should make us careful. We must weigh the risks and benefits, be certain that we know the output intensities of the Doppler devices we employ, and obtain informed consent from every patient and the approval of a Human Investigation Committee (HIC) or Institutional Review Board (IRB).

When the subject of ultrasound intensity is discussed, definitions become important, since "intensity" can mean almost anything we want it to mean. The most widely quoted intensity measurement is the spatial peak temporal average (SPTA). This is most easily related to the total energy absorbed by the tissue and hence is best related to the heating induced by insonation. It is assumed that heating is a major potential cause of bioeffects from insonation. Perhaps this is because other possible mechanisms of action are less well understood. Nevertheless, there is the real concern that high-intensity Doppler devices with SPTAs approaching 1 W/cm^2 (2) could induce sufficient heating of the embryo to produce teratogenic effects (17,29). However, the responsible physician can render negligible the potential risks by choice of the appropriate equipment, allowing the many advantages of pelvic Doppler examination to be employed for clinical diagnosis without hazard.

The FDA has shown great concern at the prospect of fetal exposure to pulsed Doppler ultrasound. In general, CW instruments, which have long been used by obstetricians to confirm fetal viability, operate at very low intensities in the range of 9 to 80 mW/cm^2 (3). This compares favorably with the statement by the Bioeffects Committee of the American Institute of Ultrasound in Medicine (AIUM) noting the absence of independently confirmed mammalian bioeffects at SPTA intensities below 100 mW/cm^2 (28). There is considerable discussion among equipment manufacturers, the AIUM, and the FDA with a view to increasing the permissible intensities for nonobstetric examinations. However, a limit seems prudent for obstetrical studies, and it forces investigators to review their power output, to consider the risk/benefit ratio, and to obtain informed consent and approval from an HIC or IRB.

TECHNIQUE

Iliac Vessels

Pelvic Doppler examination is complementary to ultrasonic imaging. Its main use is to aid tissue characterization and to provide information on the functional activity of the pelvic organs, especially the ovaries and uterus. In all of our studies, we have used an ATL 600 with the attenuator permanently reduced by −9 dB to yield an *in*

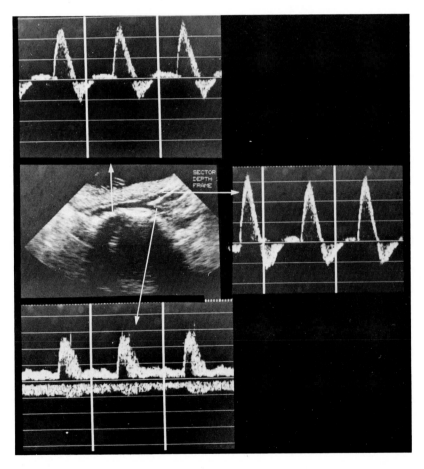

FIG. 1. Montage to show bifurcation of the common iliac arteries into the internal and external iliac arteries. Note the corresponding time–velocity spectrum. The common iliac waveform is similar to that of the aorta and external iliac. It demonstrates plug flow with a reverse component. In contrast, the internal iliac shows filling in of the waveform envelopes indicating the presence of parabolic flow in a relatively small vessel.

situ intensity of less than 40 mW/cm² at the target organ. When other instruments, capable of emitting higher intensities, are used, it is essential to know the power output of the equipment for each transducer and power setting. Some devices start up at maximum power. The operator must know what this maximum is and reduce the power control to a prudent level within the FDA guidelines. After starting at minimal power, the gain can then be increased until a satisfactory signal is obtained. The power should only be increased if the signal-to-noise ratio is adequate. A frequency of 3 MHz is used both for imaging and for Doppler evaluation, and a sample volume of 3 mm is optimal both for the best signal-to-noise ratio and for the isolation of each vascular signal.

As in all pelvic sonography, a full bladder is mandatory and in Doppler examination allows easy access to the common, internal, and external iliac vessels (Fig. 1) in addition to the uterine and ovarian vessels (Figs. 2 and 3). The iliac arteries, lying

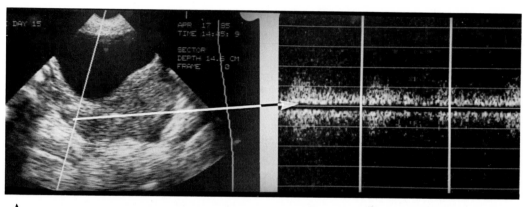

A

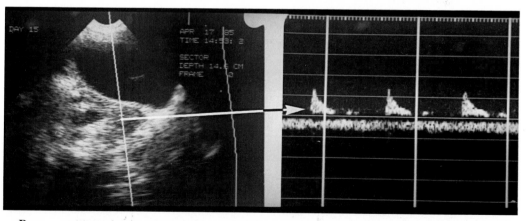

B

FIG. 2. A: Transverse scan of the pelvis showing the right ovary. A low-impedance waveform is seen following ovulation, with marked diastolic flow indicating a low-impedance ovarian vasculature on day 15 of the cycle. This is typical of the functioning corpus luteum. **B:** The inactive left ovary shows a high-impedance signal bereft of diastolic flow. Note ovarian venous flow as a continuous waveform below the line, indicating flow away from the transducer.

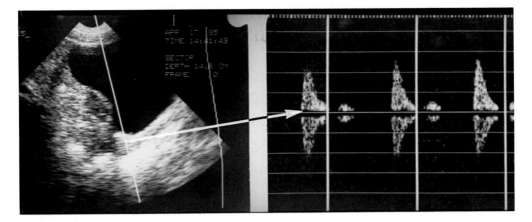

FIG. 3. Longitudinal section of the uterus. A cursor in the lateral part of the cervix shows a high-impedance flow with a small hump during diastole. The waveform is of a high-impedance pattern and is consistant with the uterine artery in both the nonpregnant state and the first trimester of pregnancy.

on each side of the pelvis, can be recognized by their pulsation, and in some patients the iliac bifurcation can clearly be seen (Fig. 1). The Doppler waveforms aid in identifying these vessels. The common and external iliac arteries show a high-impedance pattern similar to that found in the aortofemoral arteries, with a window under the time–velocity waveform because of the presence of plug flow and a diastolic reversal of flow considered in previous chapters. In contrast, the internal iliac artery, usually clearly seen just deep to the ovary, shows spectral broadening because of parabolic flow, with a small hump in late diastole (Fig. 1). In our initial experiments, we compared the waveforms obtained at surgery from all of the pelvic vessels with those obtained percutaneously to ensure that they correlated well (31,32).

The corresponding iliac veins can be seen using the same technique, and deep venous thrombosis can be excluded (Fig. 4). With a larger sample volume, both

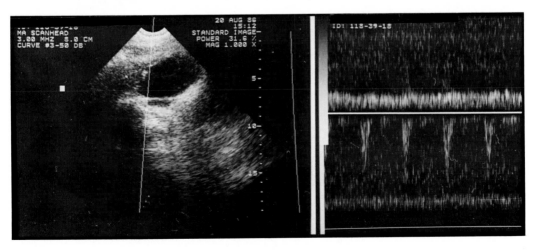

FIG. 4. External iliac arterial and venous waveforms in a patient with deep vein thrombosis of the femoral vein. This demonstrates patency of the iliac vein.

arterial and venous signals may be observed simultaneously, with the waveforms on opposite sides of the zero line because of the opposing directions of flow.

The wall filter is usually placed as low as possible (50–100 Hz). However, where there is a considerable "wall thumping," the wall filter can be increased to 200 Hz. Particularly when looking for low-velocity flow, for example, in the ovarian artery, it is important for the wall filter to be as low as possible. Flow in these small vessels seldom returns frequencies above 500 Hz, so an 800-Hz wall filter, or higher, removes all such signals.

Ovarian Vessels

The ovaries develop high in the retroperitoneum and, like the testes, descend carrying their blood supply with them. Thus, the ovarian arteries arise from the upper aorta, pass down the retroperitoneum, and enter the pelvis through the infundibulopelvic ligament on the side wall of the pelvis. The ovarian vessels can often be seen in this position. The internal iliac artery lies just below the ovary, making it imperative that a small sample volume be used, not exceeding 3 mm. Initially, the sample volume is placed just lateral to the ovary. If no signal is detected, the sample volume is brought into the ovary, and the area is interrogated until a low-amplitude signal is appreciated. The angle of the transducer is manually adjusted to optimize the amplitude of the signal, which is monitored both by ear and by the waveform on the spectrum analyzer. As can be seen from our later studies, the waveform shape varies with the functional activity of the ovary. This functional activity affects volume flow to the ovary and increases the amplitude of the signal, since the amplitude varies with the number of reflectors (red cells). Thus, an inactive ovary is a difficult organ from which to elicit signals, whereas an active ovary gives rise to signals that are easily detected.

Six volunteers with regular menstrual cycles were serially examined with duplex Doppler ultrasound during three consecutive cycles. Early in the cycle (days 1–7), both ovaries showed similar waveforms consisting of a high-impedance signal of low amplitude and without evidence of diastolic flow (Fig. 5). By day 9, the ovary developing the dominant follicle showed diastolic flow and also increased amplitude, making it easier to detect. The amplitude in that ovary continued to increase through ovulation and into the functioning period of the corpus luteum, becoming maximal around day 21 (Fig. 5). After day 23, the waveform rapidly changed back to the inactive, high-impedance pattern seen on day 1. Throughout this cycle, the contralateral ovary showed the same low-amplitude, high-impedance signals without diastolic flow. Usually, the inactive ovary became active the following month.

These cyclic changes can be summarized using a pulsatility index (PI) to quantitate the ovarian impedance, which is inversely related to flow. Here we have used the Stewart PI (Chapter 4), which is the systolic frequency over the diastolic frequency (Fig. 6). The conclusion from these studies is that blood flow to the functioning ovary is greatly increased and that this change is reflected in the decreased impedance (low PI).

Prior to the development of duplex Doppler technology, there had been few studies of ovarian flow in humans. However, there are many previous reports on luteal flow

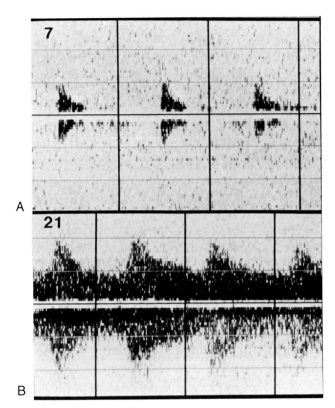

FIG. 5. A: Waveform on the seventh day of the cycle demonstrates a high-impedance signal without evidence of diastolic flow. **B:** Same ovary on day 21 demonstrates an increased number of scatterers (the intensity of the trace), increased velocity, and increased diastolic flow compared with the inactive ovary on day 7. All these characteristics indicate increased flow associated with the functioning of the corpus luteum.

in domestic and farm animals. Blood flow has been shown to vary during the estrous cycle in the ewe, cow, and other mammals, being highest during the luteal phase and lowest during the follicular phase (7,13,15,24). Various noninvasive and invasive techniques have been used including the use of microspheres (16), direct blood collection (6), and implantation of Doppler flowmeters (4) and electromagnetic flowmeters in cows (13). These techniques have shown that 80 to 90% of the blood flow to the ovary is supplied to the corpus luteum (1,5). In rabbits and sheep, luteal blood flow has been shown to be more than ten times that of surrounding tissues (8,23). This increased blood flow results from the production of new blood vessels, similar to those observed around the growing edges of tumors. This high blood supply is necessary for the supply of the precursors of steroidogenesis and for the removal of synthesized progesterone. There is a rapid decrease in ovarian blood flow accompanying luteolysis (8,18). Prostaglandin $F_{2\alpha}$ is reported to be the active luteolysin, and a reduction of 90% in luteal flow has been reported following administration of prostaglandin $F_{2\alpha}$ (21).

In patients with stimulated cycles and bilateral ovulating ovaries, these active changes with a low-impedance signal are seen bilaterally. If pregnancy occurs, then the corpus luteum maintains its function for the first trimester of pregnancy, and the active waveforms persist during this period. Pregnancy is known to be dependent on a functioning corpus luteum, and Doppler ultrasound is an excellent means by which to identify this activity. A most important conclusion follows: the absence of

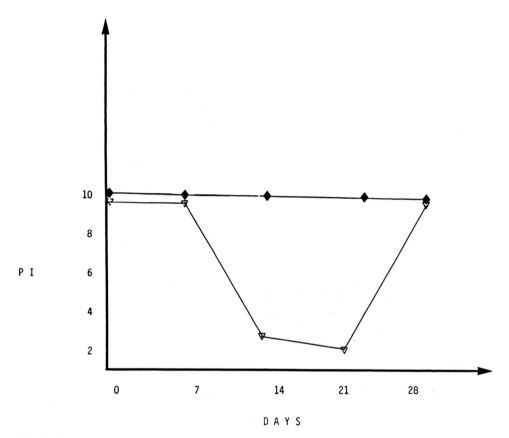

FIG. 6. Sequential changes in the impedance of the ovarian arteries during the menstrual cycle. The left ovary demonstrates a high impedance throughout the cycle. The right ovary demonstrates a marked lowering of impedance in the ovulating ovary, with minimal impedance around day 21, before returning to a high-impedance state. The pulsatility index used here is the Stewart index (systolic frequency over diastolic frequency). The disadvantage of this index is that the PI is theoretically infinite when there is zero diastolic flow. However, this is indicated as a PI exceeding 10 on the graph. (Reprinted with permission from Taylor et al., ref. 33.)

a functioning corpus luteum indicates a nonviable pregnancy, whether normotopic or ectopic. The important clinical applications that follow from this statement are considered further later in this chapter.

Doppler examination may be used simplistically to characterize tissue. Figure 7 shows a clinical example. A mass was seen contiguous with the uterus and apparently part of it and was assumed to be a fibroid. However, the possibility was raised that it might be merely the right ovary in contact with the uterus. A Doppler examination demonstrated low-impedance flow, characteristic of an active ovary. In a similar way, Doppler ultrasound can be used to demonstrate the functional activity of an ovarian cyst. Functioning cysts displaying typical luteal flow are often associated with prolonged amenorrhea and premenstrual discomfort. In contrast, nonfunctioning cysts exhibit high-impedance flow characteristics (Fig. 8). The technique has been helpful in excluding torsion of the ovary. Usually vessels can be easily located on the surface of a cyst and interrogated for arterial and venous signals. In the presence of normal vascularity, torsion is highly unlikely.

Doppler examination has also been valuable in the diagnosis of a functioning ovarian tumor in a postmenopausal patient (27). The following case report illustrates this application. A 78-year-old woman presented with increasing baldness of the male pattern. Laboratory investigation disclosed elevated serum androgen levels, and she was referred for an ultrasound scan of her pelvis. Duplex ultrasound demonstrated a left ovary, enlarged to 3 cm, that gave signals resembling those of a corpus luteum (Fig. 9). The presence of functional ovarian flow in a postmenopausal woman with hirsuitism allowed the correct preoperative diagnosis of a hilar cell tumor, formerly called an arrhenoblastoma. Surgery confirmed the presence of a 3-cm hilar cell tumor (Fig. 10).

The ability to display luteal flow is important (33). It allows the diagnosis of abortion in patients presenting with a threatened abortion and excludes the possibility of a viable ectopic pregnancy in many patients presenting emergently with the possibility of an ectopic pregnancy. Figure 11 shows scans of two patients from the infertility clinic who presented with bleeding after 5 weeks of amenorrhea. The differential diagnosis lay among a threatened abortion, an ectopic pregnancy, and an abortion. Both ovaries were examined with Doppler ultrasound. The right ovary in both patients was slightly enlarged, usually a sign that it bears the corpus luteum.

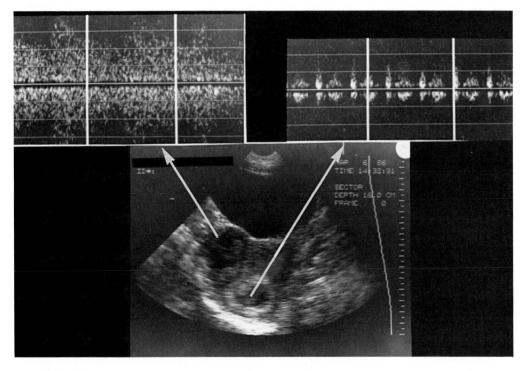

FIG. 7. An early gestational sac with a homogeneous mass contiguous with the side of the uterus. The position of the gestational sac raised the possibility of a cornual pregnancy, whereas the homogeneous mass was considered to be a fibroid on the first ultrasound scan. Repeat clinical examination showed no evidence of a fibroid, and the patient was referred back for further sonographic study. The addition of Doppler examination demonstrated the typical low-impedance corpus luteal flow in the mass contiguous with the uterus. Fetal viability was confirmed by Doppler ultrasound. The patient elected abortion.

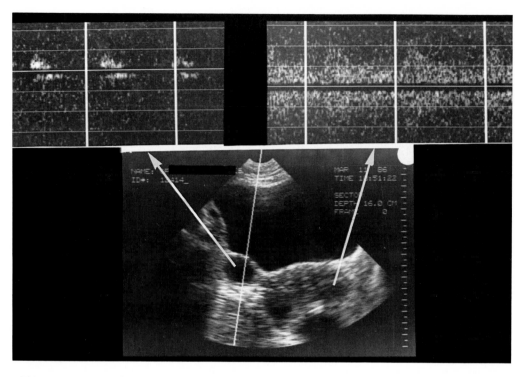

FIG. 8. A patient with a 5-week pregnancy and a right cystic adnexal mass. Although sonographically this is most likely to be a luteal cyst, Doppler examination demonstrates high-impedance signals, indicating a nonfunctional retention cyst. In contrast, the corpus luteum was located in the left ovary and was identified by its specific signal.

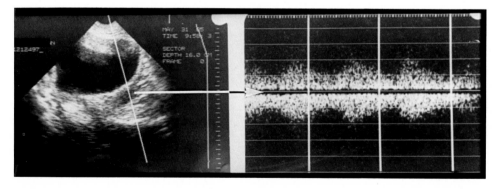

FIG. 9. Transverse scan to demonstrate an enlarged left ovary in a 78-year-old patient. This ovary measured 3 cm. The clinical history of increasing baldness of the male pattern suggested a functioning tumor. Doppler evaluation demonstrated a low-impedance flow similar to that seen in a corpus luteum. In a 78-year-old patient with hirsuitism, these appearances indicate an androgen-secreting tumor, a hilar cell tumor or arrhenoblastoma. (Reproduced with permission from Russell et al., ref. 27.)

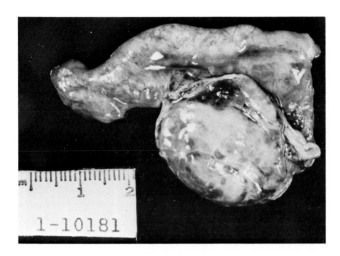

FIG. 10. Surgical specimen demonstrating a 3-cm solid ovarian tumor, which histologically proved to be a hilar cell tumor.

In one patient, a high-impedance signal was seen in both ovaries (Fig. 11A). The absence of a functioning corpus luteum suggested correctly that the pregnancy was nonviable. In contrast, the presence of a functioning corpus luteum in the other patient indicated that the pregnancy could still be viable (Fig. 11B). In fact, this pregnancy went to term.

It is important to appreciate the limitations of these observations. Luteal flow may be seen despite fetal death when, for example, there has been fetal demise as a result of fetal abnormality. Luteal flow is seen bilaterally after clomid therapy when the ovulating dose of hCG induces a chemical pregnancy. Thus, the technique is of no value in these patients. However, the absence of a corpus luteum is highly significant since a pregnancy must have a corpus luteum to support it through the first trimester.

This conclusion has importance in the diagnosis or exclusion of an ectopic pregnancy. To date, we have documented the presence of luteal flow in 12 consecutive ectopic pregnancies. Conversely, we now believe that the absence of luteal flow allows an ectopic pregnancy to be excluded. Most patients with clinical suspicion of ectopic pregnancy present to the emergency room with pelvic pain, vaginal bleeding, and no idea of their LMP. Nearly 70% of them do not have amenorrhea. Thus, the single most valuable piece of information required for appropriate clinical management is whether or not they are pregnant. Because of the high sensitivity of the hCG test, a negative result virtually excludes the possibility of an ectopic pregnancy. Unfortunately, the test result is never available with the speed required for patient management, so ultrasound is invariably requested without the benefit of the hCG result.

B-mode ultrasound may be helpful when an intrauterine sac or definite extrauterine sac can be identified. More frequently, an adnexal mass is seen, and it is unclear whether this is the corpus luteum or luteal cyst, an ectopic pregnancy, or whether the patient is not pregnant at all and it is merely a retention cyst of the ovary. In our experience, Doppler examination may be useful in several ways. First, Doppler ultrasound allows positive identification of a corpus luteum or functioning luteal cyst (Fig. 11B). Secondly, the absence of luteal flow indicates absence of a viable pregnancy, and finally, Doppler examination may help in the specific identification of an extrauterine fetal heart (Fig. 12).

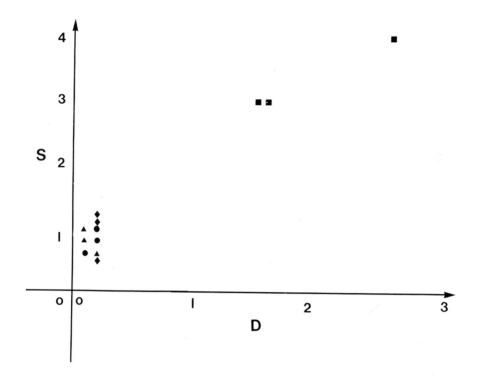

FIG. 15. Plot of peak systolic Doppler shift frequency, S (kHz), against the end-diastolic frequency, D, in the uterine arteries: ◆, nongravid; ●, normal first trimester; ▲, abortion but clinical suspicion of GTN; ■, proven GTN. There is a clear separation between patients with and without gestational trophoblastic neoplasia. (Reproduced with permission from Taylor et al., ref. 34.)

4 to 10%. About 2% of them require chemotherapy. In contrast, complete moles lack a fetus, are diploid (96% are XX and 4% are XY, being derived from one or two paternal sets of chromosomes). Persistent trophoblastic disease occurs in 15 to 20% of complete moles, and 10% require chemotherapy (10,30). To minimize the tumor burden, early diagnosis is desirable.

Hitherto, diagnostic imaging of molar disease has been inadequate. The typical molar appearances are nonspecific as described above. The patient illustrated in Fig. 13 had been treated for 9 months following an abortion, had undergone dilatation and curettage on three occasions, and had two ultrasound scans and a head and total-body CT scan, all without diagnosis. The functional activity, rapidly displayed by Doppler examination, was diagnostic. Although our experience is limited by the rarity of this disease in our population, we believe that duplex Doppler examination will prove to be of great importance for this diagnosis by showing functional activity in addition to the morphologic appearance shown by ultrasonic imaging.

CONCLUSION

Doppler evaluation of the pelvis, especially in the first trimester of pregnancy, is clearly only in its infancy. Bioeffect considerations threaten to overshadow this valuable modality. However, highly sensitive instrumentation is available, and useful diagnostic data can be obtained at low intensities within the rather stringent FDA guidelines. There is a need, however, for even more sensitive devices that can be employed at even lower outputs.

REFERENCES

1. Abdul-Karim, R. W., and Bruce, N. W. (1973): Blood flow to the ovary and corpus luteum at different stages of gestation in the rabbit. *Fertil. Steril.*, 24:44–47.

2. *Acoustical Data for Diagnostic Ultrasound Equipment* (1985). American Institute of Ultrasound in Medicine, Bethesda.

3. *Biological Effects of Ultrasound: Mechanisms and Clinical Implications* (1983). National Council on Radiation Protection and Measurements, Bethesda.

4. Brown, B. W., Emery, M. J., and Mattner, P. E. (1980): Ovarian arterial blood velocity measured with Doppler ultrasonic transducers in conscious ewes. *J. Reprod. Fertil.*, 58:295–300.

5. Bruce, N. W., and Hillier, K. (1974): The effect of prostaglandin F on ovarian blood flow and corpora lutea regression in the rabbit. *Nature*, 249:176–177.

6. Bruce, N. W., and Meyer, G. T. (1981): Ovarian blood flow and progesterone secretion in anaesthetized rats at day 16 of gestation, and the effects of haemorrhage. *J. Reprod. Fertil.*, 61:419–423.

7. Bruce, N. W., and Moor, R. M. (1975): Ovarian blood flow and function. *Bibliogr. Reprod.*, 25:581–586, 695–697.

8. Bruce, N. W., and Moor, T. J. (1976): Capillary blood flow to ovarian follicles, stroma and corpora lutea of anesthetized sheep. *J. Reprod. Fertil.*, 46:299–304.

9. Campbell, S., Diaz-Recasens, J., Griffin, D. R., Cohen-Overbeek, T. E., Pearce, J. M., Willson, K., and Teague, M. J. (1983): New Doppler technique for assessing uteroplacental blood flow. *Lancet*, 1:675–677.

10. Dodson, M. G. (1983): New concepts and questions in gestational trophoblastic disease. *J. Reprod. Med.*, 28:741–749.

11. FitzGerald, D. E., Stuart, B., Drumm, J. E., and Duignan, N. M. (1984): The assessment of the feto-placental circulation with continuous wave Doppler ultrasound. *Ultrasound Med. Biol.*, 10:371–376.

12. Fleischer, A., Schulman, H., Farmakides, G., Bracero, L., Grunfeld, L., Rochelson, B., and Koenigsberg, M. (1986): Uterine artery Doppler velocimetry in pregnant women with hypertension. *Am. J. Obstet. Gynecol.*, 154:806–813.

13. Ford, S. P., and Chenault, J. R. (1981): Blood flow to the corpus luteum-bearing ovary and ipsilateral uterine horn of cows during oestrous cycle and early pregnancy. *J. Reprod. Fertil.*, 62:555–562.

14. Friedman, D. M., Rutkowski, M., Snyder, J. R., Lustig-Gillman, I., and Young, B. K. (1985): Doppler blood velocity waveforms in the umbilical artery as an indicator of fetal well-being. *L. Clin. Ultrasound*, 13:161–165.

15. Hossain, M. I., Lee, C. S., Clarke, I. J., and O'Shea, J. D. (1979): Ovarian and luteal blood flow, and peripheral plasma progesterone levels in cyclic guinea-pigs. *J. Reprod. Fertil.*, 57:167–174.

16. Janson, P. O., Damber, J. E., and Axen, C. (1981): Luteal blood flow and progesterone secretion in pseudopregnant rabbits. *J. Reprod. Fertil.*, 63:491–497.

17. Lele, P. P. (1975): *Second World Congress on Ultrasonics in Medicine*, edited by M. de Vlieger, D. N. White, and V. R. McCready, pp. 22–27. Excerpta Medica, Amsterdam.

18. Magness, R. R., Christenson, R. K., and Ford, S. P. (1983): Ovarian blood flow throughout the estrous cycle and early pregnancy in sows. *Biol. Reprod.*, 28:1090–1096.

19. Matsuura, J., Chiu, D., Jacobs, P. A., and Szulman, A. E. (1984): Complete hydatidiform mole in Hawaii: an epidemiological study. *Genet. Epidemiol.*, 1:271–284.

20. Munyer, T. P., Callen, P. W., Filly, R. A., Braga, C. A., and Jones, H. W., III (1981): Further observations on the sonographic spectrum of gestational trophoblastic disease. *J. Clin. Ultrasound*, 9:349–358.

21. Nett, T. M., and Niswender, G. D. (1981): Luteal blood flow and receptors for LH during PGF_{2a}-induced luteolysis: Production of PGF_{2a} and PGF_{2a} during early pregnancy. *Acta Vet. Scand. [Suppl.]*, 77:117–130.

22. Niswender, G. D., Moore, R. T., Akbar, A. M., Nett, T. M., and Diekman, M. A. (1975): Flow of blood to the ovaries of ewes throughout the estrous cycle. *Biol. Reprod.*, 13:381–388.

23. Novy, M. J., and Cook, M. J. (1973): Redistribution of blood flow by prostaglandin F_{2a} in the rabbit ovary. *Am. J. Obstet. Gynecol.*, 117:381–385.

24. Reid, M. H., McGahan, J. P., and Oi, R. (1983): Sonographic evaluation of hydatidiform mole and its look-alikes. *Am. J. Roentgenol.*, 140:307–311.

25. Roberts, D. K., Wells, M. M., and Horbelt, D. V. (1986): Dysgerminoma in the differential diagnosis of hydatidiform mole. *Obstet. Gynecol.*, 67:92S–94S.

26. Romero, R., Horgan, J. G., Kohorn, E. I., Kadar, N., Taylor, K. J. W., and Hobbins, J. C. (1985): New criteria for the diagnosis of gestational trophoblastic disease. *Obstet. Gynecol.,* 66:553–558.

27. Russell, J. B., Lambert, S. J., Taylor, K. J. W., and DeCherney, A. H. (1987): Androgen-producing hilus cell tumor of the ovary. Detection in a postmenopausal woman by duplex Doppler scanning. *JAMA,* 257:962–963.

28. *Safety Considerations for Diagnostic Ultrasound* (1984). American Institute of Ultrasound in Medicine, Bethesda.

29. Shimizu, T., and Shoji, R. (1975): In: *Second World Congress on Ultrasonics in Medicine,* edited by M. de Vlieger, D. N. White, and V. R. McCready, pp. 28. Excerpta Medica, Amsterdam.

30. Szulman, A. E. (1984): Syndromes of hydatidiform moles: Partial vs complete. *J. Reprod. Med.,* 29:788–791.

31. Taylor, K. J. W., Burns, P. N., Wells, P. N. T., Conway, D. I., and Hull, M. G. R. (1985): Ultrasound Doppler flow studies of the ovarian and uterine arteries. *Br. J. Obstet. Gynecol.,* 92:240–246.

32. Taylor, K. J. W., Burns, P. N., Woodcock, J. P., and Wells, P. N. T. (1985): Blood flow in deep abdominal and pelvic vessels: Ultrasonic pulsed Doppler analysis. *Radiology,* 154:487–493.

33. Taylor, K. J. W., Grannum, P. A. T., and DeCherney, A. H. (1987): Research lessons for maternal-fetal research from reproductive system studies. In: *Doppler Ultrasound Measurement of Maternal-Fetal Hemodynamics,* Report of a NICHD Research Planning Workshop, edited by D. Maulik and D. McNellis. Perinatology Press, New York.

34. Taylor, K. J. W., Schwartz, P. E., and Kohorn, E. I. (1987): Diagnosis of persistent trophoblastic disease by duplex Doppler. *Radiology (in press).*

35. Woo, J. S. K., Wong, L. C., Hsu, C., and Ma, H. K. (1983): Sonographic appearances of the partial hydatidiform mole. *J. Ultrasound Med.,* 2:261–264.

9 / *Doppler Ultrasound in Obstetrics*

Peter N. Burns

Department of Diagnostic Radiology, Yale University School of Medicine, New Haven, Connecticut 06510

Ultrasound imaging has established its preeminence in noninvasive antenatal diagnosis by depicting anatomical change and hence following fetal growth. Doppler ultrasound, in contrast, by virtue of its ability to detect and quantify blood flow, offers the potential to study functional and hence physiological change.

The earliest, and still the most common, application of Doppler ultrasound in obstetrics is the fetal cardiotocograph (8), in which a low-frequency, weakly focused continuous-wave transducer is strapped to the maternal abdomen, and the fetal heart rate is calculated from the strong Doppler-shifted echoes originating from moving solid cardiac structures. Although some early hopes that such a measurement might be a useful prognostic indicator in pregnancy have not been realized (60), the fetal cardiotocograph today finds routine use in the monitoring of fetal well-being during labor and delivery. Other early uses of Doppler ultrasound in the fetus included the detection of fetal breathing movements (3) and of fetal cardiac valve motion (58). In 1977, Fitzgerald and Drumm (21) reported the detection of umbilical artery waveforms in the human fetus and suggested that the reduction of diastolic flow velocity was related to some cases of prematurely ruptured membranes and maternal hypertension. More recently, Doppler ultrasound has been used to investigate intracardiac flow rates in the fetus (51), fetal cardiac arrhythmias (44), cardiovascular congenital anomalies (44), and intratrachial flow during breathing movements (10). In this chapter, specific attention is given to the study of blood flow in the uterine and fetoplacental circulation.

Although the role of feto- and uteroplacental blood flow is of clear relevance to the understanding of pregnancy in general and those pregnancies complicated by such conditions as intrauterine growth retardation, diabetes, or maternal hypertension in particular, until quite recently there have been no reliable techniques available with which to make blood flow measurements noninvasively. As a result, the bulk of present knowledge of fetal and placental blood flow, in both normal and complicated pregnancies, is derived from animal studies using methods based on, for example, the use of radioactive microspheres (18,61). During the past two decades, however, a number of newer invasive techniques have been applied to human pregnancy. These include radiolabeled blood and blood-borne tracers (38), electromagnetic flowmeters (1), thermometry (4), and thermodilution (67). Some preliminary data are already becoming available to suggest that as well as offering the advantages of being wholly noninvasive, reproducible, and suited for use in a clinical environment, Doppler ultrasound measurements are confirming in humans patterns of pathological change already reported for blood flow in experimentally induced growth retardation, suggesting promise for Doppler ultrasound as a new diagnostic tool in clinical obstetrics.

EXPERIMENTAL BLOOD FLOW MEASUREMENTS IN PREGNANCY

Uteroplacental Perfusion

With intrauterine growth retardation (IUGR), widespread pathological structural changes have been described in the uteroplacental circulation. These include changes in the trophoblasts of the placenta, obliterative endarteritis of the fetal stem arteries, and narrowing of the lumen of the arteriolar branches of the uterine spiral vessels (39,65). Such changes are likely to increase the total resistance in both the fetal and maternal–placental circulations and hence decrease overall blood flow. The inference that decreased uterine blood flow may compromise fetal nutrition and hence be one factor contributing to the high risk associated with small-for-gestational-age pregnancies has led to a persistent interest in the measurement of placental blood flow. Early experimental attempts to detect such flow changes in the human, however, showed ambiguous results. It has been suggested by Jones and Fox (39) that this may be because of a superposition of hypertension and other complications in the study population.

Jansson (38) made one of the earlier attempts to measure mean myometrial capillary blood flow in human pregnancy by injecting a ^{133}Xe solution into the anterior uterine wall and estimating blood flow from the clearance rate of the radioisotope. This was done without specific knowledge of the location of the placenta. Kaar et al. (42) used a different radionuclide technique, in which the intervillous flow was estimated from the washout rate of ^{133}Xe injected into the left antecubital vein. Unlike the previous study, this method included establishing the location of the placenta using B-mode ultrasound scanning so that activity could be monitored by a scintillation camera placed over the volume of interest. These workers obtained values for the mean intervillous blood flow rates in a number of different groups. They were highest in normal pregnancies (140 ± 53 ml/min·100 ml) and lowest in preeclampsia (99 ± 27 ml/min·100 ml) and severe (class B–E) forms of diabetes (89 ± 19 ml/mi·100 ml).

Lunell et al. (47) used an intravenous bolus of ^{133m}In, a nondiffusible radioactive tracer, accompanied by careful analysis of the rate of isotope accumulation in the placenta to exclude errors from the variation in intervillous blood volume between patients. They used this method to estimate relative uteroplacental flow in eight pregnancies complicated by IUGR and 11 normal controls. In spite of the considerable variation in both groups (which they attributed to biological variance) and their inability to correct for uterine volume, they observed a dramatic decrease in mean uteroplacental flow in the IUGR group, one-quarter of that in the control group. This was one of the earliest indications that abnormal uteroplacental flow rates might be related to clinically diagnosed IUGR. They also noted that there was no direct relationship between uteroplacental blood flow rate and birth weight and that uteroplacental flow remains relatively constant per unit weight of placenta throughout gestation. This latter observation was also confirmed by Jansson (38) and Assali et al. (1) in invasive experiments using electromagnetic flowmeters.

Nylund et al. (56,57) used a similar technique in a group of 56 women, 30 of whom had growth-retarded fetuses. The median uteroplacental flow index in the IUGR group was less than half that in the control group. Interestingly, the index was as low in the six women who gave birth to infants with congenital malformation as in the other 24 women in whom the growth retardation was caused by maternal factors. They suggested that this might lend credence to the hypothesis that maternal–placental flow is regulated in part by the fetus. It should be noted that in all of these studies, the technical limitation of the use of a γ camera confined the technique to patients with anterior placentas.

Finally, Maini et al. (48) have refined the ^{113m}In method of Lunnell et al. and with it the overall precision. The total error in the placental flow measurement in their study was predicted to lie between 12 and 16%. In the 19 IUGR patients studied, the placental flow was reduced to an average of 55% of the normal level. Again, there was statistical significance in the results but conspicuous overlap between the two groups. Several normal fetuses had flow values that were as low as some of the IUGR patients, whereas one fetus with extensive malformations and impaired growth showed normal flow. This led Maini et al. to warn that blood flow measurements could not, and should not, be taken to predict the outcome of a pregnancy in terms of the weight at birth, a warning that has been echoed recently in relation to Doppler measurements. Growth retardation clearly covers a wide range of factors that are capable of affecting fetal development and well-being. These may include low growth potential resulting from such conditions as chromosomal abnormality or an intrauterine infection. Limitations of nutrient supply to the fetus may be brought about by changes in placental permeability and metabolism, in maternal substrate concentration, as well as in placental perfusion itself. In many cases a number of these influences will be interrelated. For this reason a perfusion measurement, whether inferred from radioactive tracer clearance or Doppler ultrasound, should be viewed as a single physiological measurement and not as a clinical diagnosis of the fetus at risk.

Fetoplacental Flow

Flow in the umbilical vein has been measured in animals by a variety of techniques and in humans using electromagnetic flowmeters at abortion (1) and thermodilution after term delivery (52,67). One of the most convincing demonstrations that changes in umbilical flow rates are indeed associated with clinical IUGR has come from Clapp et al. (11). They induced growth retardation in fetal lambs by embolizing the uteroplacental bed with microspheres. Using implanted transducers to measure pressure and flow, they were able to calculate resistance in the placental circulation. In most of the cases studied, embolizing the uterine circulation resulted in a decrease in flow in both the uterine and umbilical sides of the placental circulation. Furthermore, IUGR resulted only if a consistent decrease in umbilical flow was seen following the embolizations. In the normal control pregnancies they noted that the umbilical flow increased steadily during the latter half of gestation and that this increase was related to a decrease in vascular resistance of the placental bed. In the fetal lambs in which IUGR had been induced, however, this progressive decrease was absent, thus offering an indication that indirect measurement of umbilical placental resistance such as that offered by Doppler ultrasound might be an aid in the diagnosis of IUGR.

In spite of the implication from morphological examination of human placentas that vasoocclusive lesions sometimes present with IUGR could alter fetoplacental as well as uteroplacental resistance, none of the methods described above are capable of the noninvasive investigation of human fetal–placental flow rates. Assali's comment in 1960 (1) that this circulation has proven "somewhat difficult to assess" has really obtained until today. Doppler ultrasound offers the first opportunity to study this circulation in detail, with both quantitative and qualitative techniques. It is perhaps this aspect of the Doppler method that, in spite of its inherent limitations, really presents an opportunity for a unique study of cardiovascular dynamics in pregnancy.

DOPPLER TECHNIQUES IN OBSTETRICS

The Fetus

Doppler signals can be obtained from the fetus at a variety of sites using pulsed Doppler duplex scanning or from the cord (and less reliably, elsewhere) using continuous-wave Doppler ultrasound without imaging. Until the end of the second trimester, 5 MHz is a suitable frequency for both imaging and Doppler; in the last trimester a Doppler frequency of 3 MHz or less is usually necessary. A variety of types of duplex scanner are available for obstetrical applications; some are illustrated in Fig. 1. These include sector scanners, which have the advantage of being suitable for both the uterine and fetal circulations but have the disadvantage that conventional systems are limited in their ability to measure volumetric flow rates. Some mechanical sector systems offer real-time imaging using a separate transducer operating at a higher frequency than that of the Doppler transducer; this can be useful where higher-resolution imaging is required for the Doppler examination of the fetal heart, for example.

Electronically steered sector scanners (or "phased arrays") offer real-time imaging at a reduced frame rate at the same time the pulsed Doppler signal is being acquired; this is often a helpful facility when pursuing a particularly active fetus for Doppler signals. In general, however, activity such as fetal breathing has such a dramatic effect on blood flow rates and time–velocity waveforms that fetal waveforms are best acquired during periods of inactivity. Linear arrays have a well-established place in obstetrical imaging, and two variations on this configuration for duplex scanning are shown in Fig. 1C,D. Both of these arrangements are capable of rapid alternation between Doppler and imaging modes, resulting in the "real-time" duplex display. The offset transducer system (Fig. 1D), although a potentially

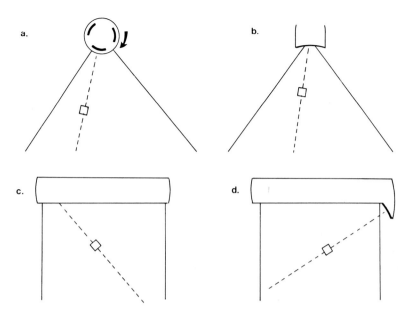

FIG. 1. Four configurations of duplex scanner suitable for obstetrical applications: (**A**) mechanical sector; (**B**) electronically steered sector; (**C**) electronically steered linear; (**D**) offset linear.

useful device for volumetric flow measurement, is quite cumbersome to use, especially for obtaining signals from the uterine artery.

Figure 2 shows some typical Doppler signals obtained from a 27-week fetus. The cord is sampled consistently from one point along its length; for consistency we choose a point as near as possible to its insertion in the placenta. Figure 2B,C illustrates how the best signal will not in general be obtained from a region in which the cord is imaged most clearly. The optimum imaging conditions obtained, of course, when the specular reflections from the vessel walls are directed back to the transducer; this occurs when the ultrasound beam is perpendicular to the axis of the vessel. With a sector scanner, this beam is also used for Doppler measurements, so the best Doppler signals are acquired when the vessel axis makes a small angle with the beam. Usually a loop of cord will provide a point at which arterial and venous velocity flow velocity signals can be heard. In the presence of oligohydramnios, this can become a surprisingly demanding examination. The umbilical artery waveform (Fig. 2C) has a typical triangular appearance derived from the relatively slow upstroke of systolic velocity, itself a consequence of the elasticity of the long arterial segment between the heart and the point of sampling. Note that at this stage of gestation there is a moderate degree of flow extending throughout diastole. The ascending aorta signal (Fig. 2D) can be obtained near the aortic root and is recognized by the rapid acceleration during systole. The pulmonary artery, which in the fetus is the vessel carrying the highest blood flow rate, can be identified from a short-axis view of the heart at the level of the great vessels; the signal is rather similar in appearance to that of the ascending aorta.

The descending aorta signal (Fig. 2E) can be obtained in the thorax just above the level of the diaphragm. This location excludes the possibility of variation caused by the major branches of the aorta, which occur in the upper abdomen. Because

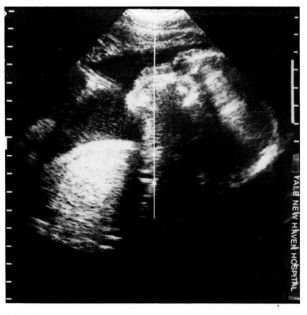

A

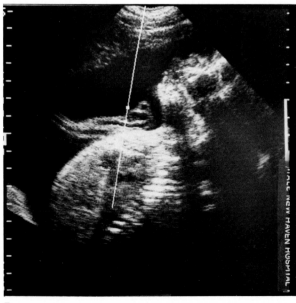

B

FIG. 2. A: Doppler signals from a typical 27-week fetus, scanned using a mechanical sector duplex scanner with 5-MHz annular array imaging and 3-MHz Doppler transducer. **B:** The sample volume positioned in umbilical cord artery. **C:** Umbilical cord artery signal. **D:** The ascending aorta. **E:** The descending aorta. **F:** The common carotid artery. **G:** Common carotid artery signal.

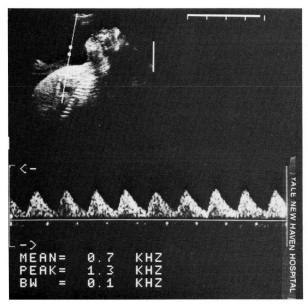

C

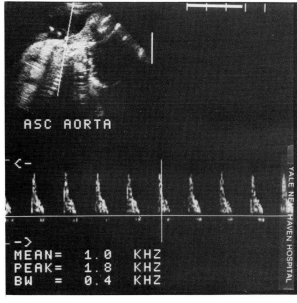

FIG. 2. (continued)

D

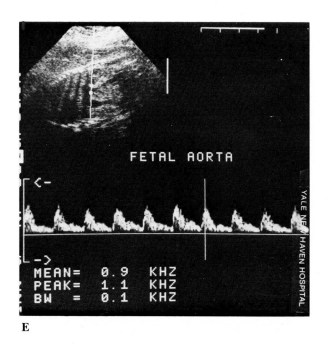

E

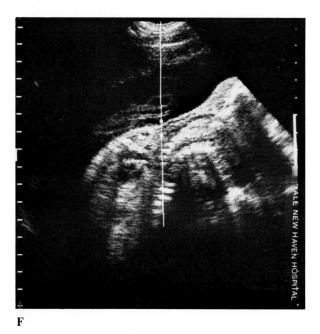

FIG. 2. (continued)

F

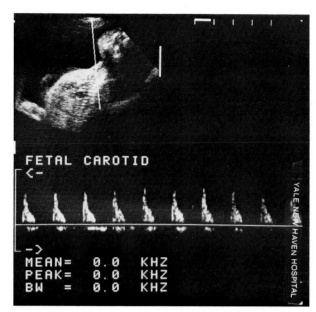

FIG. 2. (continued)

G

the course of the aorta usually lies parallel to the maternal skin surface, it is often difficult to obtain a good Doppler angle without using an offset system such as the linear arrays shown in Fig. 1. Note that in the signal shown in Fig. 2E, there is already an indication of variation in velocity profile over the cardiac cycle, with plug flow occurring in systole and blunted parabolic flow in diastole. Figure 1F,G illustrates a signal from the common carotid artery of the fetus. This is not as difficult an examination as it may seem. In our series of 98 fetal carotid examinations, the technical success rate was approximately 80%. Signals can also be obtained from the intra-abdominal portion of the umbilical vein (see Fig. 13). Doppler examination of the umbilical cord vessels is possible in nearly all cases from early in the second trimester onward. Figure 3 shows typical cord artery and vein signals using an electronically steered duplex scanner in a fetus of between 15 and 17 weeks' gestation. Note that there is relatively low flow at the end of diastole in the cord artery signal.

The Uterine Circulation

Doppler signals may be obtained from the uteroplacental circulation at the level of the uterine or arcuate arteries. To detect uterine arterial signals transabdominally, a parasagittal plane following the uterine wall in the lower segment is employed. Alternatively, a vaginal approach is possible using a CW probe positioned in the lateral fornix, although the confusion of pelvic vessels lying within the transducer beams can make the identification of signals difficult (68).

Figure 4 shows the iliac bifurcation together with the distinctive Doppler signatures of the major pelvic vessels. The common and external iliacs show the reverse flow component in diastole typical of a high-impedance distal circulation; the internal iliac (Fig. 4D) has a small amount of forward flow in diastole with a marked notch at the

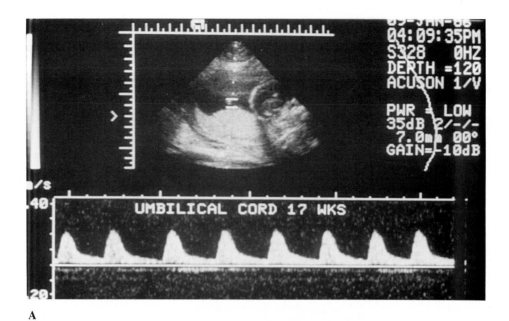

A

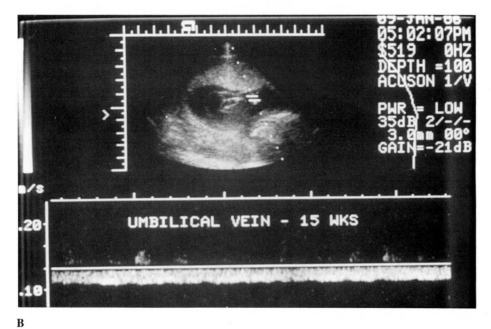

B

FIG. 3. Umbilical cord signals at 15 to 17 weeks using an electronically steered sector scanner at 3.5 MHz: **(A)** artery; **(B)** vein.

end of systole. The normal uterine artery, on the other hand, has a marked forward diastolic flow component with no notch (Figs. 4E and 22A). With duplex scanning one can trace the uterine artery anteriorly from its origin with the internal iliac and superiorly to obtain signals from the uterine wall, believed to originate from flow in the arcuate vessels (9) (Fig. 5).

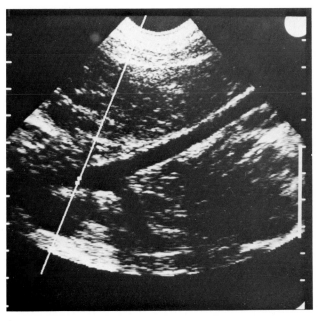

A

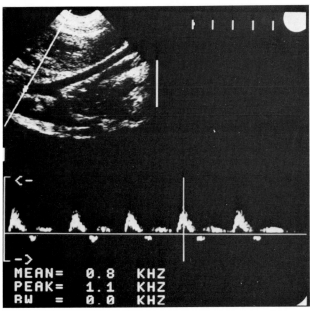

B

FIG. 4. The pelvic vessels in pregnancy at 32 weeks: (**A**) the bifurcation of the common iliac artery; (**B**) the common iliac artery signal; (**C**) the external iliac artery signal (note the reversed diastolic flow); (**D**) the internal iliac signal; (**E**) the uterine artery signal (note the high diastolic flow).

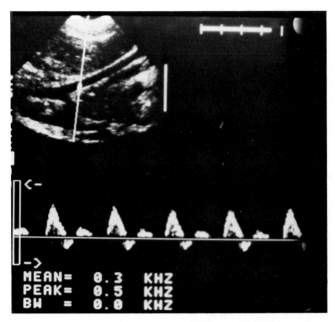

MEAN= 0.3 KHZ
PEAK= 0.5 KHZ
BW = 0.0 KHZ

C

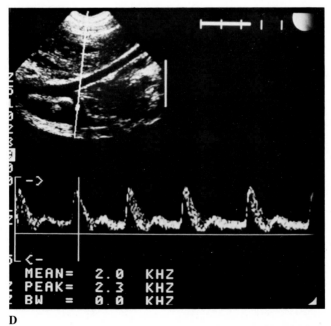

MEAN= 2.0 KHZ
PEAK= 2.3 KHZ
BW = 0.0 KHZ

FIG. 4. (continued)

D

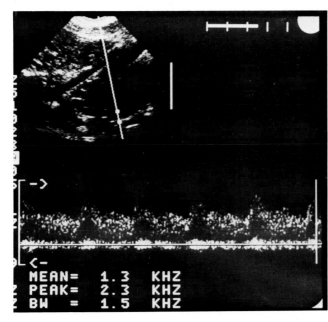

MEAN= 1.3 KHZ
PEAK= 2.3 KHZ
BW = 1.5 KHZ

FIG. 4. (continued)

E

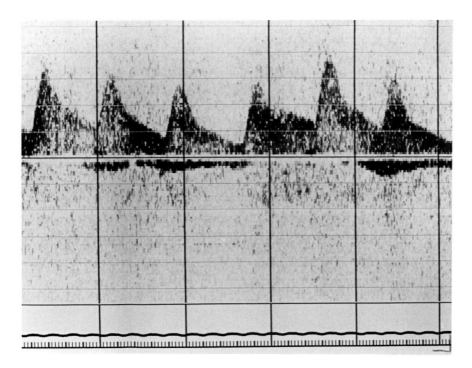

FIG. 5. Arcuate artery signal from normal 33-week pregnancy. The modulation of the Doppler shift is an effect of maternal respiration.

The characteristics of the normal uterine flow signal in the second and third trimesters render it unique in the pelvis and therefore relatively easy to identify. Even with duplex scanning, it is often necessary to rely on these Doppler characteristics in order to identify the vessel, as visualization using real-time ultrasound imaging is frequently poor, and the anatomical relationship of the vessels changes as the uterus enlarges. The distinctive signatures of these vessels have encouraged users of CW Doppler to perform uterine Doppler examinations transabdominally without imaging guidance (23,63,72,74). Although it is relatively easy to obtain uterine artery signals in this fashion from the second trimester onwards, a problem arises in the identification of vessel sites in patients with abnormal characteristics. In particular, the abnormal uterine artery waveform looks remarkably similar to the normal internal iliac waveform (*vide infra*). For this reason it is an essential component of any examination in which a signal appearing to originate from an abnormal uterine artery is seen to obtain a separate signal from the internal iliac artery. This procedure seems most straightforward to perform using pulsed Doppler duplex scanning. Arcuate vessels are easier to see, as they run a less tortuous path; a linear array is probably best for this. The example of Fig. 5 shows marked beat-to-beat variation, which is probably associated with changes in abdominal pressure with maternal respiration. Both the relative diastolic flow velocity and the peak systolic velocity increase in the uterine artery toward the end of pregnancy: a signal from a normal 39-week uterus is shown in Fig. 6. The high Doppler shifts with a substantial continuous component are indicative of a high-flow, maximally vasodilated circulation.

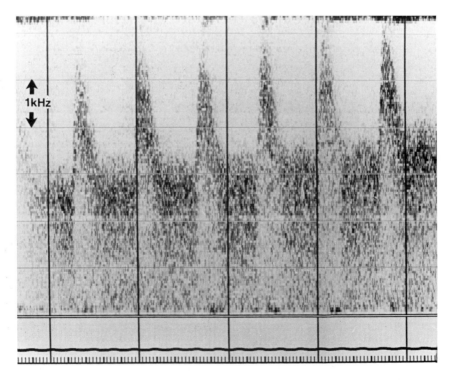

FIG. 6. Normal uterine artery signal near term (39 weeks). Both the systolic and diastolic Doppler shifts are unusually high. The ultrasound frequency is 3 MHz.

Fetal Exposure and Safety Using Pulsed Doppler Ultrasound

Although over one million pregnant women now receive at least one diagnostic ultrasound imaging examination each year, and several hundred investigations of bioeffects on plant and animal tissue have been undertaken, there is still some uncertainty as to the nature of potential risk to the fetus during a clinical ultrasound examination. This uncertainty has become more pronounced with the application of pulsed Doppler ultrasound to the fetus. There are several possible reasons for this. First, the acoustic intensity averaged over time (the spatial peak temporal average intensity, SPTA) is considerably higher in pulsed Doppler mode with many duplex scanners than in most imaging instruments. One survey (55) reports values up to 750 mW/cm^2, but some pulsed Doppler systems are known to deliver SPTA intensities as high as 1,000 to 2,000 mW/cm^2. Second, the beam in a Doppler examination is stationary and may insonate a target area for a period of minutes, in contrast to an imaging beam that moves quite rapidly through a much larger volume of tissue. Finally, it is widely felt that of all tissues, those of the fetus are likely to be among the most sensitive to biological effects of ultrasound. At present, the U. S. Food and Drug Administration has not approved the marketing of any single-gate pulsed Doppler duplex system for fetal use, bringing questions to many users' minds as to whether this modality is indeed safe for clinical use.

There are two classes of interaction of ultrasound with tissue that it is relevant to consider. Heating is a consequence of the progressive absorption of ultrasound energy as it travels through tissue. Heat production is affected by the tissue type as well as the form and frequency of the ultrasound beam, with higher frequencies associated with more rapid absorption. Although fetal tissue is sensitive to heat, it is generally assumed that induced temperature changes that are less than those of normal diurnal variation (about 1°C) are of no consequence. Local temperature rise will increase with the SPTA intensity but will also be affected by physiological factors such as local blood flow.

Nonthermal effects in tissue can be caused by the growth of oscillating microbubbles in tissue fluids, stimulated by the presence of the ultrasound field. Such stable cavitation can modify cell function or destroy cells. However, stable cavitation requires relatively long "on" times of the ultrasonic field. These are found in continuous-wave but not pulsed Doppler systems. Finally, the more dangerous phenomenon of transient cavitation is certainly capable of destroying tissue but can only occur at high instantaneous (that is, spatial peak temporal peak, SPTP) intensities. Transient cavitation is not known to take place in tissue at diagnostic intensities. Furthermore, conventional imaging employs higher SPTP intensities than pulsed Doppler, so that if there is a risk it will be greater for ultrasound imaging than for pulsed Doppler.

It would be fair to conclude, then, that concern over the use of pulsed Doppler systems in the fetus centers on the possibility of temperature rise in tissue. By reducing both SPTA intensity and exposure time, the likelihood of such an effect taking place can be minimized. As long as there is the possibility of subtle effects on tissue from ultrasound exposure, however, it seems prudent to employ as low an ultrasound intensity and as short an examination time as are consistent with obtaining clinically useful data. At present, there have been no independently confirmed significant biological effects noted in mammalian tissues exposed to ultrasound SPTA intensities below 100 mW/cm^2. At our institution we limit exposure level of all examinations to below this value. Current indications are that if the FDA does decide to approve instruments for fetal Doppler examination, the maximum exposure intensities that they will specify are likely to be considerably above this value. However, as fetal Doppler is still an experimental method, our own research protocols are approved by our institutional Human Investigations Committee, whom we also keep informed of the changing state of discussion on the issues involved. At present, written informed consent is obtained from all patients who participate in our obstetrical Doppler studies.

Calibration of machine intensity is not a trivial procedure. Fortunately, the FDA requires calibration of all ultrasound instruments before they are marketed in the United States, so these data are known by the manufacturer and should be made available to the user. With the help of these, it is a simple matter to reduce the output of the Doppler system to the desired level. Using modern machines, it is our experience that all obstetrical Doppler examinations can be performed easily at SPTA exposure levels of less than 100 mW/cm^2 without noticeable loss in signal quality. Sensitive pulsed Doppler systems are able to function well at exposure levels below those of ultrasonic fetal heart monitors now in routine use.

In summary, concern over the use of fetal Doppler is a consequence of the relatively high acoustic output of some duplex scanners designed for peripheral vascular use rather than of any known risk of hazard. By adjusting the output of such systems to as low a value as possible and reducing Doppler examination time, such potential risk may be minimized without prejudice to signal quality.

VOLUME FLOW MEASUREMENT IN THE FETOMATERNAL CIRCULATION

The invasive and animal studies described above suggest an obvious role for a method capable of the noninvasive measurement of flow in the human feto- and uteroplacental circulations. Here it is the physiological quantity of volumetric flow, preferably normalized with respect to fetal weight, that it is desired to measure. Early attempts (15) using rather crude methodology were quickly refined into an ultrasonic technique that has found application in circulations outside pregnancy (29,30,50). In fact, much of the development of Doppler volume flow calculations has taken place in the context of the fetus. Furthermore, the clinical results of the volume flow estimations performed to date lay a foundation for the use of the more accessible technique of time–velocity waveform shape analysis, which is described in the next section.

All clinical studies of obstetrical flow measurement reported to date have employed a variation of the even-insonation technique described in Chapter 4. Although the basic principles of the technique are simple, practical applicability is constrained by some inherent limitations, which are mostly physical in origin. At present, these confine the method to selected vessels in the fetal circulation.

The principle of the even-insonation method is illustrated in Fig. 7. The mean velocity of blood flowing at one point in a vessel is measured using the Doppler system and multiplied by the lumen cross-sectional area, yielding volume flow.

For this measurement, then, three parameters are required. First, the mean Doppler shift is calculated from the Doppler power spectrum and averaged over time.

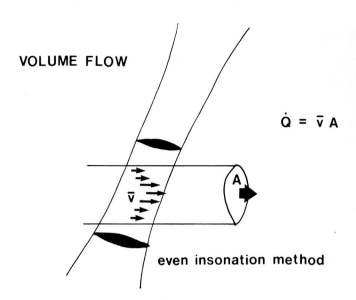

VOLUME FLOW

$$\dot{Q} = \bar{v} A$$

even insonation method

FIG. 7. The principle of the even-insonation method for the measurement of volume flow. The volume flow rate $\dot{Q}$ is equal to the product of the spatial mean velocity $\bar{v}$ and the lumen area A.

Then, the beam–vessel angle must be measured in order to solve the Doppler equation and calculate the mean velocity $\bar{v}(t)$. Finally, the cross-sectional area A of the vessel must be estimated.

Beam–Vessel Angle

For a given Doppler shift frequency and blood flow in a large vessel, it is a simple matter to solve the Doppler equation for velocity using an estimate of the beam–flow angle obtained from the two dimensional image. Most duplex scanners provide a cursor for the direct measurement of this angle. However, as discussed in Chapter 4, the error in the estimate of velocity resulting from the uncertainty of angle measurement is strongly dependent on the magnitude of the angle itself. For angles less than about 30°, the error will be reduced to practical insignificance. For larger angles, the cosine term in the Doppler equation causes a small uncertainty in the measurement of the angle, which results in a large error in velocity estimation; the technique should probably not be used for angles greater than about 55°. Looking at Fig. 1 and considering a vessel lying parallel to the maternal abdomen, it is apparent that a satisfactory angle of insonation requires an offset Doppler system, such as a linear array with a Doppler transducer mounted on the end or attached to an articulated arm. The sector scanners with their Doppler beam originating from the apex of the field of view are the most difficult in this respect. An example of a scan using a linear array with an offset Doppler signal is shown in Fig. 8. Recently, linear array scanners that use phased array technology to direct an oblique beam within the rectangular image field of view (Fig. 1C) have allowed transducer arrays that are not specifically modified for Doppler to be used instead of the offset configuration. Alternatively, a sector or linear array scanner may be modified to allow the addition of an offset Doppler transducer attached by an articulated arm (Fig. 9). This configuration has the advantage of a variable approach angle for the Doppler beam and the opportunity to choose the optimum characteristics for the dedicated Doppler

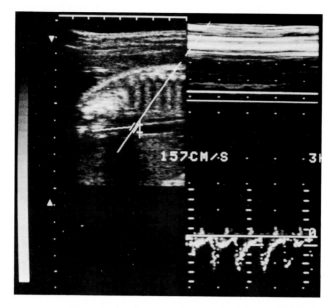

FIG. 8. Volume flow calculation of the thoracic fetal aorta using a linear array with fixed offset Doppler transducer.

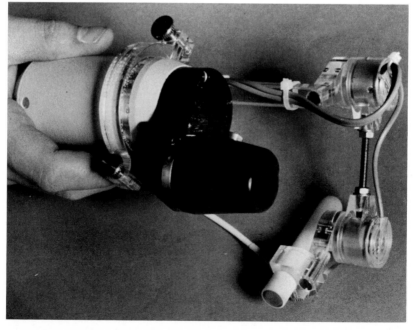

FIG. 9. Example of custom-made duplex device for volume flow measurement. The offset Doppler transducer operates at a lower frequency than the imager, and the angle of approach is optimized using the articulated arm with position sensors.

transducer. Whatever method is used, the need to measure the angle of insonation confines this method to vessels whose axis lies in the same plane for a few centimeters of its course. Excluded, therefore, are the umbilical cord vessels and the maternal uterine arteries, both of which follow a helical or very curved path. Two suitable vessels for ultrasound volume flow measurements are the fetal descending aorta and the intraabdominal umbilical vein (7).

Cross-Sectional Area

The most common method for the estimation of the cross-sectional area of the vessel orifice is to measure its diameter and assume circular symmetry. Because of the quadratic dependence of area on diameter, the percentage error in diameter measurement will cause an error of approximately double that figure in the flow estimate. For example, a 1-mm uncertainty in the measurement of a 6-mm vessel will produce a 33% variation in the flow calculation. To minimize such errors, a variety of methods have been proposed. Eik-Nes et al. (16), for example, described an M-mode tracking device that follows the moving echoes from arterial walls. The limiting factor, however, remains the performance of the imaging system. Once again, the requirements for high-resolution imaging of the vessel lumen are at variance with those for adequate Doppler signals. Early studies employed a linear array system with relatively poor resolution for such a measurement; later workers used higher-resolution imaging or M-mode. The further question of which echoes one should choose in order to measure the vessel lumen diameter is one that cannot be answered by *in vitro* calibration: an invasive *in vivo* comparison with a reliable flow-measuring standard is needed to resolve such questions. The problem is that such a standard does not exist: even if an electromagnetic or ultrasonic transit time flow-meter yields an accurate flow rate in a dissected vessel, the ultrasonic tissue path (which affects the imaging contrast resolution) will inevitably have been altered in such an experiment. In practice, the best one can do is make a careful measurement using a consistent technique, preferably with an M-mode beam operating at a high ultrasound frequency and intersecting the precise location of the Doppler sample volume.

The cross-sectional area of fetal vessels varies considerably over the cardiac cycle: Fig. 10 shows a 5-mm fetal aorta varying 20% in diameter—that is, 40% in cross-sectional area—between systole and diastole. For such distensible vessels, it would be better to calculate the instantaneous area and multiply by the instantaneous mean flow value, but this is rarely possible. For the situation of the highly distensible vessel with appreciable diastolic flow, such as the fetal descending aorta, Eik-Nes et al. (16,17) have estimated that by averaging the area from ten diameter measurements on a frozen real-time scan, they introduce an error of approximately 10% in the flow calculation. Further errors result if the vessel, particularly the umbilical vein, is not circulate in cross section. Here real-time imaging could be used, but there remains the difficulty of ensuring that the image plane is perpendicular to the flow axis. Figures 11 and 12 show how with nondedicated equipment these errors can accumulate to the point that the method may be incapable of detecting any difference between flow rates in normal and IUGR fetuses. These considerations alone probably limit the usefulness of such measurements in small vessels such as those found in the fetus without recourse to specially designed equipment (30).

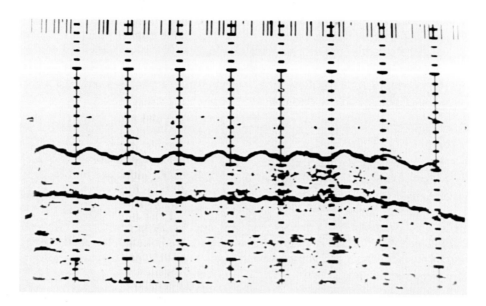

FIG. 10. An M-mode representation of the diameter of the thoracic aorta of a 28-week fetus, showing diameter variation over the cardiac cycle. Each vertical marker represents 1 mm. The 20% variation between systolic and diastolic diameter shown here corresponds to an approximately 40% variation in lumen area over the cardiac cycle.

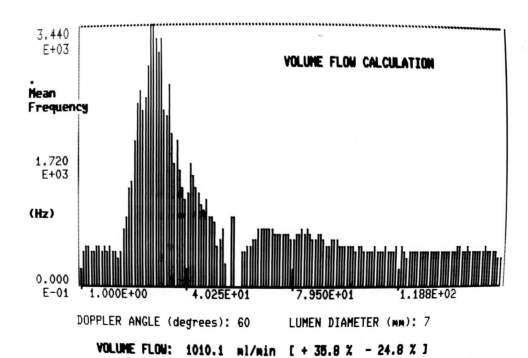

FIG. 11. A typical volume flow measurement from a sector duplex scanner applied to the fetal aorta, with estimated errors. The final value is averaged over ten heartbeats.

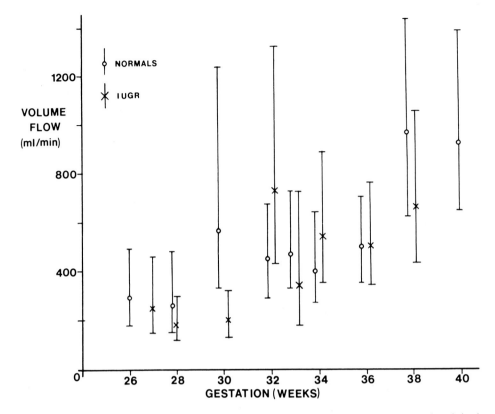

FIG. 12. Volume flow results from normal and IUGR patients measured using conventional duplex equipment in the thoracic descending aorta. The error bars represent the estimated sum of systematic and random uncertainties. Note that these obscure any difference between normal and IUGR pregnancies.

Mean Doppler Shift Frequency

The mean Doppler shift frequency, calculated as the normalized first moment of the Doppler power spectrum, corresponds to the average velocity of the scatterers moving within a volume of uniform insonation. This is the quantity needed to measure volume flow. If the beam is sufficiently uniform and the sample volume length sufficiently long, the mean Doppler shift frequency corresponds to the average velocity within a vessel lumen. Once this spatial mean velocity is estimated, an average value over several, perhaps ten, cardiac cycles is calculated. In practice this is, however, one of the more difficult parameters to tackle using Doppler ultrasound (19,29).

Unlike the maximum velocity, detecting the mean velocity requires measurement of flow elements that extend over a large volume. In a large vessel, the flow profile is likely to contain slow-moving elements near the vessel walls; in smaller vessels a parabolic flow profile contains a different velocity at every point across the lumen diameter. If the mean velocity is to be determined accurately, all these must contribute equally to the Doppler signal. The beam should not vary in intensity over the sensitive volume, and the receiver should not vary in sensitivity over the duration of the sample gate or for different Doppler shift frequencies. Additionally, the sample volume should embrace the entire lumen of the vessel, both axially and laterally. In reality these requirements are unattainable (19).

As discussed above, the cross-sectional area measurement is only reliable in larger vessels, so that those duplex scanners that use the same beam for Doppler ultrasound and imaging are unlikely to have a beam with sufficient lateral extent to insonate the entire lumen. The solution is to use lower-frequency dedicated Doppler transducers such as that illustrated in Fig. 9 designed to produce a beam whose lateral extent is as large as possible. Special techniques, such as the use of annular arrays, can be used to flatten a Doppler beam profile (7), but it remains difficult to create a uniform sensitivity over the lateral extent of the beam. The sensitivity of the receiver to different Doppler frequencies is modified by a high-pass filter designed to reject the clutter signals described earlier. Excluding low Doppler frequencies introduces an error into the mean velocity estimate, which varies with the flow velocity profile.

Calculation of the mean Doppler shift itself can be made using a variety of techniques, both analog (29) and digital (2). The first moment is sensitive to spurious contributions of very low or very high frequency; these may come from clutter from pulsating solid structures, e.g., those of the fetal heart, or from equipment noise. Digital systems have the potential advantage that they can be programmed to restrict the influence of such artifacts. A calculation using one such system is shown in Fig. 11. The relatively high estimated error in this measurement is a consequence of using a duplex sector scanner; note that the angle of insonation is high.

Some workers have been tempted to dispense with the calculation of the mean frequency altogether, relying on a visual inspection of the spectral display to give the maximum Doppler shift frequency. Unfortunately, this will only bear a predictable relationship to the mean frequency if the velocity profile remains constant throughout the cardiac cycle (53). Figure 2E shows that in the fetal aorta, at least, this is not the case, so an empirically derived "calibration factor" is unlikely to be satisfactory. In parabolic flow, the maximum Doppler shift frequency is double the mean frequency, so that ignoring this difference can lead to errors of up to 100%. Griffin et al. (35) dispensed with the calculation of the mean frequency, instead estimating the mean frequency from the subjective appearance of gray levels in the spectral display. This is a rather precarious matter, however. The gray scale in a display bears a nonlinear relationship (usually square-root or logarithmic) to the spectral power and can therefore be misleading to the operator.

Finally, an appropriate sample gate must be chosen to insonate the selected volume of blood. Gill (28) has shown that for low beam–flow angles, a gate length that actually exceeds the width of the vessel will serve to compensate in part for the inadequacies of the beam width. Unfortunately, in the case of the fetal aorta in particular, this may cause clutter from the fetal heart or interference from the fetal inferior vena cava to enter the sample volume.

Clinical Studies

In spite of the methodological difficulties outlined above, which have been noted by several investigators (7,16,28), a number of measurements of fetal flow rates have been made using ultrasound Doppler techniques. The first studies were made in 1979 by Gill in Australia using a modified eight-transducer water-path system (29,30) and by Eik-Nes in Norway using a linear array with offset Doppler scanner (15). Among subsequent measurements of fetal umbilical venous and descending aorta flow are those by Kurjak and Rajhrajn (45), Jouppila and Kirkinen (40,41), Griffin et al. (35,36), Marsal et al. (49), and van Lierde et al. (75) (Table 1). A typical measurement from the umbilical vein of the 28-week fetus is shown in Fig. 13. First, the diameter of the vessel is measured using the B-scan or M-mode image. The Doppler signal is then acquired, and the beam–vessel angle is measured. The mean velocity is calculated from the temporal integral of the first moment of the Doppler power spectrum, the product of this value and the lumen area yielding the volume flow estimate. The accumulated systematic errors in such a measurement depend on ultrasonic parameters that are likely to vary from patient to patient as well as from instrument to instrument.

The most systematic approach to the development of dedicated instrumentation for fetal blood flow measurement has been that of Gill (29–31). Using the "Octoson" system, Gill et al. (32,33) employ eight transducers arranged in a water bath below the patient (Fig. 14). The transducers are used to obtain a compound B-scan, from which the umbilical vein diameter measurement is made. A transducer is then selected to give the optimum angle of insonation with respect to the axis of the vessel and is connected to the pulsed Doppler system. A frequency of 1.5 or 3 MHz is chosen according to the vessel size, the larger beam of the lower-frequency system being used to ensure even insonation of vessels beyond 7 mm in diameter. An analog processor is used to estimate the mean Doppler shift frequency, an average over 5 sec of which is then fed into the volume flow calculation. The final flow value may then be corrected for fetal weight, which is estimated using standard biometric techniques.

With such specialized instrumentation and careful attention to the analysis of physical sources of error, Gill estimates that he achieves systematic errors of less than 10%, with random errors slightly in excess of this figure (31). However, using

TABLE 1. *Normal fetal volume blood flow rates estimated using doppler ultrasound*[a]

First author	Reference		Technique	Gestational age (wks)	N	Volume flow rate (ml/min · kg)	
						Umb v	Thoracic Ao
Gill	30	1979	Octoson	25–40	12	104	
Eik-Nes	15	1980	Linear with offset	32–41	26	110	191
Gill	33	1981	Octoson	26–35	27	120	
Gill	33	1981	Octoson	35–40	20	106	
Jouppila	41	1981	Linear with offset	30–36	101	108	
Kurjak	45	1982	Sector	30–41	63	107	
Griffin	35, 36	1983	Linear with offset	24–42	45	122	246 ($n = 75$)
Lindblad	46	1984	Linear with offset	Term	6	100	220
Marsal	49	1984	Linear with offset	27–40	64		240
Van Lierde	75	1984	Linear with offset	37–40	20	117	216
Assali	1	1960	EM at abortion	10–28	10	114	
Stembera	67	1965	Thermodilution	Term	17	75	
Rudolph	62	1971	Microspheres at abortion	10–20	11	110	

[a] N, number of patients studied; umb v, umbilical vein; Ao, aorta.

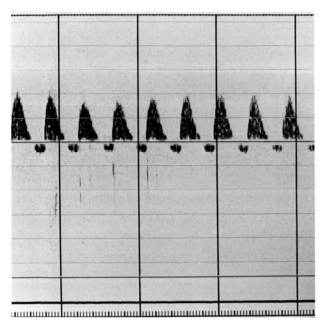

A

FIG. 20. A: Fetal distress. Note reverse flow in the umbilical artery. B: Regurgitant flow persists throughout diastole in the fetal thoracic aorta and can be traced through the ductus arteriosis into the pulmonary circulation.

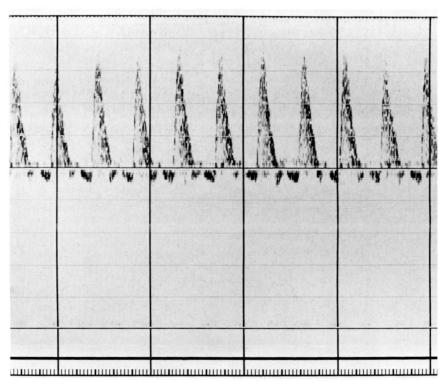

B

cord PI decreases correspondingly, as first reported by Stuart et al. (66) and shown in Fig. 17. Cord measurements are made most reliably with a pulsed Doppler sample volume length comparable to the diameter of the cord artery, so as to avoid sampling umbilical venous flow or flow from the body of the placenta. Many workers, however, employ continuous-wave Doppler ultrasound, some with the benefits of duplex imaging guidance, others not. The descending aorta flow signals (Fig. 2E) show blunted parabolic flow with a shorter rise time, with flow again persisting throughout diastole. Only approximately 50% of this flow is destined for the placenta (35), and PIs from this vessel, measured just above the diaphragm, show more variation than do those of the umbilical cord artery. A normal range is shown in Fig. 18.

It might be speculated that if the low fetoplacental flow rates observed by Gill and others in cases of IUGR result from an increase in resistance to flow in the placenta, then low flow may be reflected by changes in the time–velocity waveform of the cord artery and hence its PI. This is indeed the case (Fig. 19). In a study of the RI in 221 patients, for example, Fitzgerald et al. (22) report a statistically significant rise in RI (greater than the mean plus two standard deviations) in 77% of patients with birth weights below the tenth centile. In 13 of the 22 IUGR fetuses, no diastolic flow was observed (Fig. 19B). In severe cases, reverse flow is seen in the cord artery and fetal descending aorta (Fig. 20). Data are accumulating to suggest that Clapp's observation that IUGR is associated with raised resistance in the fetoplacental bed also holds for human IUGR. Giles et al. (27), for example, undertook a pathological correlation between Doppler signals and IUGR placentas and observed a higher count of small muscular arterials (less than 90 μm diameter) in the tertiary stem villi of placentas in patients who had a high Doppler *A/B* ratio. The control group of "at-risk" pregnancies, on the other hand, with normal *A/B* ratio had the same modal small vessel count as normal pregnancies. The authors concluded that abnormal time–velocity waveforms in the umbilical artery identify placentas with a high rate of obliteration of the tertiary stem villi. They also noted that the clinical outcome correlated with the antenatal Doppler study, with high *A/B* ratio accompanying high morbidity in the neonatal study population.

This time–velocity domain approach to the analysis of waveforms has been pursued in the umbilical circulation by Thomson et al. (69), who examined a variety of approaches to the comparison of normal and abnormal waveforms and suggested that one of them, the relative flow rate index, may be a useful supplement to a ratio intended to reflect resistance. This index is defined as the ratio of the mean of the maximum Doppler shift frequency taken before peak systole and the mean of the maximum Doppler shift frequency taken after peak systole. Because the index is affected by the acceleration of the blood in systole, they suggest that it should reflect fetal cardiac contractability as well as relative diastolic flow. It is certainly likely that mechanisms for compensation of cardiac output exist in the face of raised fetoplacental resistance and that future efforts in the interpretation of umbilical waveforms may result in the explanation of these as diagnostic signs.

Waveform Analysis in the Uterine Circulation

The relatively small diameter and tortuous course of the uterine vessels at present render them unsuitable for volume flow measurement using Doppler flow ultrasound.

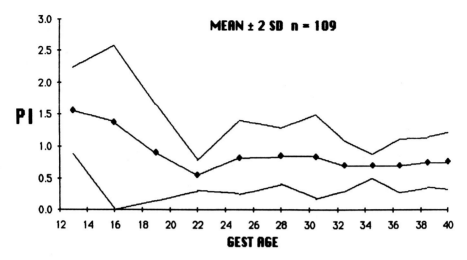

FIG. 21. Normal range of pulsatility index in the maternal uterine artery measured near its origin with the internal iliac. (From Burns, P. N., Grannum, P. A. T., Copel, J., and Hobbins, J. A., *unpublished data*, 1986.)

However, much of the evidence of flow changes associated with growth retardation points to uteroplacental perfusion, and it seems likely that analysis of the time-velocity waveforms here will be of clinical interest, as they reflect a fundamental aspect of the evolution of the placental circulation in pregnancy.

By about the 20th week of normal gestation, the trophoblast invades the placenta and migrates through the course of the spiral arteries. One effect of this invasion is to destroy the smooth muscle lining of these vessels and hence control of their tone by the maternal vasomotor system. From this point onward, these vessels are effectively at a point of maximal vasodilation, and this presumably accounts for the unusually low resistance of the uteroplacental bed. The PI for the uterine artery measured in normal subjects from 13 to 40 weeks, taken at its origin from the internal iliac artery (Fig. 21), shows a marked drop in pulsatility from about 14 to 20 weeks, from which point the PI remains fairly constant at about 0.8 to 1.0. This is consistent with the physiological process described above.

Where the trophoblastic invasion is ineffective or incomplete, normal vasomotor tone results in an abnormally high resistance of the distal uterine circulation. Pathological examination of the placenta may reveal thrombotic and other vasoocclusive lesions in the uterine spiral arteries (14). The result is decreased uteroplacental perfusion, which may lead to intrauterine growth retardation (IUGR). That this chain of events is probably related to toxemia of pregnancy is suggested by the work of Brosens (5,6), who examined placental bed biopsies in patients with pregnancy-induced hypertension and found that in all cases the trophoblastic invasion had failed or was incomplete. Furthermore, 50% of normotensive patients with IUGR showed only superficial placental invasion, indicating that IUGR may itself be a consequence of a primary problem of impaired uteroplacental flow.

Gerretsen et al. (25) looked at 93 biopsies from the placentas of a group that included 30 preeclamptic patients. They confirmed the physiological change observed by Brosens in the normal arteries and its absence in preeclampsia. In addition, they documented a relationship between the degree of invasion and the neonatal

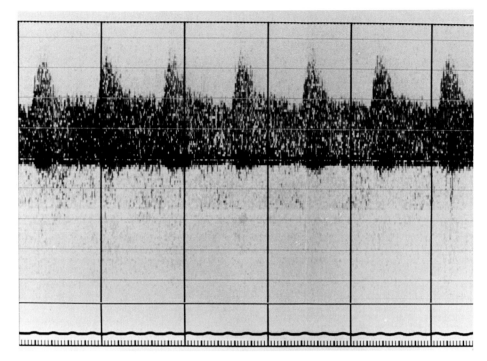

A

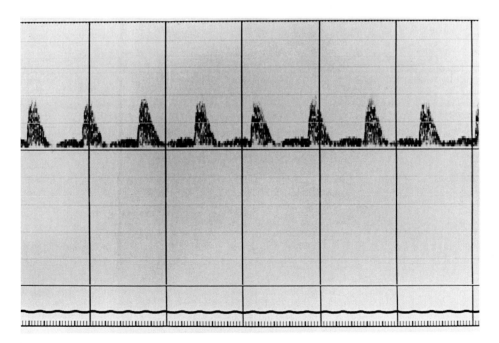

B

FIG. 22. A: Uterine artery signal from a normal 33-week pregnancy. **B:** Uterine artery signal from a 33-week patient with toxemia of pregnancy. Note high pulsatility.

outcome, with 70% of the patients in whom the change was completely absent giving birth to infants weighing less than the 2.5th centile. They hypothesized that hypertension in pregnancy is a consequence of failure of the spiral arteries to undergo these adaptive changes. Either the elevation of blood pressure succeeds as a mechanism of compensation, in which case uteroplacental perfusion is preserved and the pregnancy progresses to a normal outcome, or the mechanism fails. It could fail, they speculate, if either the rise in blood pressure is limited or the hypertension gives rise to side effects such as vasospasm or thrombosis; in both cases the result is fetal growth retardation. Thus, a subset of patients with raised uteroplacental resistance would be predicted to bear IUGR babies. Trudinger (73,74) has suggested that it may be of value to proceed on the basis of an abnormal uterine artery waveform to an umbilical artery waveform measurement, thus determining whether there may, in fact, be fetal compromise.

The existence of such mechanisms of compensation has also been proposed for the fetus itself: of Gill's patients (32) in whom pathological placentas were diagnosed with ultrasound, only a proportion went on to suffer poor outcome, and these corresponded to the low-flow group. This certainly would help to explain why placental pathology is not a particularly good predictor of fetal well-being (24).

Clinical Doppler examination with Doppler ultrasound bears out both the normal physiological change in uterine vascular resistance and the abnormally high resistance of some toxemic patients. An example of a uterine artery signal from a patient

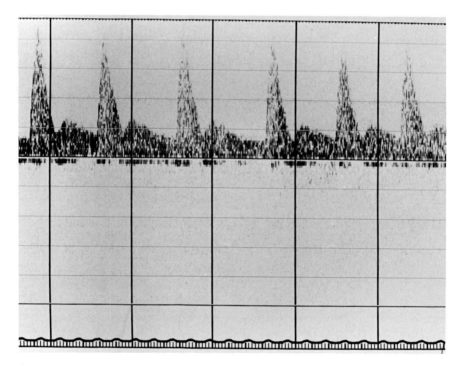

FIG. 23. Uterine artery signal in the nongravid patient. Note the similarity in waveform shape to that of Fig. 22B.

with toxemia of pregnancy is shown in Fig. 22. Here the PI is higher than two standard deviations above the mean for that gestational age but within the normal range for both the early or nongravid uterine artery and the normal internal iliac artery (68), supporting the notion that the normal physiological change has not taken place. The waveform also looks remarkably similar to that of the nonpregnant uterine artery (Fig. 23). This also serves to illustrate the potential pitfall of a CW technique for this application: although the normal uterine artery may be identified when it is present, a solitary signal looking like that of Fig. 22 may not be distinguished from that of the normal internal iliac artery, which lies close by. In the situation in which only signals such as these are found, it therefore seems best to use duplex scanning to obtain signals from both the internal and external iliac arteries and demonstrate that these originate from separate locations before concluding that the signals obtained are indeed abnormal uterine artery waveforms.

Cohen-Overbeek et al. (12) used duplex scanning to study 53 patients with complicated pregnancies. They divided them on the basis of the form of the "frequency index profiles" (FIP) for the arcuate arteries. The FIPs were considered abnormal if more than two points fell outside the nomogram. Those patients with abnormal Doppler signals had a higher incidence of proteinuric hypertension, were delivered earlier, of smaller babies, and with greater frequency by cesarian section.

Trudinger et al. (72) studied 91 complicated pregnancies, obtaining signals from what they considered to be the uterine arteries using a 4-MHz CW Doppler scanner. Of the 25 small-for-gestational-age (SGA) infants born, 15 had a B/A ratio (see Fig. 14) of less than 0.5, which constituted the approximate fifth centile for the last trimester. Nine out of the 12 patients with severe hypertension had abnormal B/A ratios consistent with a high uteroplacental resistance. One patient with lipidemia and diabetes showed a particularly low B/A ratio of less than 0.4. In this study umbilical artery waveforms were examined at the same time. SGA infants were found with abnormal uterine waveforms only (6/25), abnormal umbilical cord waveforms only (5/25), or abnormal uterine and umbilical waveforms (9/25). The preponderance of hypertension in the first of these groups lends weight to the notion that IUGR can be primarily of fetal origin or can be associated with some form of uteroplacental insufficiency. The potential of uterine Doppler examination to help distinguish these groups presents an encouraging prospect for the technique in spite of its lack of susceptibility to quantitation. More recently it has been pointed out that features of the waveform other than the relative diastolic flow rate, for example, a visible "notch" at the end of systole (63), may be helpful adjucts to the assessment of the uterine time–velocity waveform shape. This might suggest that other frequency-domain methods for the characterization of waveform shape probably deserve investigation. The fact that the physiological vascular changes occur late in the second trimester has also led to the suggestion that it may be practicable to screen hypertensives for abnormal uterine signals at a point early in the final trimester.

Although there is some recent indication that abnormal umbilical artery waveforms may anticipate traditional diagnostic criteria by as much as 3 weeks (37), the time course of Doppler signals in abnormal pregnancy and their relation to conventional indicators of fetal well-being and neonatal outcome have yet to be described fully. Until this is known, it would be difficult to predict the effect of changing the management of a patient on the basis of placental Doppler waveform analysis alone.

CONCLUSIONS

Doppler ultrasound offers a relatively simple, inexpensive, and noninvasive means of assessing fetal and uterine blood flow in pregnancy. The measurements most likely to be of clinical value in the study of blood flow are both quantitative and semi-quantitative. First, volumetric flow rate may be estimated in the descending fetal aorta, fetal umbilical vein, and maternal ascending aorta. It is improbable that useful estimates of uteroplacental flow rate can be made with present ultrasound methods. Although these measurements are based on a simple principle, their practical implementation is complicated by a number of physical problems that must be taken into account. These restrict both the number of sites in the vascular system at which volume flow measurements can be made and the precision of the results obtained. The most reliable volume flow measurements have been made with specially designed Doppler instrumentation, which is not widely available at present.

Interpretation of arterial time–velocity waveforms, in spite of the availability of only semiquantitative methods of analysis, can extend the role of Doppler to assess of the uterine circulation. In general, waveform shape analysis may be used to follow changes in downstream arterial resistance in situations in which the proximal circulation is relatively stable. Examples are the fetal umbilical artery, fetal descending thoracic aorta, and maternal uterine and maternal arcuate arteries. These waveforms show dramatic changes with intrauterine growth retardation. The use of pulsatility indices may, for example, help elucidate the relationship between some of the changes in intervillous flow known to accompany growth retardation and the onset of morphological and clinical signs in the fetus.

In spite of a number of studies using various noninvasive and pathological techniques, relatively little is known of the relationship between fetal and intervillous flow rate and placental resistance. Because of the more active regulation in the fetal circulation, it seems reasonable to suppose that resistance will be more stable and predictable in the uterine vessels than in the fetus. It is surprising, perhaps, that there has only been one study of the relative clinical efficacy of waveform analysis and umbilical volume flow in the same population (26). The somewhat inconclusive results of this study probably reflect the large number of physical and physiological variables involved. In spite of this, the established data showing intervillous flow reduction in IUGR combined with the evidence for a relationship between utero-placental resistance and Doppler time–velocity pulsatility in the uterine artery point to an unexplored and rather exciting new area for clinical investigation.

Until prospective studies are undertaken to assess the impact of managing patients on the basis of Doppler information from the placental circulation, it is difficult to define the precise clinical role for this technique. However, it seems certain that some form of Doppler assessment will form an indispensible part of the obstetrician's future armamentarium of diagnostic methods.

ACKNOWLEDGMENTS

The author is grateful to Drs. P. A. T. Grannum, J. A. Hobbins, and J. Copel, of the Department of Obstetrics, Yale University Medical School, for their advice and collaboration.

REFERENCES

1. Assali, N. S., Ranramo, L., and Peltonen, T. (1960): Measurement of uterine blood flow and uterine metabolism. *Am. J. Obstet. Gynecol.*, 79:86–98.

2. Atkinson, P., and Woodcock, J. P. (1982): *Doppler Ultrasound and Its Use in Clinical Measurement*. Academic Press, London.

3. Boyce, E. S., Dawes, G. S., Gough, J. D., and Poore, E. R. (1976): Doppler ultrasound method for detecting human fetal breathing *in utero*. *Br. Med. J.*, 2:17.

4. Brettes, J. P., Renaud, R., and Gauder, R. (1976): A double blind investigation into the effects of ritodrine on uterine blood flow during the third trimester of pregnancy. *Am. J. Obstet. Gynecol.*, 124:164–168.

5. Brosens, I. (1977): Morphological changes in the utero–placental bed in pregnancy hypertension. *Clin. Obstet. Gynecol.*, 4:573–594.

6. Brosens, I., Dixon, H. G., and Robertson, W. E. (1977): Fetal growth retardation and the arteries of the placental bed. *Br. J. Obstet. Gynaecol.*, 84:656–636.

6a. Burns, P. N. (1987): Doppler flow estimations in the fetal and maternal circulation: principles, techniques and some limitations. In: *Doppler Ultrasound Measurement of Maternal-Fetal Hemodynamics*, edited by D. Maulik and D. McNellis. Perinatology Press, Ithaca, New York.

7. Burns, P. N., and Jaffe, C. C. (1985): Quantitative flow measurements with Doppler ultrasound: Techniques, accuracy, and limitations. *Radiol. Clin. North Am.*, 23(4):641–657.

8. Callagan, D. A., Rowland, T. C., and Goldman, D. E. (1964): Ultrasonic Doppler observation of the fetal heart. *Obstet. Gynecol.*, 23:637.

9. Campbell, S., Diaz-Recasens, J., Griffin, D. R., Cohen-Overbeek, T., Pearce, J. M. F., Willson, K., and Teague, M. J. (1983): New Doppler technique for assessing uteroplacental blood flow. *Lancet*, 1:675–677.

10. Chiba, Y., Utsu, M., Kanzaki, T., and Hasegawa, T. (1985): Changes in venous flow and intra-tracheal flow in fetal breathing movements. *Ultrasound Med. Biol.*, 11:43–49.

11. Clapp, J. F., Szeto, H. H., Larrow, R., Hewitt, J., and Mann, L. I. (1980): Umbilical blood flow response to embolization of the uterine circulation. *Am. J. Obstet. Gynecol.*, 138:60–67.

12. Cohen-Overbeek, T., Pearce, J. M., and Campbell, S. (1985): The antenatal assessment of utero-placental and feto-placental blood flow using Doppler ultrasound. *Ultrasound Med. Biol.*, 2:329–339.

13. Dawes, T. S. (1968): *Fetal and Neonatal Physiology*. Yearbook Medical Publishers, Chicago.

14. Sheppard, B. L., and Bonnar, J. (1976): The ultrastructure of the arterial supply of the human placenta in pregnancy complicated by growth retardation. *Br. J. Obstet. Gynaecol.*, 83:948–959.

15. Eik-Nes, S. H., Bruback, A. O., and Ulstein, M. K. (1980): Measurement of human fetal blood flow. *Br. Med. J.*, 280:283–284.

16. Eik-Nes, S. H., Marsal, K., and Kristoffersen, K. (1984): Methodology and basic problems related to blood flow studies in the human fetus. *Ultrasound Med. Biol.*, 10:329–337.

17. Eik-Nes, S. H., Marsal, K., Kristoffersen, K., and Vernesson, E. (1981): Transcutaneous measurement of human fetal blood flow. Methodological studies. In: *Recent Advances in Ultrasound Diagnosis, Vol. 3*, edited by A. Kurjak and A. Kratochwil, pp. 209–219. Excerpta Medica, Amsterdam.

18. Eriksson, U. J., and Jansson, L. (1984): Diabetes in pregnancy: Decreased placental blood flow and disturbed fetal development in the rat. *Pediatr. Res.*, 18:735–738.

19. Evans, D. H. (1982): Some aspects of the relationship between instantaneous volumetric blood flow and continuous wave Doppler ultrasound recordings. I: The effect of ultrasonic beam width on the output of maximum, mean and rms frequency processors. *Ultrasound Med. Biol.*, 8:605–615.

20. Evans, D. H., Barrie, W. W., Asher, M. J., Bentley, S., and Bell, P. R. F. (1980): The relationship between ultrasonic pulsatility index and proximal arterial stenosis in a canine model. *Circ. Res.*, 46:470–475.

21. Fitzgerald, D. E., and Drumm, J. E. (1977): Noninvasive measurement of human fetal circulation using ultrasound: A new method. *Br. Med. J.*, 2:1450–1451.

22. Fitzgerald, D. E., Stewart, B., Drumm, J. E., and Duignan, N. M. (1984): The assessment of the feto–placental circulation with continuous wave Doppler ultrasound. *Ultrasound Med. Biol.*, 10:371–376.

23. Fleischer, A., Schulman, H., Farmakides, G., Bracero, L., Grunfeld, L., Rochelson, B., and Koenigsberg, M. (1986): Uterine artery Doppler velocimetry in pregnant women with hypertension. *Am. J. Obstet. Gynecol.*, 154:806–813.

24. Fox, H. (1978): *Pathology of the Placenta*. W. B. Saunders, London.

25. Gerratsen, G., Huisjes, H. J., and Elema, J. D. (1981): Morphological changes of the spiral arteries in the placental bed in relation to pre-eclampsia and growth retardation. *Br. J. Obstet. Gynaecol.*, 88:876–881.

26. Giles, W. B., Lingman, G., Marsal, K., and Trudinger, B. J. (1986): Fetal volume blood flow and umbilical artery flow velocity waveform analysis: A comparison. *Br. J. Obstet. Gynaecol.*, 93:461–465.

27. Giles, W. B., Trudinger, B. J., and Baird, P. J. (1985): Fetal umbilical artery flow velocity waveforms and placental resistance: Pathological correlation. *Br. J. Obstet. Gynaecol.*, 92:31–38.

28. Gill, R. W. (1982): Accuracy calculations for ultrasonic pulsed Doppler blood flow measurements. *Aust. Phys. Eng. Sci. Med.,* 5:51–57.

29. Gill, R. W. (1979): Performance of the mean frequency Doppler demodulator. *Ultrasound Med. Biol.,* 5:237–247.

30. Gill, R. W. (1979): Pulsed Doppler with B-mode imaging for quantitative blood flow measurement. *Ultrasound Med. Biol.,* 5:223–235.

31. Gill, R. W. (1985): Measurement of blood flow by ultrasound: Accuracy and sources of error. *Ultrasound Med. Biol.,* 11:625–641.

32. Gill, R. W., Kossoff, G., Warren, P. S., and Garrett, W. J. (1984): Umbilical venous flow in normal and complicated pregnancy. *Ultrasound Med. Biol.,* 10:349–363.

33. Gill, R. W., Trudinger, B. J., Garret, W. J., Kossoff, G., and Warren, P. S. (1981): Fetal umbilical venous flow measured in utero by pulsed Doppler and B-mode ultrasound. 1: Normal pregnancies. *Am. J. Obstet. Gynecol.,* 139:720–725.

34. Gosling, R. G., and King, D. H. (1975): Ultrasound angiology. In: *Arteries and Veins,* edited by A. W. Marcus and L. Adamson, pp. 61–98. Churchill Livingstone, Edinburgh.

35. Griffin, D., Cohen-Overbeek, T., and Campbell, S. (1983): Fetal and utero-placental blood flow. *Clin. Obstet. Gynaecol.,* 10:565–602.

36. Griffin, D. R., Teague, M. J., Tallet, P., Willson, K., Bilardo, C., Massini, L., and Campbell, S. (1985): A combined ultrasonic linear array scanner and pulsed Doppler velocimeter for the estimation of blood flow in the fetus and adult abdomen. 2: Clinical evaluation. *Ultrasound Med. Biol.,* 11:37–41.

37. Hackett, G. A., Campbell, S., Gansu, H., Cohen-Overbeek, T., and Pearce, J. M. F. (1987): Doppler studies in the growth retarded fetus and prediction of neonatal necrotizing enterocolitis, hemorrhage, and neonatal morbidity. *Br. Med. J.,* 294:13–16.

38. Jansson, I., (1969): Forearm and myometrial blood flow in diabetic pregnancy studied by venous occlusion plethysmography and ^{133}Xenon clearance. *Acta Obstet. Gynecol. Scand.,* 48:322–338.

39. Jones, C. J. P., and Fox, H. (1976): Placental changes in gestational diabetes. An ultrastructural study. *Obstet. Gynecol.,* 48:274–280.

40. Jouppila, P., and Kirkinen, P. (1984): Umbilical vein blood flow in the human fetus in cases of maternal and fetal anemia and uterine bleeding. *Ultrasound Med. Biol.,* 10:365–370.

41. Jouppila, P., Kirkinen, P., Eik-Nes, S., and Koivula, A. (1981): Fetal and intervillous blood flow measurements in late pregnancy. In: *Recent Advances in Ultrasound Diagnosis 3,* edited by A. Kurjak and A. Kratochwil, pp. 226–233. Excerpta Medica, Amsterdam.

42. Kaar, K., Jouppila, P., Kuikka, J., Luotola, H., Toivanen, J., and Rekonon, A. (1980): Intervillous blood flow in normal and complicated late pregnancy measured by means of an intravenous ^{133}Xe method. *Acta Obstet. Gynecol. Scand.,* 59:7–10.

43. Kirkinen, P., Jouppila, P., and Eik-Nes, S. H. (1983): Umbilical vein blood flow in rhesus iso-immunization. *Br. J. Obstet. Gynecol.,* 90:640–643.

44. Kleinman, C. S., Weinstein, E. M., and Copel, J. A. (1986): Pulsed Doppler analysis of human fetal blood flow. In: *Clinics in Diagnostic Ultrasound, Vol. 17, Basic Doppler Echocardiography,* edited by J. Kisslo, D. Adams, and D. B. Mark, pp. 173–185. Churchill Livingstone, New York.

45. Kurjak, A., and Rajhvajn, B. (1982): Ultrasonic measurements of umbilical blood flow in normal and complicated pregnancies. *J. Perinat. Med.,* 10:3–16.

46. Lindblad, A., Marsal, K., Vernersson, E., and Renck, H. (1984): Fetal circulation during epidural analgesia for caesarian section. *Br. Med. J.,* 288:1329–1330.

47. Lunnell, N. O., Sarby, B., Lewander, R., and Nylund, L. (1979): Comparison of uteroplacental blood flow in normal and intra-uterine growth retarded pregnancy. *Gynecol. Obstet. Invest.,* 10:106–118.

48. Maini, C. L., Rosati, P., Galli, G., Bellati, U., Bonetti, M. G., and Moneta, E. (1985): Noninvasive radioisotopic evaluation of placental blood flow. *Gynecol. Obstet. Invest.,* 19:196–206.

49. Marsal, K., Lindblad, A., Lingman, G., and Eik-Nes, S. H. (1985): Blood flow in the fetal descending aorta: Intrinsic factors affecting fetal blood flow, i.e., fetal breathing, movements, and cardiac arrythmia. *Ultrasound Med. Biol.,* 10:339–348.

50. Madjar, H., Gill, R. W., Griffith, K. A., and Kossoff, G. (1985): Liver function tested by pulsed Doppler measurements of portal venous flow fasting and following a standard meal. In: *Proceedings 4th Meeting World Federation for Ultrasound in Medicine and Biology,* edited by R. W. Gill and M. J. Dadd, p. 70. Pergamon Press, Sydney.

51. Maulik, D., and Nanda, N. C. (1985): Fetal Doppler echocardiography. *Echocardiography,* 2(4):377–391.

52. McCallum, W. D. (1977): Thermodilution measurement of human umbilical blood flow and delivery. *Am. J. Obstet. Gynecol.,* 127:491–496.

53. McDonald, D. A. (1974): *Blood Flow in Arteries,* second ed., pp. 64–69. Edward Arnold, London.

54. Namekawa, K., Kasai, C., and Omoto, R. (1983): Real-time two-dimensional bloodflow imaging using ultrasound Doppler. *J. Ultrasound Med.,* 2:10.

55. National Council on Radiation Protection and Measurements (1983): *Biological Effects of Ultrasound: Mechanisms and Clinical Implications.* Report No. 74,266, Bethesda.

56. Nylund, L., Lunell, N. O., Lewander, R., Persson, B., Sarby, B., and Thornstrom, S. (1982): Uteroplacental blood flow in diabetic pregnancy: Measurements with Indium 113*m* and a computer-linked gamma camera. *Am. J. Obstet. Gynecol.,* 144(3):298–302.

57. Nylund, L., Lunell, N. O., Lewander, R., and Sarby, B. (1983): Uteroplacental blood flow index in intrauterine growth retardation of fetal or maternal origin. *Br. J. Obstet. Gynaecol.,* 90:16–20.

58. Organ, L. W., Bernstein, A., Rowe, I. H., and Smith, K. C. (1973): The pre-ejection period of the fetal heart: Detection during labor with Doppler ultrasound. *Am. J. Obstet. Gynecol.,* 115:369–376.

59. Planiol, T. H., and Pourcelot, L. (1974): Doppler effect study of the carotid circulation. In: *Ultrasonics in Medicine,* edited by M. Vlieger, D. N. White, and V. R. McCready, pp. 104–111. Excerpta Medica, Amsterdam.

60. Robinson, J. P., and Shaw-Dunn, J. (1973): Fetal heart rates as determined by sonar in early pregnancy. *J. Obstet. Gynaecol. Br. Commonw.,* 80:805–809.

61. Rosenfeld, C. R., Barton, H. D., and Meschia, G. (1976): Effects of epinephrine on distribution of blood flow in the pregnant ewe. *Am. J. Obstet. Gynecol.,* 124:156–163.

62. Rudolph, A. M., Heymann, M. A., Teramo, K. A. W., Barnett, C. T., and Raiha, N. C. R. (1971): Studies on the circulation of the previable human fetus. *Pediatr. Res.,* 5:452–465.

63. Schulman, H., Fleischer, A., Farmakides, G., Bracero, L., Rochelson, B., and Grunfeld, L. (1986): Development of uterine artery compliance in pregnancy as detected by Doppler ultrasound. *Am. J. Obstet. Gynecol.,* 155:1031–1036.

64. Schulman, H., Fleischer, A., Stern, W., Farmakides, G., Jagani, N., and Blattner, P. (1984): Umbilical velocity wave ratios in human pregnancy. *Am. J. Obstet. Gynecol.,* 148:985–990.

65. Shepherd, B. L., and Bernard, J. (1976): The ultrastructure of the arterial supply of the human placenta in pregnancy complicated by fetal growth retardation. *Br. J. Obstet. Gynaecol.,* 83:948–959.

66. Stewart, B., Drumm, J., Fitzgerald, D. E., and Duigan (1980): Fetal blood velocity waveforms in normal pregnancy. *Br. J. Obstet. Gynecol.,* 87:780–785.

67. Stembera, Z. K., Modr, J., Ganz, V., and Fronek, A. (1964): Measurement of umbilical cord blood flow by local thermodilution. *Am. J. Obstet. Gynecol.,* 90:531–536.

68. Taylor, K. J. W., Burns, P. N., Wells, P. N. T., Conway, D. I., and Hull, M. G. R. (1985): Ultrasound Doppler flow studies of the ovarian and uterine arteries. *Br. J. Obstet. Gynaecol.,* 92:240–246.

69. Thompson, R. S., Trudinger, B. J., and Cook, C. M. (1986): Doppler ultrasound waveforms in the fetal umbilical artery: Quantitative analysis technique. *Ultrasound Med. Biol.,* 11:707–711.

70. Trudinger, B. J., and Cook, C. M. (1985): Umbilical and uterine artery flow velocity waveforms in pregnancy associated with major fetal abnormality. *Br. J. Obstet. Gynaecol.,* 92:666–670.

71. Trudinger, B. J., Cook, C. M., Jones, L., and Giles, W. B. (1986): A comparison of fetal heart rate monitoring and umbilical artery waveforms in the recognition of fetal compromise. *Br. J. Obstet. Gynaecol.,* 93:171–175.

72. Trudinger, B. J., Giles, W. B., and Cook, C. M. (1985): Utero-placental blood flow velocity time waveforms in normal and complicated pregnancy. *Br. J. Obstet. Gynecol.,* 92:39–45.

73. Trudinger, B. J., Giles, W. B., Cook, C. M., Bombardieri, J., and Collins, L. (1985): Fetal umbilical artery flow velocity waveforms and placental resistance: clinical significance. *Br. J. Obstet. Gynaecol.,* 92:23–30.

74. Trudinger, B. J., Warwick, B., Giles, M. B., and Cook, C. N. (1985): Flow velocity waveforms in the maternal uteroplacental and fetal umbilical placental circulation. *Br. J. Obstet. Gynaecol.,* 152(2):155–161.

75. Van Lierde, M., Oberweis, D., and Thomas, K. (1984): Ultrasonic measurement of aortic and umbilical blood flow in the human fetus. *Obstet. Gynecol.,* 63:801–805.

spite reports in the literature to the contrary, we believe that few Doppler systems are capable of discriminating reliably between the left and right ACAs, which are usually only 1 to 2 mm apart at this point. The larger branch of the internal carotid artery, the MCA, may be insonated through the thin temporal bone between the orbit and the upper part of the earlobe, where a zero Doppler angle will also be obtained, although this is more reliably achieved when a duplex system is used (7,8).

SIGNAL ANALYSIS

Conclusions of many early reports analyzing signals from these arteries using the Pourcelot index of resistance are likely to have been confounded by the many influences of Doppler waveform shape other than vascular resistance and blood flow (see above). Animal experiments in which the potent cerebral vasodilator CO_2 was used to manipulate cerebral perfusion suggested that the time-averaged mean Doppler shift (corresponding to the area under the curve or mean veocity) was proportional to total cerebral perfusion and was a more useful measurement to make providing the Doppler angle was kept constant (6,14). For mean cerebral artery velocity to be proportional to cerebral perfusion, we must assume that the arteries themselves do not alter in caliber, which appeared to be the case in the animal experiments. However, there is substantial evidence from other animal work that the major cerebral arteries are in fact vasoactive, particularly in response to perfusion pressure changes, where they may be involved in the process of autoregulation (1,20). It may be unwise to assume that mean cerebral artery velocity is proportional to the volume of blood flowing within these arteries.

VOLUMETRIC METHODS

A different approach that we have used (9) makes no such assumptions and provides volumetric data on blood flow to the head and neck. At present, however, the difficulty of achieving accuracy probably makes it a technique more appropriate for research than clinical use. A duplex scanner interfaced to a microcomputer (ATL Mk 600 and Apple IIe) is used to measure blood flowing around the aortic arch using the method based on the product of mean velocity and lumen area. Blood flow to head, neck, and arms is calculated as the difference between aortic flow measured proximal and distal to the great arch vessels. About 75 to 80% of this flow supplies the brain in the adult. It may be expected that in infancy this proportion will be even higher because of the high brain-to-body weight ratio. Systematic error, largely arising from preferential central stream sampling, is minimized in this system by laboratory calibration using a pulsatile flow rig and artificial vessels of varying diameters. The system makes no assumptions about flow profile since the mean velocity is calculated digitally from the full Fourier spectrum. Random error in the measurement of vessel diameter and Doppler angle (13) is minimized by making multiple recordings from each site and by using the technique to study populations of infants rather than drawing conclusions from a single subject.

Using this method to perform sequential studies during the first 48 hr of life, we have found no overall change in cerebral perfusion either in healthy full-term infants or in a heterogeneous group of preterm infants born at less than 33 weeks of gestation.

Blood flow velocity in both ACA and MCA, however, increased substantially over the same period, especially in the preterm infants. We interpret these findings of increasing velocity but constant flow as indicating that the cerebral arteries themselves reduce their caliber over this period, further evidence that these vessels have vasoactive properties. The relative vasodilation in the hours immediately following delivery in preterm infants may be of etiological significance in the pathogenesis of intracerebral hemorrhage, which largely occurs in the first 48 hr of life and is quite uncommon after 72 hr of age. We have speculated that this progressive constriction of the cerebral arteries may be part of the autoregulatory response to rising cerebral perfusion pressure over the same period. If this hypothesis is supported by further work, then possible intervention to reduce the incidence of cerebral hemorrhage may be suggested.

MEASURING HEMODYNAMIC LABILITY

Transient arterial pressure variations applied to delicate vasodilated cerebral vascular beds may be the major cause of cerebral hemorrhage in the preterm infant. If this is so, then Doppler studies of the short-term lability of the neonatal circulation may provide a prognostic index of risk for hemorrhage. The coefficient of variation of the area under successive ACA Doppler waveforms is one way of assessing this lability and has been shown to be higher in infants who go on to develop cerebral hemorrhage (23). It has also been shown to be reduced when these high-risk ventilated infants were paralyzed. Paralysis in these infants was also associated with a reduced incidence of hemorrhage (21). We have also shown that this variability is greatest very shortly after delivery, which may be a further factor in the observed early incidence of neonatal cerebral hemorrhage. Whether this Doppler velocity waveform method has advantages over the assessment of the central arterial pressure waveform, which is easier to obtain and to monitor continuously, is not clear. In the future, the simultaneous analysis of arterial pressure and cerebral artery velocity may provide useful information on the short-term pressure/velocity and autoregulatory characteristics of the prejudiced cerebral circulation.

ASPHYXIA AND HYDROCEPHALUS

Cerebral Doppler ultrasound may provide useful clinical information following perinatal asphyxia and in the detection of raised intracranial pressure from hydrocephalus. Following severe perinatal asphyxia, cerebral Doppler waveforms tend to be less pulsatile, and this observation may be of prognostic help (4). Convulsions from any cause also decrease cerebral waveform pulsatility and increase the mean Doppler frequency shift. It is possible, therefore, that in some asphyxiated infants with decreased cerebral arterial pulsatility, subtle convulsions may have been the cause (24). In rapidly progressive hydrocephalus, particularly posthemorrhagic hydrocephalus, there is an increase in cerebral artery pulsatility index and a decrease in mean frequency shift (16). These changes rapidly reverse following drainage of a small quantity of cerebrospinal fluid by lumbar puncture (8). It may be that measuring the cerebral artery pulsatility index as well as real-time measurement of ventricular size will be of assistance in deciding whether to perform drainage procedures.

ASSESSMENT OF LEFT-TO-RIGHT DUCTAL SHUNTS

Persistence of left-to-right shunting is a major cause of morbidity in preterm infants. The large flow of blood through the ductus arteriosus into the pulmonary circulation decreases lung compliance, increases the work of breathing, delays weaning from respiratory support, and may contribute to the genesis of chronic lung disease (10,11). The increased circulatory load may precipitate cardiac failure exacerbated by myocardial ischemia caused by the diastolic ductal run-off (17). Finally, if left ventricular output does not rise adequately to compensate for the ductal shunt, there may be tissue hypoperfusion, particularly of kidney, gut, and brain (19,22,25). Estimation of the size of left-to-right ductal shunts is of great importance when considering either the pharmacological or surgical closure of the duct. Clinical methods of assessing ductal size either by loudness of murmur or by pulse pressure are notoriously unreliable, and echocardiographic methods dependent on left atrial distension are not specific (28). Doppler ultrasound offers an objective and potentially quantitative method of assessment (26). Our own studies are the only quantitative ones I know and are currently in press (9).

Qualitative or semiquantitative Doppler methods of assessing ductal shunt rely on the effect of ductal flow on the Doppler waveform in either the pulmonic or systemic circulations or on the detection of flow within the ductus itself. Quantitative assessment may be performed by measuring volume flow within the aorta before and after the level of the duct in a similar manner to that described above for the measurement of flow to head, neck, and arms.

EFFECT OF DUCTAL FLOW ON ARTERIAL WAVEFORMS

Systemic

In the absence of a ductal shunt, aortic diastolic flow proximal to the duct is very low entirely because of the elastic recoil within the ascending aorta. A ductal shunt elevates this diastolic flow. These changes may be quantified using an index of pulsatility (Fig. 2).

The Doppler waveform beyond the ductus, in the absence of a patent ductus, is very similar to that before the ductus with perhaps just a flick of diastolic reversed flow. However, a ductal shunt causes significant and often biphasic reversed flow of blood during diastole. Again, these changes may be quantified using an index of pulsatility or a ratio of reversed to forward flow (26). Similar increases in the waveform pulsatility with ductal shunts may be found throughout the systemic arterial system, but because the waveform shape peripherally is more influenced by vascular resistance, there are few advantages to Doppler sampling distal to the descending aorta.

Pulmonary

Within the pulmonary artery (Fig. 3), spectral analysis reveals that there is continuous turbulent flow in the presence of a ductal shunt, and with a precordial ap-

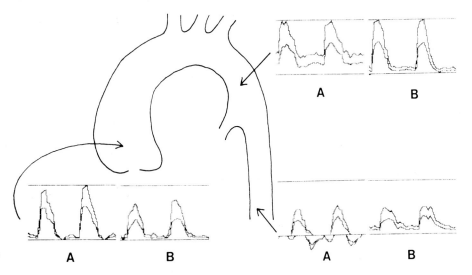

FIG. 2. Superimposed maximum and mean Doppler waveforms from the ascending preductal and postductal aorta before and after closure of the ductus arteriosus. These waveforms were obtained from a term infant at 1 hr (A) and 48 hr (B) of age. Because of variation in Doppler angle and pulse repetition frequency, the *y* axis Doppler shift frequencies are not necessarily comparable.

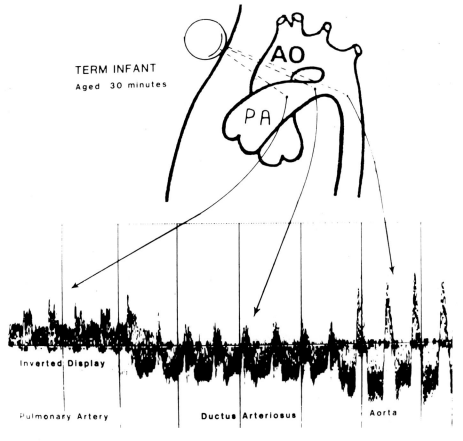

FIG. 3. Pulsed Doppler recording made precordially as the sample volume was moved from pulmonary artery through the patent ductus into the postductal aorta. This recording was made in a term infant within 1 hr after birth.

proach, a diastolic ductal jet will be detected (27). Early diastolic curtailment of the ductal jet is indicative of pulmonary hypertension. It is frequently possible to pass the Doppler sample volume through the duct itself when using a duplex system from the suprasternal window, but this is less easy and less reliable than assessing the effects of the ductal shunt on the aortic and pulmonary waveforms.

VOLUMETRIC ASSESSMENT OF DUCTAL FLOW

Volumetric assessment of ductal flow, as described above, necessitates taking the mean value of a number of recordings to achieve sufficient accuracy and is therefore more time consuming. It does, however, provide the most useful noninvasive measure of the size of a ductal shunt. Figure 4 demonstrates the different time course

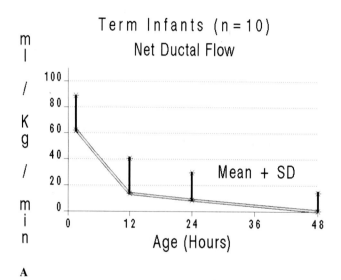

A

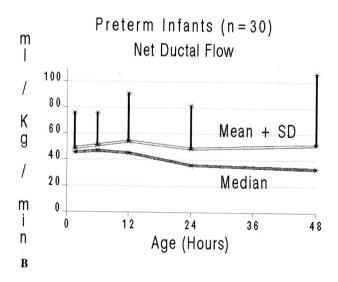

B

FIG. 4. Ductal closure. **A:** In full-term infants ductal flow decreases rapidly within the first 12 hr after birth. **B:** In preterm infants (<33 weeks of gestation), mean ductal flow does not change significantly over the first 48 hr of life, although the median flow rate does decrease while the standard deviation increases. This indicates that there is a tendency toward ductal closure in the majority of preterm infants, but the ductal shunt increases in a small number of infants.

in the closure of the duct in a group of healthy full-term infants and a group of infants of less than 33 weeks' gestation. During the 48 hr of this study, no ductal murmur was audible in any of the infants. Much higher ductal flows were recorded later in those preterm infants who went on to develop clinically significant ductal shunts during the second week of life. Although an accurate volumetric assessment of ductal flow may be an extremely important piece of clinical information, it is only one of several clinical factors that need to be considered before deciding to attempt closure of the ductus.

CARDIAC OUTPUT

If measurement of cardiac output were easier, it would perhaps be the most useful clinical index of the circulatory state of critically ill infants and children in the intensive care unit. In practice, clinicians rely on indirect indicators, arterial blood pressure, and clinical assessment of peripheral perfusion. Accurate measurement of arterial blood pressure in small children is itself difficult, and vascular compensatory mechanisms make it a very insensitive measure of circulatory adequacy. Peripheral perfusion assessment is frequently more useful but is influenced by many factors other than cardiac output, such as pain, drugs, and blood viscosity, and is difficult to do objectively. Doppler ultrasound offers the first viable noninvasive method for measuring cardiac output in the intensive care unit.

The challenge is to reduce errors in the measurement to clinical insignificance. Some of the sources of these errors in childhood have been discussed in the early part of this chapter. Most can be reduced either by *in vitro* calibration of the particular Doppler system or by taking the mean of serial measurements (random errors decrease with the square root of the number of observations) (13). In the future, systems that are under development that are independent of vessel size, flow profile, and Doppler beam angle may provide the best solution for routine use in relatively unskilled hands. However, currently available systems, if used with care, can yield invaluable results.

Doppler cardiac output data both from normal infants and from infants in pathological situations have been reported (2,3,29–31). In most instances, these studies have failed to guard against the systematic errors described above. Thus, absolute flow values need to be interpreted with caution (2). The values obtained from some modern duplex scanners may be particularly suspect (12). In clinical application, the absolute values of cardiac output may be less important if data are available for normal infants using the same system or if trends with time or following treatment are to be observed.

DETECTION OF AV MALFORMATIONS AND SHUNTS

Arteriovenous malformations are uncommon in childhood. However, they occur most often in the brain, particularly involving the posterior cerebral artery and the great vein of Galen, and may be of major clinical significance, causing focal neurologic symptoms, hydrocephalus, cardiac failure, and cerebral hemorrhage (18). The effect of a large arteriovenous shunt on the arterial Doppler signal is to produce a high-velocity, low-pulsatility waveform characteristic of a low peripheral vascular

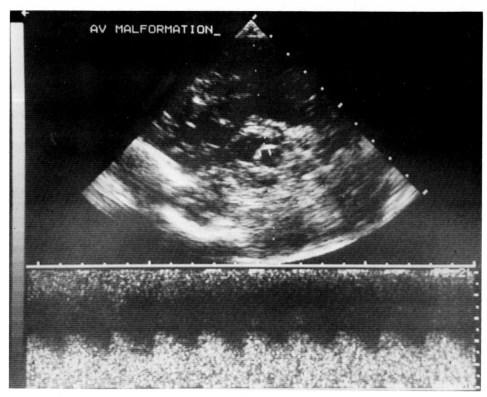

A

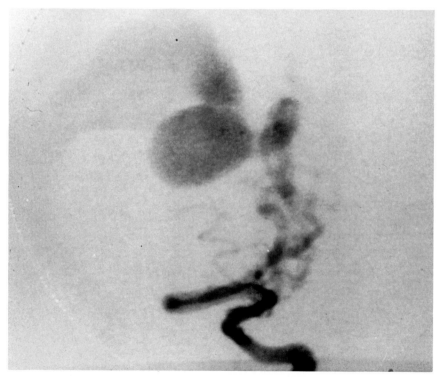

B

314

impedance (Fig. 5). Within the venous system adjacent to the malformation, there is disturbed pulsatile flow. In these situations Doppler ultrasound is a useful adjunct to the auscultation of bruits and provides much more precise anatomical detail of the site of shunt. The major value of Doppler examination is that it permits differentiation between vascular masses and nonvascular cysts in the region of the tectum. Such avascular masses may require no further evaluation.

CONCLUSION

As with any new technology or application of an old technology in a new field, the underlying physical and physiological principles must be well understood and results and conclusions carefully validated before unwarranted conclusions are drawn. The application of Doppler ultrasound within the field of pediatrics is in its infancy, but the great potential for noninvasive cardiovascular diagnosis will certainly lead to a succession of new applications. The enormous developmental changes in the circulation, particularly in the perinatal period, have been poorly understood because they have been difficult to study but are undoubtedly of clinical importance for the sick and preterm infant. Doppler ultrasound is filling these gaps in our knowledge. Its use is already well established in the fields of research and diagnostic cardiology. It is likely that improved equipment and techniques will allow it to find an expanding role in the clinical care of sick infants and children.

REFERENCES

1. Abboud, F. M. (1981): Special characteristics of the cerebral circulation. *Fed. Proc.*, 40:2296–2300.
2. Alverson, D. C., Eldridge, M., Dillon, T., Yabek, S. M., and Berman, W. (1982): Noninvasive pulsed Doppler determination of cardiac output in neonates and children. *J. Pediatr.*, 101:46–50.
3. Alverson, D. C., Eldrige, M. W., Johnson, J. D., Burstein, R., Papile, L., Dillon, T., Yabek, S., and Berman, W., Jr. (1983): Effect of patent ductus arteriosus on left ventricular output in premature infants. *J. Pediatr.*, 102:754–757.
4. Archer, L. N. J., Levene, M. I., and Evans, D. H. (1986): Cerebral artery Doppler ultrasonography for prediction of outcome after perinatal asphyxia. *Lancet*, 2:1116–1118.
5. Bada, H. S., Hajjar, M. S., Chua, C., and Sumner, D. S. (1979): Noninvasive diagnosis of neonatal asphyxia and intraventricular hemorrhage by Doppler ultrasound. *J. Pediatr.*, 95:775–779.
6. Batton, D. G., Hellmann, J., Hernandez, M. J., and Maisels, J. M. (1983): Regional cerebral blood flow, cerebral blood velocity, and pulsatility index in newborn dogs. *Pediatr. Res.*, 17:908–912.
7. Drayton, M. R., and Skidmore, R. (1986): Doppler studies of the neonatal cerebral circulation. In: *Recent Advances in Ultrasound Diagnosis 5*, edited by A. Kurjack and G. Kossoff, pp. 113–127. Excerpta Medica, Amsterdam.
8. Drayton, M. R., and Skidmore, R. (1986): Doppler ultrasound in the neonate. *Ultrasound Med. Biol.*, 12:761–772.
9. Drayton, M. R., and Skidmore, R. (1987): Vasoactivity of the major intracranial arteries in newborn infants. *Arch. Dis. Child.*, 62:236–240.
10. Dudell, G. G., and Gersany, W. M. (1984): Patent ductus arteriosus in neonates with severe respiratory disease. *J. Pediatr.*, 104:915–920.
11. Edwards, D. K., Dyer, W. M., and Nathway, W. H. (1977): Twelve years' experience with bronchopulmonary dysplasia. *Pediatrics*, 59:839.
12. Evans, D. H. (1985): On the measurement of the mean velocity of blood flow over the cardiac cycle using Doppler ultrasound. *Ultrasound Med. Biol.*, 11:735–741.

FIG. 5. Arteriovenous malformation of the great vein of Galen. **A:** Doppler signals characteristic of an arteriovenous communication are detected within an echo-free area near the third ventricle. Note that the venous signal is modulated at the cardiac rate. **B:** Arteriogram from the same patient.

13. Gill, R. W. (1985): Measurement of blood flow by ultrasound: Accuracy and sources of error. *Ultrasound Med. Biol.*, 11:625–641.

14. Hansen, N. B., Stonestreet, B. S., Rosenkrantz, T. S., and Oh, W. (1983): Validity of Doppler measurements of anterior cerebral artery blood flow velocity: Correlation with brain blood flow in piglets. *Pediatrics*, 72:526–531.

15. Hattle, L., and Angelsen, B., eds. (1985): *Doppler Ultrasound in Cardiology: Physical Principles and Clinical Applications*. Lea & Febiger, Philadelphia.

16. Hill, A., and Volpe, J. J. (1982): Decrease in pulsatile flow in the anterior cerebral arteries in infantile hydrocephalus. *Pediatrics*, 69:4–7.

17. Hoffman, J. I. E. (1978): Factors affecting shunting and the development of heart failure. In: *The Ductus Arteriosus*, edited by M. A. Heyman and A. M. Rudolph, pp. 69–72. Ross Laboratories, Columbus.

18. Huttenlocher, P. R. (1983): Cerebral vascular diseases. In: *Nelson Textbook of Pediatrics*, 12th ed., edited by R. E. Behrman and V. C. Vaughan, pp. 1592–1593. W. B. Saunders, Philadelphia.

19. Kitterman, J. A. (1975): Effects of intestinal ischemia. In: *Necrotizing Enterocolitis in the Newborn Infant*, edited by T. D. Moore, pp. 38–40. Ross Laboratories, Columbus.

20. Mchedlishvili, G. (1980): Physiological mechanisms controlling cerebral blood flow. *Stroke*, 11:240–248.

21. Perlman, J. M., Goodman, S., Kreusser, K. L., and Volpe, J. J. (1985): Reduction in intraventricular hemorrhage by elimination of fluctuating cerebral bloodflow velocity in preterm infants with respiratory distress syndrome. *N. Engl. J. Med.*, 312:1353–1357.

22. Perlman, J. M., Hill, A., and Volpe, J. J. (1981): The effect of patent ductus arteriosus on flow velocity in the anterior cerebral arteries: Ductal steal in the premature infant. *J. Pediatr.*, 99:767–771.

23. Perlman, J. M., McMenamin, J. B., and Volpe, J. J. (1983): Fluctuating cerebral blood flow velocity in respiratory distress syndrome. *N. Engl. J. Med.*, 309:204–209.

24. Perlman, J. M., and Volpe, J. J. (1982): The effects of seizures (Sz) on cerebral blood flow velocity (CBFV), intracranial pressure (ICP) and systemic blood pressure (BP) in the preterm infant. *Pediatr. Res.*, 16:339A.

25. Serwer, G. A., Armstrong, B. E., and Anderson, P. A. W. (1980): Noninvasive detection of retrograde descending aortic flow in infants using continuous wave Doppler ultrasonography. *J. Pediatr.*, 97:394–400.

26. Serwer, G. A., Armstrong, B. E., and Anderson, P. A. W. (1982): Continuous wave Doppler ultrasonographic quantitation of patent ductus arteriosus flow. *J. Pediatr.*, 100:297–299.

27. Stevenson, J. G., Kawabori, I., and Guntheroth, W. G. (1980): Pulsed Doppler echocardiographic diagnosis of patent ductus arteriosus: Sensitivity, specificity, limitations, and technical features. *Cathet. Cardiovasc. Diagn.*, 6:255–263.

28. Valdes-Cruz, L. M., and Dudell, G. G. (1981): Specificity and accuracy of echocardiographic and clinical criteria for diagnosis of patent ductus arteriosus in fluid-restricted infants. *J. Pediatr.*, 98:298–305.

29. Walther, F. J., Siassi, B., King, J., and Wu, P. Y.-K. (1985): Cardiac output in infants of insulin dependent mothers. *J. Pediatr.*, 107:109–114.

30. Walther, F. J., Siassi, B., Ramadan, N. A., and Wu, P. Y.-K. (1985): Cardiac output in newborn infants with transient myocardial dysfunction. *J. Pediatr.*, 107:781–785.

31. Walther, F. J., Siassi, B., Ramadan, N. A., Ananda, A. K., and Wu, P. Y.-K. (1985): Pulsed Doppler determinations of cardiac output in neonates: Normal standards for clinical use. *Pediatrics*, 76:829–833.

11 / Evaluation of Lower Extremity Occlusive Disease with Doppler Ultrasound

Marsha M. Neumyer and Brian L. Thiele

Vascular Studies Section, Department of Surgery, The Milton S. Hershey Medical Center, The Pennsylvania State University, Hershey, Pennsylvania 17033

The evolution of Doppler technology is important for the evaluation of peripheral vascular occlusive disease since it demonstrates the hemodynamic consequences produced by disease, and the development of symptoms correlates with these hemodynamic disturbances. Indirect techniques were initially used, as in the noninvasive study of carotid arterial disease. Later refinements permitted better localization of the disease process.

The initial evaluation of a patient with peripheral vascular disease must begin with an accurate history of the patient's complaints and a physical examination of the entire peripheral vascular system. After such an evaluation, it may be determined whether the symptoms are ischemic in origin and whether the peripheral pulse volume is diminished. The evaluation may also disclose abnormality in an asymptomatic area.

After initial clinical evaluation, laboratory tests should be ordered. The routine use of a large battery of tests on all patients is to be deplored. The vascular laboratory examinations provide confirmation that the hemodynamic changes present are consistent with claudication, or ischemic pain at rest, and with the anatomic locations of these changes. For intermittent claudication, treadmill testing is required, whereas rest pain may be evaluated using resting studies alone. Such selective evaluation minimizes patient discomfort associated with protracted examinations and at the same time focuses attention on the most relevant part of the study. To employ such a selective approach, it is mandatory that the specific advantages of each study be understood.

Many devices and techniques for vascular evaluation have evolved within the past two decades and have yielded data shown to be highly sensitive, accurate, and reproducible (5,6,10,17,22). The most widely applied and evaluated of these techniques employ Doppler ultrasound. The complexity of Doppler instrumentation ranges from pocket-sized continuous-wave (CW) Doppler devices to sophisticated pulsed-wave duplex systems combining B-mode ultrasound imaging with Doppler velocity spectral analysis. The CW instruments are not range specific and detect Doppler shift frequencies from motion at any depth within the range of the instrument, which is dependent on the operating frequency. With pulsed Doppler devices, the arterial velocity profile can be sampled at any site located on the B-scan tomogram, allowing characterization of flow patterns at any site within the vessel lumen.

INDIRECT MEASUREMENT OF ARTERIAL PRESSURES

Continuous-wave directional Doppler velocity detectors have been the most commonly used noninvasive devices for assessment of peripheral arterial disease (10,11,13,14). These instruments permit qualitative evaluation of the audible or analog velocity signal at various points along the artery in addition to ankle and segmental blood pressure measurements. They also permit determination of the ankle blood pressure response to exercise or postocclusive reactive hyperemia. After these studies, it should be possible to decide if there is hemodynamic abnormality present and the arterial segments involved.

The ankle systolic pressure measurement, obtained using a pneumatic cuff with a Doppler velocity detector placed over a distal vessel, has been the single most valuable test for assessing the adequacy of the lower limb arterial circulation. In the absence of proximal arterial occlusive disease, the ratio of ankle systolic pressure to brachial systolic pressure is always >1.0, with a mean value of 1.11 ± 0.10 (22). This "ankle pressure index" has been correlated with angiographic assessment of arterial disease in patients with intermittent claudication and those with severe rest pain. In general, limbs with a single diseased segment have indices >0.5, and limbs with multisegmental disease have indices <0.5 (5,7,17). Yao has shown that in limbs with impending gangrene, the mean pressure index has a mean value of 0.05 ± 0.08 (22).

LOCALIZATION OF DISEASE

The ankle pressure index cannot localize adequately proximal arterial disease or define the relative contribution of a hemodynamic disturbance caused by multilevel disease. Segmental pressure measurements may aid in the localization and semiquantitation of occlusive disease. Systolic pressures are obtained at the high thigh (HT), above the knee (AK), below the knee (BK), and at ankle levels (Fig. 1).

Measurements of systolic pressures at multiple locations down the leg provide a means of localizing disease. In normal individuals, there should be less than a 20 mm Hg difference in systolic pressures between any two adjacent levels on the leg. An abnormal gradient between the HT and AK levels indicates superficial femoral arterial disease. An abnormal gradient between the AK and BK segments results from distal superficial femoral and/or popliteal disease. A disproportionate BK-to-ankle gradient reflects the presence of tibioperoneal lesions. The horizontal gradients between any two corresponding segments of the limb must also be noted to indicate the presence of occlusive disease, with differences in systolic pressure exceeding 20 mm Hg considered to be significant.

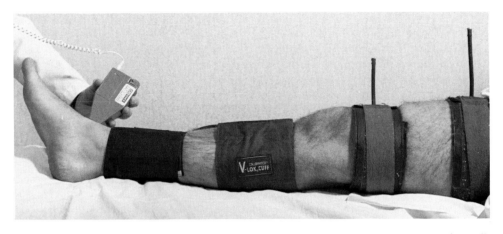

FIG. 1. Pneumatic cuff placement and technique for measuring lower extremity segmental systolic blood pressures by Doppler ultrasound.

The clinical need to evaluate the hemodynamic significance of lesions in the aortoiliac vessels and the inadequacy of HT measurements stimulated interest in analysis of the Doppler velocity signals recorded from the common femoral artery. Several features of the time–velocity waveform have increased the overall sensitivity and specificity of the examination. The Gosling and King pulsatility index (PI, the peak-to-peak velocity difference divided by the mean velocity) is relatively independent of the probe-to-vessel angle and is easily obtained (Fig. 2). Thiele et al. (19) compared the pulsatility index from the common femoral artery with intra-arterial pressure measurements and found a PI > 4.0 to be very predictive of a hemodynamically normal aortoiliac segment. A PI < 4.0, with patency of the superficial femoral artery established, indicated a hemodynamically significant aortoiliac lesion. The presence of occlusive disease in the superficial femoral artery, however, mark-

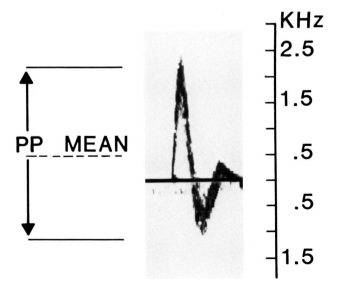

KHz

2.5

1.5

.5

.5

1.5

FIG. 2. A velocity spectral waveform demonstrating calculation of the peak-to-peak pulsatility index (PI).

edly decreases the diagnostic sensitivity of this index and precludes its use in this instance.

In limbs with normal arteries, blood flow increases in response to exercise or postocclusive reactive hyperemia by a factor of five to ten as a result of vasodilation of the peripheral resistance vessels. This increase in flow occurs with little or no drop in the ankle systolic pressure. However, when occlusive lesions are present in the main vessels, the collateral vessels that maintain distal perfusion pressure are frequently inadequate. Pressure gradients develop when flow rates are increased in response to exercise, providing a sensitive method for detecting mild arterial occlusive disease when little or no hemodynamic effect is observed at rest (Fig. 3).

Arterial pressure measurements and Doppler velocity waveforms, used to detect changes downstream from more proximal diseased segments, have provided valuable hemodynamic information but do have limitations (4,11,15,21). It is difficult to lo-

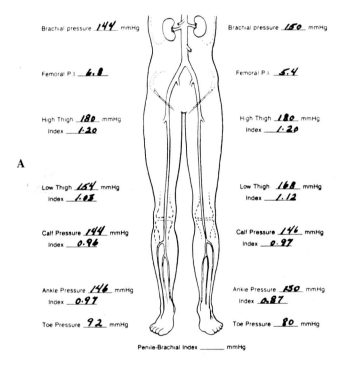

A

Brachial pressure *144* mmHg	Brachial pressure *150* mmHg
Femoral P.I. *6.8*	Femoral P.I. *5.4*
High Thigh *180* mmHg	High Thigh *180* mmHg
Index *1.20*	Index *1.20*
Low Thigh *154* mmHg	Low Thigh *168* mmHg
Index *1.05*	Index *1.12*
Calf Pressure *144* mmHg	Calf Pressure *146* mmHg
Index *0.96*	Index *0.97*
Ankle Pressure *146* mmHg	Ankle Pressure *130* mmHg
Index *0.97*	Index *0.87*
Toe Pressure *92* mmHg	Toe Pressure *80* mmHg

Penile-Brachial Index _____ mmHg

B

○ Right
△ Left

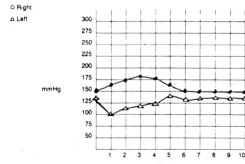

mmHg

Minutes

FIG. 3. Peripheral arterial evaluation using indirect measurement of arterial pressures. **A:** Lower extremity resting systolic pressure data. Resting pressures and indices do not indicate a significant arterial stenosis in the left leg. **B:** A graph of postexercise ankle pressures demonstrates an immediate drop in pressure, indicating inadequate perfusion from collaterals.

calize disease precisely or to distinguish near-total from total occlusion, which may be important in identifying patients who are suitable for percutaneous transluminal angioplasty (PTA). Since these techniques rely on pressure and flow changes distal to stenotic sites, they may fail to detect minimal disease or assess reliably the significance of multilevel occlusive disease. Quantification of velocity changes is difficult with the indirect procedures because the angle of the incident sound beam in relation to the vessel cannot accurately be determined.

The development of duplex scanning has allowed many of the difficulties associated with the measurement of blood pressure and flow to be overcome. Anatomic and physiologic data from any desired location within the vascular system from the level of the abdominal aorta to the calf can be obtained. Thus, it is now possible to localize the sites of occlusive disease precisely, characterize lesion morphology, and quantitate the velocity changes that result from stenosis (3,12).

INSTRUMENTATION

The duplex systems used in our laboratory (ATL UltraMRK8, UltraMRK4, and 450PV, Advanced Technology Laboratories, Inc., Bothell, WA) combine a real-time B-mode ultrasound image with a pulsed Doppler unit for the detection of velocity information. These devices employ mechanically rotating transducer frequencies (3, 5, 7.5, or 10 MHz) with a 3- or 5-MHz Doppler transducer. The two-dimensional image may be "frozen" on the video monitor and updated by demand during pulsed

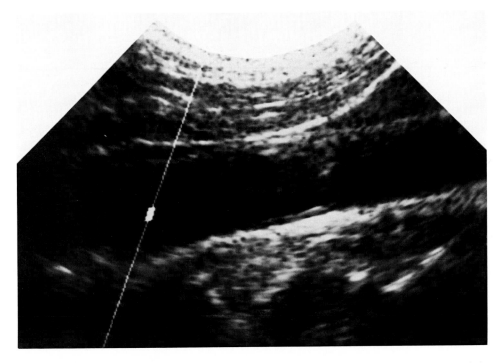

FIG. 4. B-mode image of common femoral artery. The path of the incident Doppler beam and the placement of the sample volume at center stream of the artery are displayed.

Doppler application. The path of the incident Doppler beam with respect to the vessel axis is indicated by a cursor superimposed on the image. The sample volume, the size of the range from which the Doppler signals are accepted, can be positioned along the incident Doppler beam and is indicated by a small bar (Fig. 4). A cursor is provided that can be aligned with the axis of blood flow to yield flow velocity directly as an alternative to the Doppler shift frequency.

The B-mode image is used to identify the artery of interest and to define anatomic variations. The presence of plaque and arterial narrowing noted on the B-mode image indicates the sites for Doppler evaluation of flow patterns. The tomographic characteristics of lesions can be differentiated and surface irregularity identified. Plaques that contain a large amount of lipid material (fatty plaque) and thrombus have an acoustic impedance similar to that of blood and therefore may be only faintly echogenic. The Doppler detection of flow disturbance must be relied on to prevent significant error, which could, in these cases, occur with the use of B-mode alone.

The amplitude or intensity of the signal in each segment is represented by a brightness level or gradation in gray scale. The range of velocities within the sample volume can be determined from the spectral bandwidth at any point in the cardiac cycle. As the arterial diameter is reduced, the velocity through the narrowed segment increases. Additionally, when stenotic disease is present, downstream turbulence may result, causing the velocity spectrum to broaden. Thus, spectral analysis permits evaluation of the two main criteria for classifying peripheral arterial disease, spectral broadening and increased velocity.

TECHNIQUE

The peripheral arterial duplex examination is performed with the patient in the supine position. Flow velocities are routinely recorded from the common and external iliac arteries, the common femoral artery, the proximal, middle, and distal superficial femoral artery, the deep femoral artery, and the popliteal artery. Additionally, velocity signals are recorded at any site where pathology is noted or flow disturbances are present.

The study begins with longitudinal imaging of the common femoral artery. The pulsed Doppler sample volume is placed in the center stream of the vessel using a standard Doppler angle of 60°. Peak systolic forward velocity, peak diastolic reverse velocity, and changes in spectral bandwidth are evaluated.

Several sources of artifacts that may affect classification of disease are apparent. If the selected sample volume size (the length of the range gate) is such that it equals the cross-sectional diameter of the vessel, the wall-to-wall velocity profile will be represented in the spectral waveform, resulting in pansystolic spectral broadening. In order to assess discrete regions of flow, a small sample volume size (1.5 mm) is used. In normal vessels, center stream flow is laminar. Care must be taken to place the sample volume center stream to avoid velocity gradients near the vessel wall. At times vessel movement caused by respiration and pulsation will cause the sample volume to vary from center stream, however, and sampling of the velocity profile along the wall will result in an increase in the spectral bandwidth.

Boundary layer separation and normal flow disturbances that occur at bifurcations must be recognized (Fig. 5). If the Doppler gain is adjusted too high, oversaturation

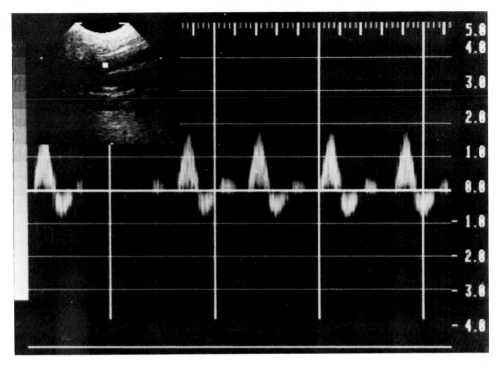

FIG. 5. Doppler waveform demonstrating spectral broadening caused by flow disturbances at the bifurcation of the superficial femoral and profunda femoris arteries.

of the returned signals precludes separation of the forward and reverse signal-processing channels. The resulting broadening may be mistaken for flow disturbance (Fig. 6).

It is important that the wall filter be set no higher than 50 or 100 Hz so that low-velocity, low-amplitude signals are not eliminated. If higher filters are selected, the reverse flow component or a low-velocity diastolic flow component may be missed (Fig. 7).

The iliac and deep femoral arteries are often tortuous. It may be difficult to maintain the standardized angle of 60° for Doppler sampling in such vessels. An acute angle of the sound beam with the blood flow vector may result in spectral broadening or an increase in recorded velocity, leading to overestimation of disease. Evaluation of the time–velocity waveforms from more proximal or distal segments may be helpful in clarifying the extent of the flow disturbance.

Calcification of anterior wall plaque frequently produces severe acoustic shadowing, which limits visualization of arterial anatomy and inhibits insonation in the area of the plaque. If the vessel is viewed in cross section to confirm that the plaque is not concentric, a more appropriate scan plane may be indicated. Velocity spectral data may need to be recorded from a location immediately distal to severely calcified lesions, as flow disturbances in peripheral vessels are often propagated for only a few centimeters beyond the stenosis.

The image will detail the arterial anatomy and permit identification of pathology at this site. The vein can be seen medial to the artery and is noted to be compressible with gentle scanhead pressure. Care must be taken to avoid exerting pressures from

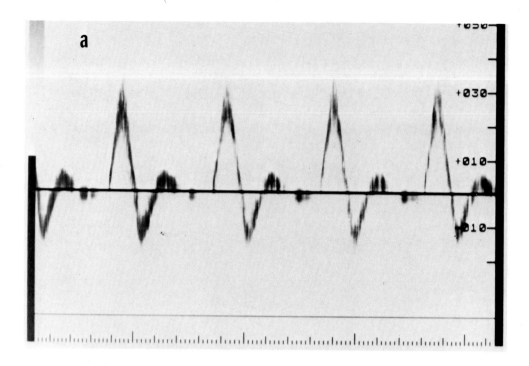

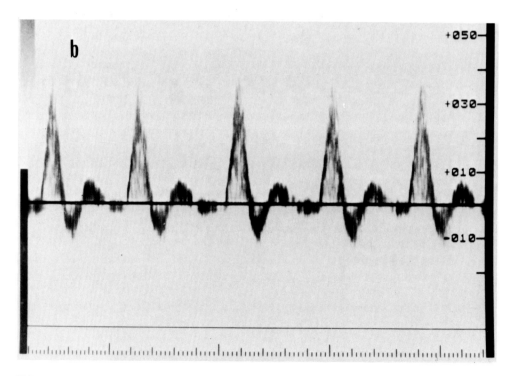

FIG. 6. Artifactual spectral broadening caused by oversaturation of the Doppler signals with use of excessive gain. **A:** Appropriate gain setting used: velocity spectral waveform indicates no evidence of a flow disturbance. **B:** Velocity waveform same as in **A.** Use of excessive gain results in mistaken impression of disturbed flow.

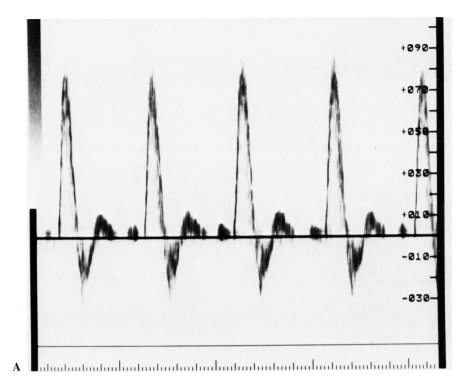

A

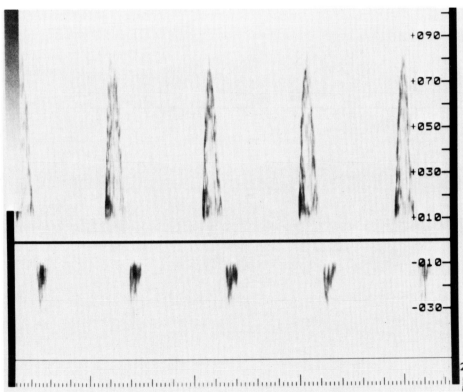

B

FIG. 7. Normal velocity waveform from the superficial femoral artery using different filters. **A:** Using a 50-Hz wall filter. The reverse flow component and forward diastolic velocity component are easily visualized. **B:** Using a 400-Hz wall filter. **C:** Using a 800-Hz wall filter.

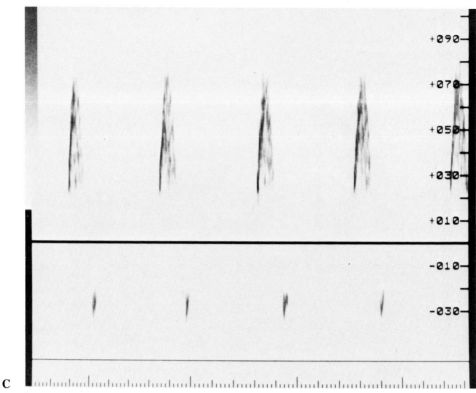

C

FIG. 7. (continued)

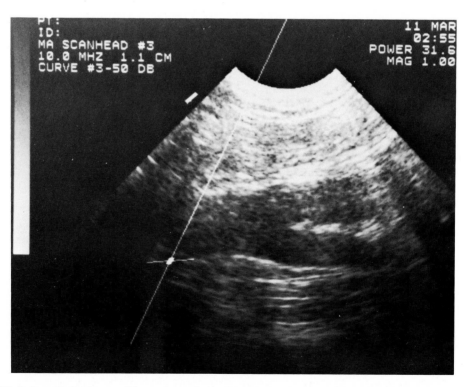

FIG. 8. Longitudinal scan of the common femoral artery showing the bifurcation into the superficial femoral and deep femoral (profunda femoris) arteries.

the scanhead on the artery, as extrinsic compression may create an artificial stenosis with a resultant flow disturbance.

The probe is moved cephalad to image the external iliac and the proximal internal iliac arteries. Doppler velocity recordings are made, and the presence of flow disturbances is noted. The probe is again moved through the common femoral artery

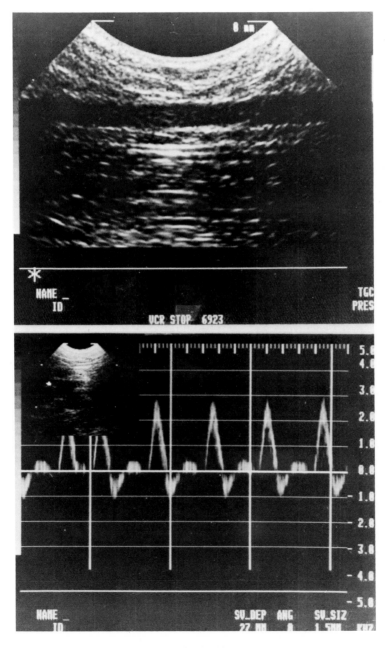

FIG. 9. Longitudinal scan and normal Doppler velocity waveform from the popliteal artery. A triphasic waveform with a narrow frequency bandwidth and systolic window is present.

to the origin of the superficial and deep femoral vessels (Fig. 8). The image is evaluated for the presence of bifurcation plaquing or anatomic variation. The sample volume is moved slowly throughout the origins of both vessels to detect flow disturbances, significant stenoses, or occlusion. The scanhead is then moved distally following the course of the superficial femoral artery to the adductor canal. The sample volume is swept through the length of the vessel in order to locate focal stenoses.

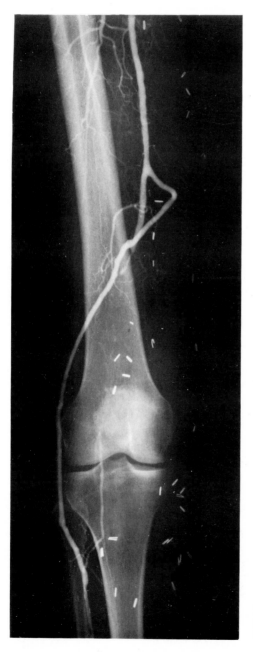

FIG. 10. Arteriogram of a femoral-to-anterior tibial vein bypass graft. *In situ* grafts may be quite superficial and are easily scanned.

The patient is then placed in the prone position with the feet elevated 20 to 30° on a pillow to facilitate evaluation of the popliteal artery. The artery lies posterior to the vein and is examined throughout its length to the popliteal trifurcation. Velocity sampling is recorded from the proximal, middle, and distal segments of this vessel (Fig. 9).

Duplex technology is also valuable for evaluation of infrainguinal vein bypass grafts (Fig. 10). The technique of examination is similar to that employed for the native arteries. Because the grafts may be quite superficial, an imaging frequency of 7.5 MHz or 10 MHz may be employed, and a 5-MHz pulsed Doppler beam is used for flow detection.

The study is begun with longitudinal imaging of the proximal anastomosis of the graft. Velocity signals are obtained at an angle of 60° proximal and distal to the anastomotic site, noting the presence of disturbed flow and increased velocities. The scanhead is moved distally following the course of the graft. Flow velocity is determined in the proximal, middle, and distal graft as well as downstream from the distal anastomosis so that impedance to outflow from the graft may be identified. Spectral waveforms must be collected along the entire course of the graft, as the

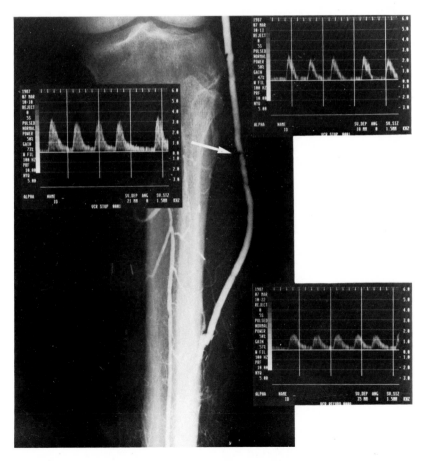

FIG. 11. Montage demonstrating 20 to 49% stenosis of a femoral-to-posterior tibial vein bypass graft. Note the narrow frequency bandwidth of the proximal and distal waveforms.

flow disturbance associated with residual vein valve cusps or wall irregularities is very focal and time–velocity waveforms may be normal immediately proximal and distal to such lesions (Fig. 11).

INTERPRETATION OF VELOCITY PATTERNS

Normal peripheral arterial velocity waveforms have a steep systolic forward velocity component followed by a reverse flow component and a second forward velocity component, which occurs during diastole (Fig. 12).

In normal arteries, the systolic peak velocity decreases between the common femoral and the proximal superficial femoral arteries. A marked drop in peak velocity can also be measured across the adductor canal between the distal superficial femoral and the popliteal arteries (Table 1). The reverse flow component from the velocity waveform recorded from the profunda femoris artery is less pronounced than that in other peripheral arterial segments because of the lower resistance in the vascular bed supplied by this vessel.

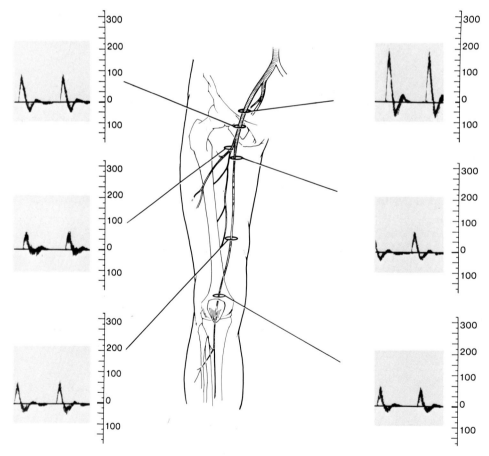

FIG. 12. Normal velocity spectral waveforms from the (**A**) common femoral artery, (**B**) profunda femoris artery, (**C**) distal superficial femoral artery, (**D**) external iliac artery, (**E**) proximal superficial artery, and (**F**) popliteal artery.

TABLE 1. *Mean values and standard deviation measured at five different arterial segments in 55 healthy subjects*[a]

Artery studied	Diameter ± SD (cm)	V_{sys} ± SD (cm/sec)	V_{rev} ± SD (cm/sec)	V_{dias} ± SD (cm/sec)
External iliac	0.79 ± 0.13	119.3 ± 21.7	41.5 ± 10.7	18.2 ± 7.5
Common femoral	0.82 ± 0.14	114.1 ± 24.9	40.6 ± 9.2	16.4 ± 8.3
Superficial femoral (proximal)	0.60 ± 0.12	90.8 ± 13.6	35.8 ± 8.2	14.5 ± 7.2
Superficial femoral (distal)	0.54 ± 0.11	93.6 ± 14.1	35.0 ± 9.8	14.6 ± 6.7
Popliteal	0.52 ± 0.11	68.6 ± 13.5	27.8 ± 9.2	9.8 ± 6.0

[a] V_{sys}, peak systolic flow velocity; V_{rev}, peak flow velocity of reverse flow component; V_{dias}, peak flow velocity of diastolic forward flow; SD, standard deviation.
From Jager et al. (8).

In healthy young subjects with marked elasticity of the vessel wall, an additional reverse flow component may be noted. With advancing age and decrease in vessel wall compliance, the peak systolic forward velocity and peak diastolic forward velocity diminish slightly, and a biphasic waveform may be found. Velocity waveforms recorded from peripheral arteries of women will generally have lower peak diastolic velocities than those from men of the same age.

A narrow frequency bandwidth is demonstrated from center stream flow in normal vessels. Spectral broadening will occur at bifurcations because of boundary layer separation and disturbed flow.

Stenosis is associated with an increase in peak systolic velocity and spectral broadening as a result of disruption of normal laminar flow patterns. Lesions that reduce the arterial diameter more than 50%, resulting in a decrease in both pressure and flow distal to the lesion, may be recognized by loss of the diastolic reverse flow component and an increase in diastolic forward velocity. The flow disturbance may be propagated only a short distance downstream from the stenosis, dependent on the degree of arterial narrowing and the length and surface morphology of the lesion.

Based on evaluation of waveform contour, the peak systolic forward velocity, the peak diastolic reverse velocity, and the presence of spectral broadening, disease can be classified into five categories: normal, <20% diameter reduction, 20 to 49% diameter reduction, 50 to 99% diameter reduction, and occlusion (16; Table 2). Waveforms typical of the classifications are shown in Fig. 13.

A normal waveform is tri- or biphasic dependent on vessel wall compliance, with a narrow frequency bandwidth. A systolic window, the clear area beneath the systolic peak, is present.

With minimal stenosis or wall irregularity, the peak systolic velocity and waveform contour remain within the normal range. The spectrum becomes broadened because of the disturbed flow and the subsequent increase in the range of velocities in the vicinity of the lesion.

As the stenosis progresses in severity from 20% to 49% diameter reduction, a 30 to 50% increase in peak systolic velocity will occur across the lesion. The reverse flow component remains and may become more pronounced because of distal resistance. Spectral broadening is marked. Flow patterns in the normal segments proximal and distal to the stenosis remain unchanged.

When arterial narrowing becomes severe (50–99% diameter reduction), peripheral resistance distal to the lesion is reduced, and the arterial waveform becomes mon-

TABLE 2. Velocity spectral classification

Angiographic category	Doppler criteria	Clinical interpretation
Normal	Tri- or biphasic waveform Systolic window present No spectral broadening	Normal No significant flow disturbance

1–19%
  diameter reduction
	Peak systolic velocity and waveform
	  within normal range
	Spectral broadening present
		Minimal disease

20–49%
  diameter reduction
	30–50% increase in peak systolic
	  velocity
	Reverse flow component present
	Marked spectral broadening
		Moderate disease

50–99%
  diameter reduction
	50–100% increase in peak systolic
	  velocity
	Reverse flow component absent
	Monophasic waveform
	Extensive spectral broadening
		Hemodynamically
		  significant disease

Occluded	No flow detected in vessel Proximal and distal flow patterns are disturbed	Occluded vessel

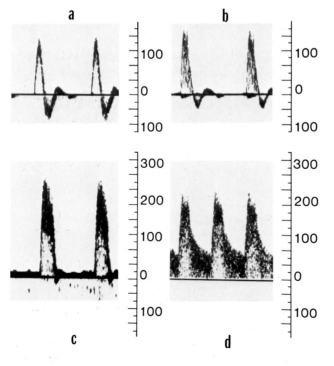

FIG. 13. Classification of velocity spectral waveforms into arteriographic categories: (**A**) normal, (**B**) <20% diameter reduction, (**C**) 20–49% diameter reduction, and (**D**) 50–99% diameter reduction.

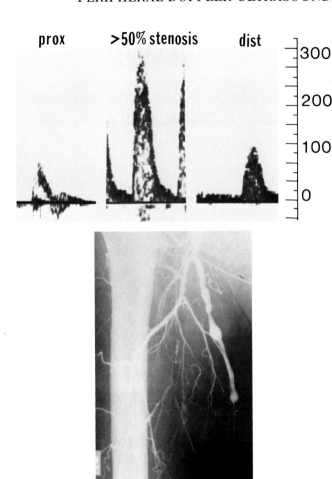

prox   **>50% stenosis**   **dist**

300
200
100
0

FIG. 14. Velocity spectral waveforms and arteriogram from a patient with a high-grade stenosis of a femoropopliteal vein bypass graft. **A:** Spectra recorded from the proximal graft (prox), just distal to the lesion (>50% stenosis), and from a point distal to the poststenotic dilatation (dist). Note marked increase in peak systolic velocity just distal to the stenosis and continued turbulence (spectral broadening) at the poststenotic recording site.

ophasic. The reverse flow component is lost, and only forward flow is present, with an increase in peak systolic velocity >100% noted. Spectral broadening is extensive because of turbulent flow immediately distal to the lesion.

In the presence of a high-grade stenosis, the peak velocity of both the proximal and distal waveform will be reduced because of diminished flow. The steepness of the systolic upstroke is short in the proximal segment and reduced distal to the lesion, resulting in a damped waveform with the peak of the reverse flow component noticeably rounded. These observations may direct the examiner to evaluate either proximal or distal arterial segments for the exact location of the stenotic lesions (Fig. 14).

With total occlusion no flow can be detected in the thrombosed section. Proximal to the occlusion, flow is disturbed, and the velocity is reduced. Distally a monophasic waveform with extensive spectral broadening is detectable (Fig. 15).

When multisegmental disease is present, the criteria for classification of stenosis remain unchanged. However, the waveform must be compared to that of the next proximal segment, maintaining a standard center stream angle of 60°.

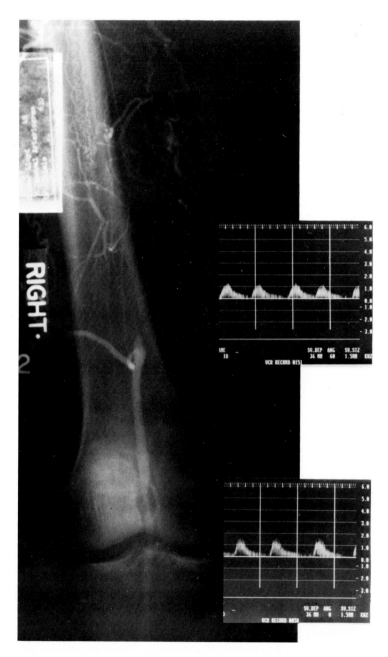

FIG. 15. Montage to show waveforms associated with proximal occlusion. **A:** A monophasic wave-form with marked spectral broadening is present distal to the occlusion. Disturbed flow is present at this site because of turbulence at the point of reentry of collaterals. **B:** Downstream flow is fairly laminar.

As noted previously, correct sample volume size, Doppler gain control settings, and choice of wall filter will reduce artifactual information in the spectral waveforms.

INDICATIONS

Unlike arteriography, which supplies only anatomic information, ultrasonic duplex scanning also provides physiologic data that may be crucial for patient management. Whereas indirect Doppler procedures detect only stenoses that produce diameter reductions in excess of 50% and cannot precisely localize disease, duplex scanning establishes the exact anatomic location of the lesion and permits accurate classification into one of five categories based on percentage obstruction (8). The anatomic and hemodynamic information available from duplex scanning may result in a more selective application of arteriography.

Unlike the carotid bifurcation, where disease is most often found at the origin of the internal carotid artery, atherosclerotic plaques may be distributed throughout all segments of the lower extremity arterial system from the level of the abdominal aorta to the tibial vessels, although there are locations where disease is more likely to be detected.

Patient management is often dictated by whether disease is found proximal or distal to the inguinal ligament. With duplex technology, Jager et al. (9) demonstrated 100% sensitivity for detection of disease in the iliac and deep femoral arteries. The ability of duplex scanning to permit evaluation of the superficial femoral bifurcation and the orifice of the profunda femoris artery make it most attractive, as arteriography is frequently limited in this area even when multiple-plane views are taken.

We have noted that the accuracy of duplex scanning is not affected by the location of disease, the degree of stenosis, or multisegmental involvement. Thus, this technique can separate normal arteries from those with wall irregularities or minimal disease and high-grade stenoses from total occlusion. Lesions that are amenable to percutaneous transluminal angioplasty (PTA) can be identified, and the immediate and long-term postdilatation results assessed easily and accurately.

In the patient who has undergone vascular reconstruction, the hemodynamics of the primary procedure can be evaluated and occurrence of restenosis identified by follow-up studies. Frequently, restenosis or thrombosis of a graft may occur without proceeding symptoms or deterioration of the ankle–brachial indices (2,16,18,20). The proximal and distal anastomoses can be evaluated with duplex scanning, and graft patency verified. Bandyk et al. (1) have shown that impending graft failure can be predicted from Doppler flow velocities recorded by duplex scanning intraoperatively and postoperatively. Velocities <40 cm/sec and the absence of diastolic forward flow have been associated with early graft failure. Serial measurements of flow velocities have been shown to be more sensitive indicators of graft stenosis than indirect evaluation of graft hemodynamics.

Studies from our institution and others have demonstrated additionally the value of duplex scanning in locating residual vein valve cusps, which may impede flow in the bypass graft, placing it at risk for thrombosis.

Not unlike duplex examination of the extracranial cerebrovascular and abdominal vessels, peripheral arterial scanning is very operator dependent and demands a great deal of technical skill. The examiner must be knowledgeable about the anatomy of the extremities, the pathophysiology of disease, and interpretation of velocity spectral patterns. A 6-month learning period is usually required for a technologist to gain competency in the examination. The results of the duplex evaluations must be compared continually with the standard contrast arteriographic studies to ensure the highest sensitivity and specificity. Jager et al. (8) have demonstrated positive and negative predictive values of 94% and 92%, respectively, for categorizing stenosis with >50% diameter reduction when compared to arteriography. The overall sensitivity was 96% with a specificity of 81%. The greatest sensitivity was shown for detection of aortoiliac stenoses. The presence of multisegmental disease did not cause reduction in the ability of duplex technology to identify and classify lesions accurately.

SUMMARY

Unlike arteriography, which yields only anatomic information, and the indirect noninvasive vascular procedures, which reflect quantitative hemodynamic measurements, duplex scanning is unique in combining both anatomic and physiologic data. This technique allows precise localization and characterization of disease as well as accurate quantitation of velocity changes resulting from stenoses. Excellent sensitivity for detection of all stages of disease has been demonstrated, making it possible to distinguish between normal vessels and those with minimal disease and between high-grade lesions and total occlusions. Disease progression can be identified. Arterial imaging of the aortoiliac segment, the origin of the profunda femoris, and superficial femoral arteries has aided in the selection of patients who may benefit from percutaneous transluminal angioplasty. The primary success rate of vascular reconstructions or dilatations, and occurence of restenosis, can be evaluated by follow-up studies. The selective use of duplex scanning in the diagnostic algorithm may enhance markedly the accuracy of noninvasive peripheral arterial testing.

REFERENCES

1. Bandyk, D. F., Cato, R. F., and Towne, J. B. (1985): A low flow velocity predicts failure of femoropopliteal and femorotibial bypass grafts. *Surgery,* 98(4):799–809.
2. Berkowitz, H. D., Hobbs, C. L., Roberts, B., Freiman, D., Oleaga, J., and Ring, E. (1981): Value of routine vascular laboratory studies to identify vein graft stenosis. *Surgery,* 90:971–979.
3. Blackshear, W. M., Jr., Phillips, D. J., and Strandness, D. E., Jr. (1979): Pulse Doppler assessment of normal human femoral artery velocity patterns. *J. Surg. Res.,* 27:73–77.
4. Carter, S. A. (1969): Clinical measurements of systolic pressures in limbs with arterial occlusive disease. *J.A.M.A.,* 207:1869–1874.
5. Carter, S. A. (1985): Role of pressure measurements in vascular disease. In: *Noninvasive Diagnostic Techniques in Vascular Disease,* 3rd ed., edited by E. F. Bernstein, pp. 513–544. C. V. Mosby, St. Louis.
6. Cutajar, C. L., Marston, A., and Newcombe, J. F. (1973): Value of cuff occlusion pressures in assessment of peripheral vascular disease. *Br. J. Med.,* 2:392–395.
7. Gosling, R. G., and King, D. H. (1974): Continuous wave ultrasound as an alternative and complement to X-rays in vascular examinations. In: *Cardiovascular Applications of Ultrasound,* edited by R. Reneman, pp. 266–282. American Elsevier, New York.
8. Jager, K. A., Ricketts, H. J., and Strandness, D. E., Jr. (1985): Duplex scanning for the evaluation of lower limb arterial disease. In: *Noninvasive Diagnostic Techniques in Vascular Disease,* 3rd ed., edited by E. F. Bernstein, C. V. Mosby, St. Louis.
9. Jager, K. A., Phillips, D. J., Martin, R. L. (1987): Noninvasive mapping of lower limb arterial lesions. *Ultrasound Med. Biol.,* 11(3):515–521.
10. Marinelli, M. R., Beach, K. W., Glass, M. J., Primozich, J. F., and Strandness, D. E., Jr. (1979):

Noninvasive testing vs. clinical evaluation of arterial disease. A prospective study. *J.A.M.A.,* 241:2031–2035.

11. Nimura, Y., Malsuo, H., Hayashi, T., Kitabatake, A., Mochizuki, S., Sakakibara, H., Kato, K., and Abe, H., (1974): Studies on arterial flow patterns—instantaneous velocity spectrums and their phasic changes with directional ultrasonic Doppler technique. *Br. Heart J.,* 36:899–903.

12. Phillips, D. J., Powers, J. E., Eyer, M. K., Blackshear, W. M., Jr., Bodily, K. C., Strandness, D. E., Jr., and Baker, D. W. (1980): Detection of peripheral vascular disease using the Duplex scanner III. *Ultrasound Med. Biol.,* 63:205–218.

13. Rushmer, R. F., Baker, D. W., and Stegall, H. F. (1966): Transcutaneous Doppler flow detection as a nondestructive technique. *J. Appl. Physiol.,* 21:554–557.

14. Satomura, S. (1959): Study of flow patterns in peripheral arteries by ultrasonics. *J. Acoust. Soc. Jpn.,* 15:151–154.

15. Strandness, D. E., Jr. (1983): Noninvasive evaluation of arteriosclerosis: A comparison of methods. *Arteriosclerosis,* 3:103–106.

16. Strandness, D. E., Jr. (1985): Exercise ankle pressure measurements in arterial disease. In: *Noninvasive Diagnostic Techniques in Vascular Disease,* 3rd ed., edited by E. F. Bernstein, pp. 575–583. C. V. Mosby, St. Louis.

17. Sumner, D. S., and Strandness, D. E., Jr. (1969): The relationship between calf blood flow and ankle blood pressure in patients with intermittent claudication. *Surgery,* 65:763–771.

18. Szilagy, D. E., Elliott, J. P., Hageman, J. H., Smith, R. F., and Dall'olmo, C. A. (1973): Biologic fate of autogenous vein implants as arterial substitutes. *Ann. Surg.,* 178:232–246.

19. Thiele, B. L., Bandyk, D. F., Zierler, R. E., and Strandness, D. E., Jr. (1983): A systematic approach to the assessment of aortoiliac disease. *Arch. Surg.,* 118:477–481.

20. Whitney, D. G., Kahn, E. M., and Estes, J. W. (1976): Valvular occlusion of the arterialized saphenous vein. *Am. Surg.,* 42:879–882.

21. Yao, J. S. T., Hobbs, J. T., and Irvine, W. T. (1969): Ankle systolic pressure measurements in arterial disease affecting the lower extremities. *Br. J. Surg.,* 56:676–678.

22. Yao, J. S. T. (1970): Hemodynamic studies in peripheral arterial disease. *Br. J. Surg.,* 57:761–766.

12 / Venous Ultrasonography of the Lower Extremities

Daniel H. O'Leary, and Robert A. Kane

Department of Radiology, New England Deaconess Hospital, Boston, Massachusetts 02215

Although deep venous thrombosis (DVT) of the lower extremities is the most common source of pulmonary emboli (16,23), clinical diagnosis of DVT is difficult and often unreliable. Approximately 50 to 60% of patients with DVT are believed to be undiagnosed clinically (6,22). Of those presenting with the clinical manifestations of DVT, only half are eventually shown to have thrombi. Failure to identify lower limb DVT leaves the patient at risk for pulmonary embolization, possibly with a fatal outcome. Conversely, a false positive diagnosis of DVT exposes the patient to medical or surgical interventions that carry their own significant hazards. In view of the limitations of clinical diagnosis, it has been recommended that all patients with suspected venous thrombosis be evaluated by objective measurements as a rational and cost-effective approach to the identification of those who require treatment and those who do not (13). B-scan ultrasound is one of the more useful tools available for this task, and the addition of Doppler techniques extends the range and reliability of the technique.

VENOUS ANATOMY

The veins of the lower extremity are divided into the deep and superficial systems. These are connected by perforating or communicating channels. The deep veins accompany the principal arteries and have the same names (Fig. 1). The deep calf veins are usually paired and lie on either side of the single posterior tibial, anterior tibial, and peroneal arteries. These paired deep calf veins drain upward into the unpaired popliteal vein, which in turn drains into the superficial femoral vein. Below the inguinal ligament at the level of the groin, the deep femoral vein and the long saphenous vein join the superficial femoral vein to form the common femoral vein. This, in turn, drains into the external iliac vein above the inguinal ligament. The long saphenous vein, the most prominent vein of the superficial system, begins at the medial malleolus and travels up the medial aspect of the calf and thigh. It is

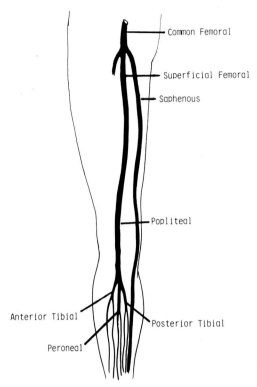

FIG. 1. Schematic of the major veins of the lower extremity.

located close to the skin surface in most individuals and is not accompanied by an artery.

The calf veins contain numerous bicuspid valves, which normally prevent retrograde flow. The veins at the level of the knee and those situated more proximally contain many fewer valves than the veins in the calf. Venous thrombi commonly form initially at the base of these valve cusps, where venous flow is relatively stagnant (26).

VENOGRAPHY

There have been a number of objective tests developed to diagnose DVT. Contrast venography, the most widely employed objective test for DVT, is the one most familiar to radiologists. When properly performed, it permits study of the calf veins and the popliteal, femoral, and external iliac veins. Because of flow defects produced by merging vessels, study of the more proximal pelvic veins usually requires insertion of a catheter at the groin.

Although it is universally accepted as the definitive test for detection of DVT, there are problems associated with venography. It is an invasive test involving the injection of contrast material into the patient. If both limbs are to be examined, each foot must be punctured. This can be painful, especially if the foot is swollen or the veins are difficult to find and multiple punctures must be attempted. Large amounts of contrast are often used. Sequential studies are seldom attempted or tolerated.

has also proven to have little utility for detecting calf thrombi, partly because of the small vessel size and partly because of their number and tortuous course. High-resolution ultrasound machines are often equipped with pulse Doppler systems, which can be useful in acquiring flow data, but the examination can be successfully performed with systems lacking Doppler capabilities.

Patients are initially examined in the supine position. It is helpful, although not necessary, to have a table that can be tilted so that the head is elevated and the legs dependent by 10 to 15° to maximize venous distension. Scanning is begun just proximal to the groin crease. Imaging is initially performed in the transverse, or short-axis, projection. This is the projection that is utilized for most of the study. The common femoral artery is usually the first vascular structure identified because of its pulsations. This provides a readily identifiable landmark for localization of the common femoral vein, which normally lies just medial to the artery. If the artery is not immediately seen, the groin can be palpated, the artery located, and the transducer moved medially.

The transducer should be held lightly on the surface of the skin to avoid collapsing normal veins. Once identified, the common femoral vein is followed distally to its bifurcation into superficial and deep portions. The deep femoral vein can only be seen for a short distance, as it rapidly moves away from the skin and is lost to view (Fig. 2). The superficial femoral vein is followed along the medial side of the thigh either to its junction with the popliteal vein or until it is lost from view. The latter often occurs at the level of the adductor canal in the lower thigh except in patients with slender lower extremities. If the vein is lost from view, it can often be relocalized by first finding its accompanying artery, which is identifiable because of arterial pulsations. A Valsalva maneuver often will enlarge the vein dramatically, particularly in the more proximal venous system, aiding in relocalization if the vein is lost from view or to distinguish the vein from an artery if uncertainty exists (Fig. 3). If pulsed

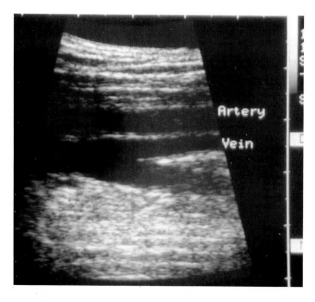

FIG. 2. B-mode ultrasound of a normal femoral artery and vein, longitudinal view. The unpaired deep femoral vein can be seen joining with the superficial femoral vein to form the common femoral vein.

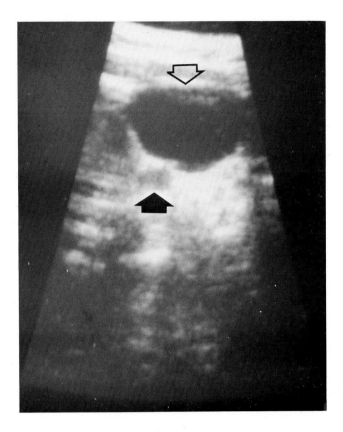

FIG. 3. Distended femoral vein, transverse view (*open arrow*), during a Valsalva maneuver. At rest, the diameter of the vein was only slightly greater than that of the accompanying artery (*solid arrow*).

Doppler equipment is available, this definitively differentiates arterial signals from venous ones.

Valvulae can occasionally be identified within the vein lumen in good-quality studies. They appear as thin, brightly echogenic structures that open and close rapidly and arise from the vessel wall. The saphenous vein can easily be seen lying more superficially just below the skin. At times it is possible to confuse the saphenous vein with the superficial femoral vein, especially in patients with large legs in whom the saphenous vein lies deeper to the skin surface. Differentiation from the superficial femoral vein can usually be made because the saphenous vein is unaccompanied by an artery.

After both limbs have been studied with the patient supine, the patient is turned to the prone position to permit examination of the popliteal veins. Patients who are on ventilators or who are otherwise unable to cooperate can be studied adequately at the knee after turning them onto their side. The popliteal artery is first sought as it exits from the adductor canal and the accompanying vein is identified. It is then followed distally to the trifurcation.

Attempts to image the calf veins have met with only limited success, and at present it is probably best to accept that B-scan ultrasound cannot reliably exclude the possibility of clot located below the level of the trifurcation. This is in part because of the small size of the calf vessels and multiple veins, paired and unpaired, which are time-consuming and difficult to visualize. Finding several normal veins in the calf does not exclude the possibility that a clot has been overlooked in a parallel channel. It is important, therefore, to pay particular attention to any site where the patient experiences local pain or tenderness, as this may indicate the presence of acute thrombus. This is true of the lower extremities in general but is particularly helpful in the calf region. Although a negative B-scan of this area may not reliably exclude pathology, a positive study is useful.

DIAGNOSTIC CRITERIA

As noted in Table 2, the principal criteria for diagnosis of DVT by ultrasound are:

1. Noncompressibility of the veins.
2. Visualization of intraluminal clot.
3. Abnormal or absent Doppler shift signal.

Minor criteria that further aid in the diagnosis of DVT include:

1. No alteration in the size of the vein during the Valsalva maneuver.
2. Absence of normal venous pulsations.
3. Absence of visible venous blood flow.
4. Absence of normal valve motion.

Not all of these findings are present in all patients with DVT, and diagnosis should not be based on minor criteria alone. However, identification of any of the three major criteria during ultrasonic examination is highly suggestive of the diagnosis of DVT.

The normal vein appears as an echo-free channel. Relative to the accompanying artery, it has very thin walls and typical venous pulsations. Veins are usually slightly larger than the accompanying arteries and should collapse easily when slight pressure is applied by the transducer (Fig. 4). Whereas a normal vein collapses with compression, a vein filled with clot does not (Fig. 5). Thus, as the probe is moved along the skin surface, pressure should be applied to the transducer every few centimeters, and collapse of the vein or its absence carefully observed. Failure of the vein to flatten completely should immediately arouse suspicion that clot is present. In our experience, this has proved to be the most useful finding in excluding DVT.

The amount of pressure required to collapse the vein is minimal in most individuals except at the level of the adductor canal, where additional pressure is usually required. Often the weight of the transducer alone on the skin surface is sufficient to collapse the vein. After scanning is initiated, the examiner should gently lift the probe off the skin so that contact is barely maintained to ensure maximum distension of the vein. In patients with elevated central venous pressure secondary to congestive heart failure or other causes, in patients with a pelvic mass obstructing venous outflow, or in patients with large muscular limbs and very deep vessels, the amount of pressure required to achieve compression will increase. If such individuals have symptoms localized to one limb, the opposite limb will serve as an internal control. Attention should also be paid to the accompanying artery. If the pressure required to collapse the vein also results in flattening of the artery, the study is abnormal.

Conversely, not all veins that appear to collapse when pressed are normal. They may contain nonocclusive thrombus or very fresh thrombus, which is still partially

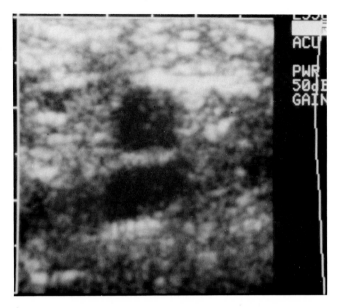

A

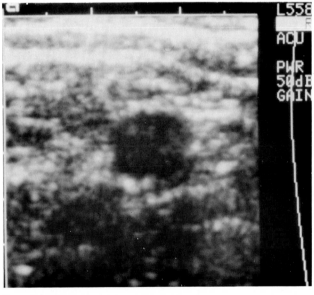

FIG. 4. A: B-mode ultrasound of a normal femoral artery and vein, transverse view. The artery lies above the vein. **B:** With compression, the vein is obliterated, and only the artery is still visualized.

B

compressible. If a vein flattens with pressure but the opposing walls do not touch, the examiner should be alert to the possibility of nonocclusive thrombus or fresh clot. When nonocclusive or nonechogenic clot is suspected, it is again critical to compare one limb with the other. The pressure required to collapse a vessel should be equal on both sides, and the degree of collapse should be similar. Any variation should at least alert the examiner to the possibility of DVT. Often, with acute thrombus, the transverse diameter of the vein will be markedly increased (Fig. 6). Marked

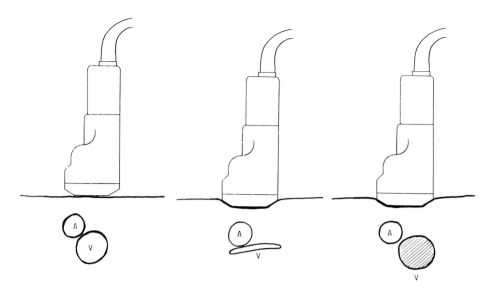

FIG. 5. Schematic of a normal and abnormal responses to compression, transverse view. The image on the **left** depicts the artery (a) and vein (v) before compression. In the **center** image, pressure has been applied, and the vein has completely collapsed; this is a normal response. In the image on the **right,** the vein does not collapse during compression; this is an abnormal response and is diagnostic of thrombus.

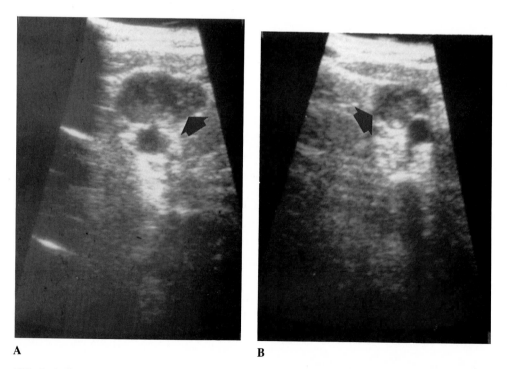

A   B

FIG. 6. A: B-mode ultrasound of the groin demonstrating echogenic thrombus in a markedly distended femoral vein (*arrow*). **B:** With compression, there is slight distortion of the vein (*arrow*), but the vessel does not collapse. Subsequent venogram confirmed the finding of extensive thrombus within the deep venous system.

enlargement of the vein may serve as an additional clue to the presence of acute clot. Under these circumstances, the addition of Doppler examination can aid in diagnosis.

Identification of clot within a vein on direct visualization is diagnostic, but differentiating between acute thrombus and normal background echoes can be difficult. Fresh thrombus may be isoechoic with flowing blood and not visible sonographically. Gain settings should be adjusted to demonstrate any low-level signals in the vessel,

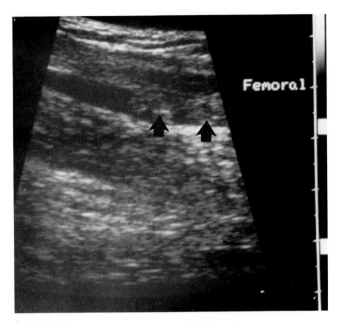

A

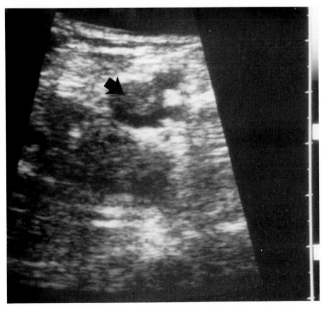

B

FIG. 7. A: B-mode ultrasound of the femoral vein, longitudinal view, showing nonocclusive echogenic thrombus floating in the vessel (*arrows*). **B:** Same vessel, transverse view, showing nonocclusive thrombus (*arrow*). Because the vessel was not completely occluded, venous Doppler response was normal in this individual.

which may represent acute thrombus. The accompanying artery can serve as the control to ensure that spurious echo patterns are not being produced. Nonocclusive thrombus is often better defined by imaging than is the far more common condition of total occlusion (Fig. 7). This is because of the clear differentiation between flowing blood and nonocclusive thrombus. With total occlusion, the echo pattern may become uniform across the entire vessel, and definition of the thrombus may be lost. In such circumstances, the use of Doppler scanning is an aid in the definitive diagnosis of total occlusion.

Low-level internal echoes sometimes visible within the normal lumen are thought to represent reflections from aggregations of relatively slowly moving red cells, although their precise origin is far from clear (24). These echoes can mimic the appearance of fresh thrombus, but whereas echoes from a thrombus are static, echoes from moving blood give the appearance of motion as they pass across the screen. Again, Doppler measurement provides a means of distinguishing static thrombus from moving blood.

Attempts have been made to link the intensity of the echo pattern with the age of the clot (21,25). This has clear applicability to processes in which multiple episodes may occur, and it may be clinically important to distinguish between old, presumably organized, clot and fresh thrombosis, which is more likely to embolize. Chronic clot usually demonstrates a hyperechoic heterogeneous pattern (3) (Fig. 8). The margins of the clot are often irregular. Also, with chronic thrombi, the vein wall may be thickened and the vessel smaller than normal in size (21).

Pulse Doppler ultrasound can be a useful adjunct to the examination. Phasic venous flow can be readily appreciated with midstream placement of the Doppler sample volume (Fig. 9). Flow decreases with inspiration, when intraabdominal pressure is elevated, and increases with expiration. Manual compression of the calf results in a surge, or augmentation, of venous outflow in normal individuals (Fig. 10). Failure to detect any flow suggests occlusion (Fig. 11). Diminished flow without

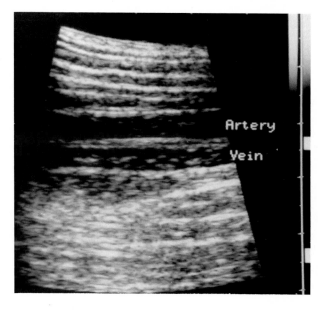

FIG. 8. B-mode ultrasound of longstanding venous thrombus, demonstrating a hyperechoic pattern.

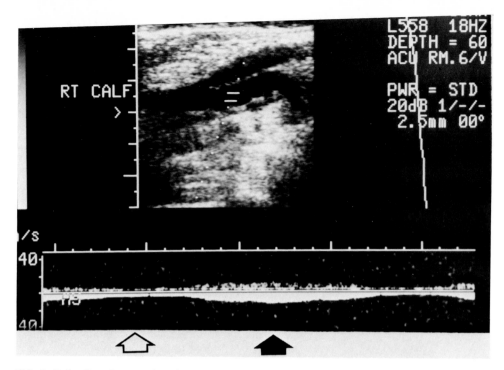

FIG. 9. Pulse Doppler sample volume has been placed in this normal vein. Normal venous flow is phasic, decreasing with inspiration (*open arrow*) and increasing with expiration (*closed arrow*).

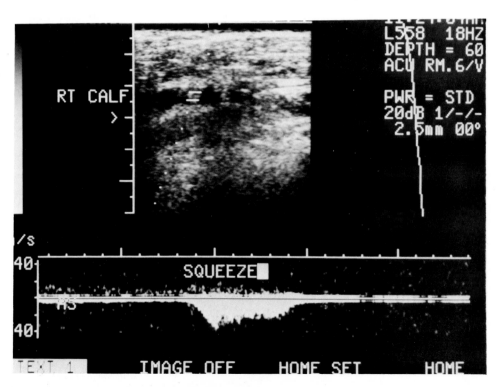

FIG. 10. With manual compression of the calf, pulse Doppler sampling detects transient increased venous flow (augmentation) in a more proximal vein.

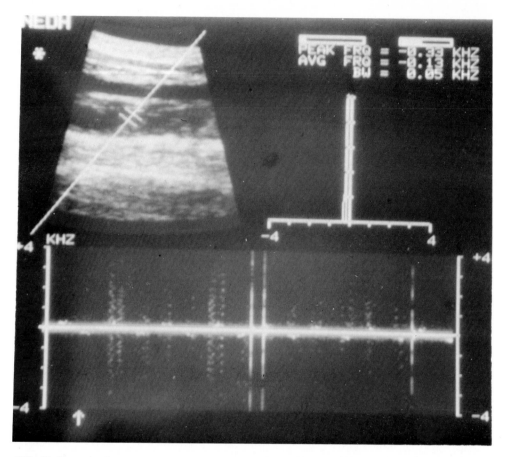

FIG. 11. B-mode ultrasound of the femoral artery and vein. The pulse Doppler sample volume has been placed in the vein, and no flow is detected. The vein is distended and demonstrates a pattern of increased echogenicity relative to the accompanying artery. The vein did not collapse on compression. This study met all major ultrasound criteria for the diagnosis of acute venous thrombosis.

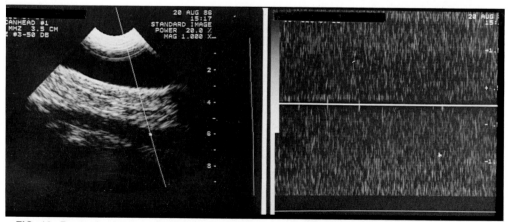

FIG. 12. Femoral vein thrombosis with nonechogenic thrombosis. In this example, lack of compressability and absence of the Doppler signal make this diagnosis.

augmentation and phasic flow in the femoral vein in the presence of a normal compression test and absence of visualized thrombus may indicate clot in the iliac veins. Venous Doppler examination cannot detect calf thrombi, as already noted, and may well appear normal even in the presence of nonocclusive clot.

Of the four minor criteria listed, venous response to the Valsalva maneuver is probably the most helpful. In normal individuals, the diameter of the veins in the extremities should increase during a Valsalva maneuver because of increased abdominal pressure and decrease with relaxation of the diaphragm. Failure of the vein to change size during a Valsalva maneuver is suggestive of thrombus. Although a normal response is helpful, failure of a vein to change in size is not, in itself, diagnostic. Many patients fail to cooperate fully in this maneuver, and this portion of the examination should be viewed with some suspicion. Also, the popliteal vein often does not respond to the Valsalva maneuver even in cooperative normal individuals.

PITFALLS

Venous ultrasound is rather simple to learn, particularly for individuals with prior training in arterial noninvasive ultrasound diagnosis. The criteria for a positive study are quite straightforward. Therefore, although undoubtedly much remains to be learned about the diagnosis of DVT by ultrasound, remarkably few pitfalls appear to be associated with the technique. When relying on imaging alone, it is important to recognize that fresh thrombus will usually be isoechoic and therefore easily missed unless compression testing is carried out. The addition of pulsed Doppler scanning will help avoid this error (Fig. 12). It is possible to make a false-positive diagnosis of clot by confusing signals reflected from aggregates of moving red blood cells in normal veins with thrombus. Although the visual display generated by signals reflected back from moving cells differs from that generated by echoes from clot, the differences may not always be appreciated by an inexperienced observer. Again, compression of the vein and utilization of pulse Doppler sampling from the visualized vessel should be sufficient to avoid this error.

In chronic or recurrent DVT, collateral channels develop to permit venous return. These may be mistaken for the normal deep venous system and thrombosed vessels thereby overlooked. The normal venous system follows the arterial system. If veins are identified without accompanying arteries in the lower extremity, the possibility that these represent collateral channels should be considered. Collaterals are tortuous or serpiginous, random, and irregular in their course. Collateral channels usually indicate chronic rather than acute DVT. When potential collateral channels are identified, the artery at that level should be located and a careful search for an adjacent thrombosed vein undertaken.

The importance of visualizing total collapse of the vein with compression has been stressed. It is possible to compress veins partially even when clot is present. This is particularly true with fresh clot or nonocclusive clot. As noted, utilization of the opposite, often uninvolved limb as an internal control can be most helpful in this setting. Overreliance on Doppler measurements to diagnose venous thrombosis, particularly in the absence of other positive findings, may well result in false-positive diagnoses. Finally, venous ultrasound has to date proven inaccurate in detecting calf thrombi.

SUMMARY

Venous ultrasound is a highly accurate technique for the detection of lower extremity DVT from the level of the groin to the upper calf. Doppler scanning is a useful but not essential adjunct to the examination. Venous ultrasound complements physiologic testing procedures already in widespread use. Because it is easily learned and quickly performed, ultrasound is rapidly becoming the initial test performed on individuals with suspected DVT. This should prove a boon to physicians and patients alike.

REFERENCES

1. Bettmann, M. A., and Paulin, S. (1977): Leg phlebography: the incidence, nature and modification of undesirable side effects. *Radiology, 122:*101–104.

2. Classen, J. N., Richardson, J. B., and Kountz, C. (1982): A three year experience with phleborheography. *Ann. Surg., 195:*800–803.

3. Coelho, J. C., Sigel, B., Ryva, J. C., Machi, J., and Renigers, S. A. (1982): B-mode sonography of blood clots. *J. Clin. Ultrasound, 10:*323–327.

4. Comerota, A. J., Cranley, J. J., Cook, S. E., and Sippel, P. J. (1982): Phleborheography—results of a ten-year experience. *Surgery, 91:*573–581.

5. Comerota, A. J., White, J. V., and Katz, M. L. (1985): Diagnostic methods for deep vein thrombosis: Venous Doppler examination, phleborheography, Iodine[125] fibrinogen uptake, and phlebography. *Am. J. Surg., 8:*14–24.

6. Cranley, J. J., Canos, A. J., and Sullivan, W. J. (1976): The diagnosis of deep venous thrombosis. *Arch. Surg., 111:*34–36.

7. Cranley, J. J., Canos, A. J., Sullivan, W. J., and Grass, A. M. (1975): Phleborheographic technique for diagnosing deep venous thrombosis of the lower extremities. *Surg. Gynecol. Obstet., 141:*331–339.

8. Cronan, J. J., Dorfman, G. S., Scola, F. H., Schepps, B., and Alexander, J. (1987): Ultrasound assessment using vein compression. *Radiology, 162:*191–194.

9. Douzat, M. M., Laroche, J. P., Charras, C., Blin, B., Domingo-Faye, M. M., Sainte-Luce, P., Domergue, A., Lopez, F. M., and Jaubon, C. (1986): Real-time B-mode ultrasonography for better specificity in the noninvasive diagnosis of deep venous thrombosis. *J. Ultrasound Med., 5:*625–631.

10. Holden, R. W., Klatte, E. C., Park, H. M., Siddiqui, A. R., Bendick, P. J., Dillery, R. S., and Glover, J. L. (1981): Efficacy of noninvasive modalities for diagnosis of thrombophlebitis. *Radiology, 141:*63–66.

11. Huisman, M. V., Buller, H. R., TenCate, J. W., and Vreeken, J. (1986): Serial impedance plethysmography for suspected deep venous thrombosis in outpatients. *N. Engl. J. Med., 314:*823–828.

12. Hull, R., Hirsch, J., Sackett, D. L., Powers, P., Turpie, A. G. G., and Walker, I. (1977): Combined use of leg scanning and impedance plethysmography in suspected venous thrombosis. *N. Engl. J. Med., 296:*1497–1500.

13. Hull, R., Hirsch, J., Sackett, D. L., and Stoddard, G. (1981): Cost effectiveness of clinical diagnosis, venography, and noninvasive testing in patients with symptomatic deep vein thrombosis. *N. Engl. J. Med., 304:*1561–1567.

14. Hull, R. D., Raskob, G. E., LeClerc, J. R., Jay, R. M., and Hirsh, J. (1984): The diagnosis of clinically suspected venous thrombosis. In: *Clinics in Chest Medicine,* edited by T. M. Hyers, pp. 439–456. W. B. Saunders, Philadelphia.

15. Hull, R. D., van Aken, W. G., Hirsch, J., Gallus, A. S., Hoicka, G., Turpie, A. G., Walker, I., and Gent, M. (1976): Impedance plethysmography using the occlusive cuff technique in the diagnosis of venous thrombosis. *Circulation, 53:*696–700.

16. Lundh, B., and Fagher, B. (1981): The clinical picture of deep vein thrombosis correlated to the frequency of pulmonary embolism. *Acta Med. Scand., 210:*353–356.

17. O'Leary, D. H., Kane, R. A., and Chase, B. A. (1987): A prospective study of the efficacy of B-scan sonography in the detection of deep venous thrombosis in the lower extremities. *J. Clin. Ultrasound. (in press).*

18. Rabinov, K., and Paulin, S. (1972): Roentgen diagnosis of venous thrombosis in the leg. *Arch. Surg.*, 104:134–144.

19. Raghavendra, B. N., Horii, S. C., Hilton, S., Subramanyan, B. R., Rosen, R. J., and Lam, S. (1986): Deep venous thrombosis: Detection by probe compression of veins. *J. Ultrasound Med.*, 5:89–95.

20. Raghavendra, B. N., Rosen, R. J., Lam, S., Riles, T., and Horii, S. C. (1984): Deep venous thrombosis: detection by high-resolution real-time ultrasonography. *Radiology*, 152:789–793.

21. Rollins, D. L., Semrow, C., Calligaro K., Friedall, M., and Buchbinder, D. (1986): Diagnosis of recurrent deep venous thrombosis using B-mode ultrasonic imaging. *Phlebology*, 1:181–188.

22. Salzman, E. W. (1986): Venous thrombosis made easy. *N. Engl. J. Med.*, 314:847–848.

23. Sevitt, S. (1962): Venous thrombosis and pulmonary embolism. *Am. J. Med.*, 33:703–704.

24. Sigel, B., Machi, J., Beitler, J. C., Justin, J. R., and Coelho, J. C. (1982): Variable ultrasound echogenicity in flowing blood. *Science*, 218:1321–1323.

25. Sullivan, E. D., Peter, D. J., and Cranley, J. J. (1984): Real-time B-mode venous ultrasound. *J. Vasc. Surg.*, 1:465–471.

26. Sumner, D. S. (1984): Venous anatgomy and pathophysiology. In: *Noninvasive Diagnosis of Vascular Disease*, edited by F. B. Hershey, R. W. Barnes, and D. S. Sumner, pp. 88–102. Appleton Davies, Pasadena.

27. Sumner, D. S. (1986): Noninvasive tests in the diagnosis and management of thromboembolic disease. *Surg. Annu.*, 18:1–28.

28. Talbot, S. R. (1982): Use of real-time imaging in identifying deep venous obstruction: a preliminary report. *Bruit*, 6:41–42.

29. Wheeler, H. B. (1985): Diagnosis of deep vein thrombosis: review of clinical evaluation and impedance plethysmography. *Am. J. Surg.*, 150:7–13.

30. Wheeler, H. B., and Anderson, F. A., Jr. (1982): Impedance phlebography: The diagnosis of venous thrombosis by occlusive impedance plethysmography. In: *Noninvasive Diagnostic Techniques in Vascular Disease*, 2nd ed., edited by E. F. Bernstein, pp. 482–496. C. V. Mosby, St. Louis.

A Doppler Glossary

P. N. Burns* and P. N. T. Wells†

*Department of Diagnostic Radiology, Yale University School of Medicine, New Haven, Connecticut 06510; and †Department of Medical Physics, Bristol General Hospital, Bristol B51 6SY, England

Acceleration   The rate of change of velocity at a given time. Acceleration is a vector quantity measured in meters per second squared.

Aliasing   The situation that arises when the Nyquist sampling limit is exceeded by the frequency of the input signal.

Amplitude   The magnitude of the wave variable, such as velocity, displacement, or acceleration.

Attack, angle of   The angle between the direction of movement of the reflector and the effective direction of the ultrasonic beam. Also known as Doppler angle.

Attenuation, compensated flowmeter   Device based on this technique does not require knowledge of the vessel cross-sectional area or Doppler angle in order to estimate blood flow rate. The specialized ultrasound beam geometries required limit of this technique to large vessels.

Autocorrelation   Multiplication of a wave by a time-shifted section of the same wave.

Backscatter   The energy reradiated by a scatterer in a direction opposite to that of the incident wave.

Base line shift (zero shift)   Control that allows the axis representing Doppler shift frequency on the spectral display to be allocated entirely to forward flow, reverse flow, or a mixture of the two. The effect is to "shift" the zero frequency axis up or down. This procedure is useful when aliasing is present in a signal representing unidirectional flow. It does not affect the Nyquist limit.

Beam shape, effective   The region within which an ultrasonic detector is able to detect the presence of reflecting or scattering targets.

Bernouilli, Daniel (1700–1782)   Swiss mathematician, sometimes referred to as the founder of mathematical physics, who unified the study of hydrodynamics under what became known later as the principle of the conservation of energy. Daniel Bernouilli was one of an extraordinary dynasty of eight mathematicians spanning three generations of the same family. Their collective contributions to mathematics and science are too numerous to list.

Bernouilli effect   The reduction in pressure that accompanies an increase in velocity of fluid flow.

Bernouilli equation   The equation that states that the total fluid energy along a streamline of fluid flow is constant. This is a form of the more general law of conservation of energy.

Boundary layer   The thin layer of stationary fluid in contact with the walls of the containing vessel.

Bruit   The name given to sounds sometimes associated with disturbed and turbulent flow. They arise from the periodic variation in shear stress on the vessel wall, which causes it to vibrate.

Center frequency   In a pulsed ultrasound system, the median frequency of the transmitted pulse, which, by its nature, comprises a range of frequencies.

Clutter   Unwanted components in the Doppler spectrum, generally caused by high-amplitude, low-Doppler-shift frequency echoes from moving solid structures such as vessel walls.

Coherence   The situation describing the degree of phase agreement among the signals making up a composite wave; if all the signals are in phase, the wave is said to be coherent.

Compliance   The rate of change of volume of a distensible vessel with pressure (''volume'' compliance); the rate of change of cross-sectional area with pressure (''area'' compliance); or the rate of change of diameter with pressure (''diameter'' compliance).

Critical Reynolds number   The Reynolds number around which the transition from laminar to turbulent flow takes place.

Critical stenosis   A stenosis of sufficient diameter reduction that flow rate and pressure are significantly affected. Sometimes called ''hemodynamically significant'' stenosis.

Decibel (dB)   Ten times the logarithm of the ratio of the powers of two signals or waves; often equal to 20 times the ratio of the amplitudes of the two signals.

Demodulation   The removal of the carrier signal from an amplitude-modulated wave to produce a signal representing the amplitude modulation.

Density   Mass per unit volume.

Diastole   The relaxation period in the cardiac cycle in which the ventricles fill and the aortic and pulmonary valves are closed. Where visible in the velocity pulse, the dicrotic notch forms a convenient point marking the beginning of diastole.

Dicrotic notch   A brief, abrupt upswing in pressure during the deceleration phase of systole, forming a ''notch'' in the pressure and velocity waveforms (Figure 28 of Chapter 3). The small undulations following the notch are known as the dicrotic wave and can be traced to reflections from the distal arterial tree. This reversal of pressure gradient is responsible for the closure of the aortic valve.

Disturbed flow   Deviations from laminar flow consisting of oscillatory variations in direction or the formation of vortices. Disturbance of blood flow may be caused by high peak velocities, by curving, branching, and divergence of vessels, or by projections into the vessel lumen.

Doppler, Christian Andreas (1805–1853)   Son of an Austrian stonemason, Doppler became Professor of Mathematics in Prague. He enunciated his principle in 1842 but unfortunately confused its interpretation (he was, it turned out, incorrectly using it to attempt to explain the color of binary stars). The acoustical Doppler effect was demonstrated in 1845 by Buys Ballot using a trumpeter riding on a steam locomotive, which was loaned for the occasion by the Dutch government.

Doppler angle   The angle between the direction of propagation of the ultrasound and the direction of flow. As an approximation, the angle between the axis of the ultrasound beam and the axis of the vessel lumen is generally used.

Doppler, pulse   A range-measuring ultrasonic system that detects Doppler-shifted signals by collecting samples, each sample corresponding to a separate ultrasonic pulse.

Doppler shift frequency, maximum   The highest Doppler shift frequency at a moment in time or in an individual Doppler spectrum. This corresponds to the fastest moving target in the Doppler sample volume. Because of the effect of noise, some form of signal conditioning is usually performed before the maximum frequency is measured.

Doppler shift frequency, mean   The average Doppler shift frequency in a given power spectrum.

Doppler shift frequency, median   The Doppler shift frequency above and below which one-half of the total power in the spectrum resides.

Doppler shift frequency, mode   The Doppler shift frequency with the greatest power in a given spectrum.

Duplex scanner   An ultrasound instrument that has real-time imaging capability with either the imaging transducer or a separate transducer used to collect continuous-wave or pulsed Doppler signals, either simultaneously with imaging or sequentially.

Energy, total fluid   The sum of the kinetic energy (associated with velocity), inertial energy (related to acceleration), potential energy (caused by pressure or gravity), and viscous energy (arising from fluid friction) in a volume of fluid. The unit of energy is the Joule.

Energy, kinetic   Energy associated with the motion of a mass. For a unit volume of fluid, it is equal to $\frac{1}{2}\rho v^2$ where ρ is density and v velocity.

Energy, potential   Energy associated with the ability to do work. Examples are the gravitational (or hydrostatic) energy of an object (or volume of fluid) raised to a height in a gravitational field and pressure in a fluid.

Energy, viscous   Energy used to overcome the internal cohesion of a liquid in order to, for example, maintain laminar flow. Energy expended in this way is converted to heat.

Ensemble   A collection of scatterers large enough to backscatter a detectable quantity of energy.

Entrance effects   The change in velocity profile experienced by flow when there is a sudden change in caliber of the lumen. Laminar flow will tend to stabilize some distance downstream; the distance over which this occurs is known as the entrance length.

Exit effects   The change in velocity profile experienced by flow when there is a sudden increase in lumen area, for example, downstream to a stenotic orifice. Flow disturbance flow can result, with accompanying energy loss.

Fast Fourier transform (FFT)   A numerical algorithm used to compute the frequency components present in a periodic function varying with, for example, time. The Doppler signal is an example of such a function: the FFT produces an estimate of the relative amplitude of each frequency component, known as the amplitude spectrum.

Field, far   The region beyond the last axial maximum of an ultrasonic beam.

Field, near   The region between a source and the last axial maximum of an ultrasonic beam.

Filter   An electronic circuit designed to allow signals of certain frequencies to pass and to stop signals of other frequencies.

Filter, high-pass   A device that allows high- but not low-frequency variations to pass through. An example is the electrical filter used in Doppler devices to elimiante low-frequency Doppler shifts caused by clutter.

Filter, low-pass   A device that allows low- but not high-frequency variations to pass through. An example is a stenosis, which has the effect of damping rapid variations in the pressure and flow waveforms.

Flow rate   The rate of change of volume of fluid with time. Measured in liters per second or milliliters per minute.

Flow separation   If a body of fluid within a vessel has a particularly high momentum (because it has entered the vessel as a jet through a small orifice, for example), its boundary will separate from the laminae of surrounding fluid. The region of flow separation is marked by a high velocity gradient and hence shear stress.

Focus   The point on the axis of an ultrasonic beam where the width of the beam has a minimum value; generally, all the waves passing through the focus are in phase in relation to the surface of the transducer or to the electronic summing point of an electronically focused array.

Focus, depth of The length of the axial region within which the ultrasonic beam is effectively in focus.

Focusing, dynamic A method for controlling the axial position of the focus of an ultrasonic beam; often realized by phase control of the signals detected by a transducer array.

Fourier, Joseph (1768–1830) Son of a French tailor who was persuaded to leave his Benedictine monastery to become a Professor of Mathematics at the age of 21. Among his many original and outstanding contributions to mathematical physics is the analytic theory of heat, which Lord Kelvin called "a great mathematical poem." Some say that his death was speeded by his insistence that heat was good for the health and his later habit of living in rooms "hotter than the Sahara desert."

Fourier analysis Mathematical technique for the representation of a periodic function (such as a time-varying waveform) as a sum of sinusoidal functions of different frequencies. Each of these constituent functions has a frequency that is an exact multiple of the same number. Fourier analysis allows the presentation of a Doppler signal in terms of the relative power of the various Doppler shift frequencies of which it is composed.

Frequency-domain processing A signal-processing scheme that operates on signals according to their frequencies.

Frequency, Doppler shift The difference between the frequencies of the transmitted wave and of the echo received from a moving target.

Frequency, lower bandwidth Frequency used in the quantitation of spectral width. The definition varies but might typically be the lowest frequency with an amplitude of -12 dB relative to that of the mean or mode frequency.

Frequency, received The frequency of the signal detected by the receiving transducer.

Frequency spectrum, instantaneous The range of frequencies present in a signal at some instant in time.

Frequency spectrum, mean The range of frequencies in a spectrum averaged over a (long) period of time.

Frequency, upper bandwidth Frequency used in the quantitation of spectral width. The definition varies but might typically be the highest frequency with an amplitude of -12 dB relative to that of the mean or mode frequency.

Huygen's principle The principle that states that any wave phenomenon can be analyzed by the addition of the contributions from some distribution of simple sources, or simple detectors, properly selected in phase and amplitude to represent the physical situation.

Image update The ability of a duplex scanner to alternate between the two functions of imaging and Doppler measurements. In systems in which the beam is moved electronically, this can be at a sufficiently rapid rate to permit real-time imaging during the same period in which the Doppler signal is acquired.

Impedance, acoustic The product of acoustic velocity and density of a medium in which sound is traveling. Discontinuities in acoustic impedance are responsible for the echoes on which ultrasound imaging and Doppler flow detection are based.

Impedance, fluid The ratio of pressure to flow rate expressed as a function of frequency in time-varying flow. Impedance summarizes the effect on flow rate of resistance, compliance, and inertia when the pressure varies with time.

Inertia The tendency of a body of fluid to resist a change in its velocity. Such a change requires a force proportional to the body's mass.

Interference The phenomenon describing the interaction between two waves of the same or different frequencies to produce a resultant wave, the amplitude of which depends on the amplitude and phase relationship of the interfering waves.

Interference, constructive The phenomenon of interference in which the resultant wave has an amplitude greater than that of either of the two interfering waves.

Interference, destructive The phenomenon of interference in which the resultant wave has an amplitude less than that of the two interfering waves.

Kelvin, Lord (1824–1907) British physicist and president of the Royal Society; exponent of the principle that heavier-than-air flying machines are impossible.

Laminar flow Flow in which there is smooth and gradual variation of velocity with position and with time. Flow may be thought of as comprising a series of individual laminae, each moving at one velocity, with viscous cohesion maintaining the flow of adjacent laminae at nearly the same velocity.

Mirror-image artifact Loss of directional resolution in a Doppler system employing phase-quadrature detection, resulting in a "mirror image" of the spectral display about the zero-frequency axis. The artifact may be seen when the signal level is too great or when the Doppler angle is near 90°.

Mixer A device that mixes two or more signals to produce products and quotients.

Monostable An electrical circuit that produces a second pulse at a known delay following the application of a triggering pulse.

Newtonian fluid A fluid in which the viscous force opposing flow is proportional to the velocity gradient.

Noise Random, and usually unwanted, signals.

Noise, electrical Noise signals arising within the electrical circuits.

Nyquist criterion The criterion that a continuously varying signal can only be unambiguously represented by instantaneous samples if the sampling rate is more than twice the maximum frequency present in the signal.

Nyquist limit The highest frequency in a sampled signal that can be represented unambiguously; equal to one-half of the sampling frequency.

Percentage window A measure of spectral broadening, integrated over systole. The measure is normalized so that 100% indicates no spectral broadening or a "clear" window. Sometimes defined as the ratio of the upper to lower bandwidth frequencies calculated at regular intervals and summed over systole.

Phase, angle of The numerical value of the angle of rotation of the vector describing a periodic wave; waves that are in phase have simultaneously occurring maxima (and zero crossings and minima); the maximum of a wave that is in antiphase with another wave occurs at the same time as the minimum of the other wave.

Phase-domain processing A signal-processing scheme that operates on signals according to their phases.

Phase quadrature A signal-processing technique depending on an input signal being available both with its original phase and shifted through 90° of phase angle.

Plug flow A region of flow with a flat velocity profile, that is, one in which all the flow is at a single velocity.

Poise The unit of viscosity. One Poise is equal to 10 Pascal seconds (Pa sec).

Poiseuille, Jean Leonard M. (1797–1869) French physician and physicist who performed the first experiments demonstrating viscosity in a fluid and its relationship to pressure gradient in a tube. Poiseuille also refined the techniques of Hales for measuring pressure in the arterial circulation.

Poiseuille's law Law stating that the fluid resistance in a long, straight tube with steady, irrotational flow is proportional to its length and viscosity and inversely proportional to the fourth power of its radius.

Power The energy delivered by a wave in unit time; measured in watts.

Power spectrum A graph showing the relative power of each frequency component in a periodic function. For a Doppler signal, the power spectrum gives the distribution of Doppler shift frequencies present in the signal.

Pressure A form of potential energy in a fluid. Pressure is defined as the force acting on each square meter of an imaginary plane facing any direction in a fluid. The unit of pressure is Pascal (Pa).

Pulsatility index A parameter used to convey the pulsatility of a time-varying waveform such as the maximum Doppler shift frequency of the signal from an artery. Indices of pulsatility are usually ratios of Doppler shift frequencies and are hence independent of Doppler angle. The most common definition of pulsatility index (PI) of a waveform such as that defined by the maximum Doppler shift frequency is the difference between the maximum and minimum value divided by the mean value of the waveform over the cardiac cycle.

Pulse pair covariance Particular type of autocorrelation processing in which signals obtained from successive pulses are correlated.

Pulse repetition frequency In a pulsed system, the number of ultrasonic pulses emitted by the transducer per second.

Pulse pressure The difference between the peak systolic and minimum diastolic pressures in the cardiac cycle.

Range, dynamic The range of values of a variable over which a change in input produces a change in output.

Range gating An electronic circuit for selecting an ultrasonic signal according to its depth along the ultrasonic beam by gating the signal with an appropriate time delay.

Rayleigh, Lord (1842–1919) Born John William Strutt in Essex, England, third baron Rayleigh was the son of a Duke and member of Parliament for Essex. Although educated at Cambridge, where he became Cavendish Professor of Physics and eventually Chancellor, he carried out much of his work in his private laboratory at his home in Terling. He received the Nobel Prize for physics in 1904 for his experimental work on the atmospheric elements but is perhaps remembered better for his classic and comprehensive treatise on the theory of sound published in 1877.

Rayleigh scattering The name given to the deflection of waves by an ensemble of targets much smaller than the wavelength of the incident radiation. Red blood cells are Rayleigh scatterers to ultrasound. The intensity of ultrasound scattered back to the transducer by the Rayleigh process is proportional to the fourth power of frequency.

Reflection, specular The phenomenon of reflection of a wave by a flat surface large in relation to the wavelength.

Resistance, fluid With steady flow, the resistance is the ratio of pressure drop to flow rate.

Resistance index An index of pulsatility defined as the difference between the maximum and minimum Doppler shifts divided by the maximum. Also known as the Pourcelot index.

Reynolds, Sir Osborne (1842–1912) English mechanical and civil engineer who pioneered the study of vortical and turbulent flow in liquids and laid the theoretical basis for subsequent study of the behavior of viscous fluids. Reynolds also built a steam engine for the determination of mechanical equivalent of heat and held patents the design of marine turbines.

Reynolds number A number expressing the balance of inertial and viscous forces acting on a flowing fluid. Reynolds numbers higher than a critical value result in disturbed or turbulent flow.

Reynolds stress The increased resistance to flow offered by a fluid in turbulence, which has its origin in viscous forces resulting from chaotically oriented velocity gradients.

Root mean square (rms) The square root of the mean value of the square of the wave amplitude.

Sample volume The region of the ultrasound beam (or beams in a CW system) sensitive to the presence of Doppler-shifted echoes. In a pulsed Doppler system, the axial position and extent of the sample volume are under control of the operator.

Scatterer A discontinuity small in relation to the wavelength that reradiates ultrasound through an angle rather than in specular fashion.